ANIMAL DISEASE RESEARCH
& DIAGNOSTIC LAB.
P.O. Box 2175
South Dakota State University
BROOKINGS, S.D. 57007

International Review of
EXPERIMENTAL PATHOLOGY

Volume 32
MOLECULAR CELL PATHOLOGY

Editorial Advisory Board

M. Bessis
Kremlin-Bicetre, France

K. M. Brinkhous
Chapel Hill, North Carolina

T. O. Caspersson
Stockholm, Sweden

F. Deinhardt
Munich, Federal Republic of Germany

E. Farber
Toronto, Canada

D. W. Fawcett
Boston, Massachusetts

Sir J. Gowans
London, England

H. Harris
Oxford, England

P. Lacy
St. Louis, Missouri

Sir G. Nossal
Melbourne, Australia

International Review of
EXPERIMENTAL PATHOLOGY

Volume 32
MOLECULAR CELL PATHOLOGY

Edited by
G. W. Richter
Department of Pathology
University of Rochester Medical Center
Rochester, New York

Kim Solez
Department of Pathology
Faculty of Medicine
University of Alberta
Edmonton, Alberta

ACADEMIC PRESS, INC.
Harcourt Brace Jovanovich, Publishers
San Diego   New York   Boston   London   Sydney   Tokyo   Toronto

This book is printed on acid-free paper. ∞

COPYRIGHT © 1991 BY ACADEMIC PRESS, INC.
All Rights Reserved.
No part of this publication may be reproduced or transmitted in any form or by any means, electronic or mechanical, including photocopy, recording, or any information storage and retrieval system, without permission in writing from the publisher.

ACADEMIC PRESS, INC.
San Diego, California 92101

United Kingdom Edition published by
ACADEMIC PRESS LIMITED
24-28 Oval Road, London NW1 7DX

LIBRARY OF CONGRESS CATALOG CARD NUMBER: 62-21145

ISBN 0-12-364932-3 (alk. paper)

PRINTED IN THE UNITED STATES OF AMERICA
91 92 93 94   9 8 7 6 5 4 3 2 1

Contents

Contributors   ix

Applications of *in Situ* Hybridization
Gerald Niedobitek and Hermann Herbst

I. Introduction   1
II. Methodology   3
III. Applications   21
IV. Practical Value for Histopathology   43
References   44

Interactions between Endothelial Cells and the Cells of the Immune System
Druie E. Cavender

I. Introduction   58
II. Interactions between Endothelial Cells and Immune System Cells in the Control of Coagulation   58
III. Lymphocyte/Endothelial Cell Interactions in Lymphocyte Recirculation   63
IV. Interactions between Endothelial Cells and Immune System Cells in the Regulation of Mononuclear Cell Migration into Inflammatory Lesions   71
V. The Role of Cytokines in the Activation of Endothelial Cells at Sites of Inflammation   79
VI. The Effects of Cytokines on Endothelial Cell Expression of MHC Antigens and Their Possible Role in Endothelial Cell Antigen Presentation   80
VII. Endothelial Cell Proliferation and Angiogenesis   85
VIII. Effects of Endothelial Cell Products on the Function of Immune System Cells   86
IX. Conclusions   87
References   88

Molecular Biology of Cytokine Effects on Vascular Endothelial Cells
Hiroshi Suzuki and Heihachiro Kashiwagi

I. Introduction   95
II. Molecular Basis of Cytokine Responsiveness of Vascular Endothelial Cells   97

III. Regulation and Induction of Endothelial Gene Expression by Cytokines   104
IV. Endothelial Gene Expression in *in Vivo* and *in Situ* Hybridization   134
V. Future Directions of Research   136
References   139

Interphase Nucleolar Organizer Regions in Cancer Cells
Massimo Derenzini and Dominique Ploton

I. Introduction   150
II. Silver Staining Techniques for the Visualization of NORs   151
III. General Factors Influencing the Specificity of the Silver Stain for NORs   155
IV. Molecular Components Responsible for Silver Staining   157
V. NORs Not Stained by the Ag-NOR Techniques   159
VI. Localization of NORs in Interphase Nucleoli   159
VII. Structure and Function of Interphase NORs   164
VIII. Nucleolar Morphology   170
IX. Interphase NOR Distribution   173
X. Distribution of Silver-Stained Interphase NORs in Neoplastic Cells   175
XI. Is the High Number of Interphase NORs a Peculiar Feature of Cancer Cells?   179
XII. Relationship between Interphase NOR Distribution and Neoplastic State of the Cell   181
XIII. Structural Changes of Ribosomal Genes in Cells Stimulated to Proliferate   188
References   189

Antineutrophil Cytoplasmic Autoantibodies: Disease Associations, Molecular Biology, and Pathophysiology
J. Charles Jennette, Linda A. Charles, and Ronald J. Falk

I. Introduction   193
II. Clinical and Pathologic Spectrum of ANCA-Associated Diseases   195
III. Elucidation of ANCA Antigen Specificity   205
IV. Pathogenetic Potential of ANCAs   212
V. Conclusion   219
References   220

Apoptosis: Mechanisms and Roles in Pathology
Mark J. Arends and Andrew H. Wyllie

I. Introduction   223
II. Morphology   226

III. Mechanisms   232
IV. Roles in Pathology   242
V. Conclusions   247
   References   251

Molecular Events in Measles Virus Infection of the Central Nervous System
Peggy T. Swoveland

I. Introduction   255
II. Clinical and Epidemiological Features   256
III. Pathology of Measles-Infected Brain Tissue   257
IV. Properties of Measles Virus   260
V. Viral Protein Expression   264
VI. Viral Gene Expression   269
VII. Role of Antibodies in Viral Persistence   271
VIII. CNS Damage by Measles Virus   272
IX. Concluding Remarks   273
   References   273

Index   277

Contributors

Numbers in parentheses indicate the pages on which the authors' contributions begin.

Mark J. Arends, Department of Pathology, University of Edinburgh Medical School, Edinburgh EH8 9AG, Scotland (223)

Druie E. Cavender, Department of Microbiology and Immunology, University of Miami School of Medicine, Miami, Florida 33101 (57)

Linda A. Charles, Department of Pathology, University of North Carolina, Chapel Hill, North Carolina 27599 (193)

Massimo Derenzini, Dipartimento di Patologia Sperimentale, 40126 Bologna, Italy (149)

Ronald J. Falk, Department of Medicine, University of North Carolina, Chapel Hill, North Carolina 27599 (193)

Hermann Herbst, Institute of Pathology, Klinikum Steglitz, Freie Universität Berlin, Berlin, Federal Republic of Germany (1)

J. Charles Jennette, Department of Pathology, University of North Carolina, Chapel Hill, North Carolina 27599 (193)

Heihachiro Kashiwagi, Department of Rheumatology, Institute of Clinical Medicine, University of Tsukuba, Ibaraki-ken 305, Japan (95)

Gerald Niedobitek, Institute of Pathology, Klinikum Steglitz, Freie Universität Berlin, Berlin, Federal Republic of Germany (1)

Dominique Ploton, Unitè de Recherche, INSERM 314, 51092 Reims, France (149)

Hiroshi Suzuki, Department of Rheumatology, Institute of Clinical Medicine, University of Tsukuba, Ibaraki-ken 305, Japan (95)

Peggy T. Swoveland, Department of Neurology, University of Maryland School of Medicine, Baltimore, Maryland 21201 (255)

Andrew H. Wyllie, Department of Pathology, University of Edinburgh Medical School, Edinburgh EH8 9AG, Scotland (223)

Applications of in Situ Hybridization

GERALD NIEDOBITEK and HERMANN HERBST

Institute of Pathology
Klinikum Steglitz
Freie Universität Berlin, Berlin, Germany

I. Introduction
II. Methodology
    A. Tissues, Fixatives, and Adhesives
    B. Probes
    C. Pretreatment and Hybridization Conditions
    D. Probe Detection
    E. Combined *in Situ* Hybridization and Immunohistology
    F. Pitfalls and Controls
    G. Sensitivity of Radioactive and Nonradioactive Techniques
III. Applications
    A. *In Situ* Hybridization for the Detection of DNA
    B. *In Situ* Hybridization for the Detection of RNA
IV. Practical Value for Histopathology
    References

I. Introduction

In recent years, progress in molecular biology has made several techniques for research and diagnosis available even to laboratories not specialized in this field. The basis of all these techniques is the ability of single-stranded nucleic acids, either deoxyribonucleic acid (DNA) or ribonucleic acid (RNA), to hybridize, i.e., to form selectively double strands with nucleic acid molecules of complementary sequence. However, prior to hybridization, most of these methods, e.g., Southern and Northern blot hybridization, require extraction of nucleic acids from tissues, restriction enzyme digestion, gel electrophoresis, and transfer of nucleic acids to membranes (Sambrook *et al.*, 1989). These are very time-consuming procedures requiring special knowledge and facilities. Another serious disadvantage of extractive techniques is that it is usually not possible to attribute a signal to a particular cell type. However, because most tissues represent a heterogeneous rather than a homogeneous assembly of cells, the sole information that a particular nucleic acid sequence is present in a given tissue is often insufficient.

Moreover, a sequence present in only a small proportion of the cells of a given tissue may be detectable by *in situ* hybridization (ISH) whereas in filter hybridization of DNA extracted from this tissue, the sequence may be diluted by the total cellular DNA to below the threshold of detection.

The introduction of *in situ* hybridization was therefore met with interest from pathologists because it provides a synthesis of classical histopathology with modern molecular biological techniques. *In situ* hybridization was first described as early as 1970 (Gall and Pardue, 1969; John *et al.*, 1969; Buongiorno-Nardelli and Amaldi, 1969). Applications, however, have been limited by the lack of probes and the availability of only radioactive reporter molecules. The steadily increasing number of cloned and sequenced genes, the advancements in oligonucleotide synthesis technology, and the development of nonradioactive probes now allow widespread use of this technique.

In the beginning, *in situ* hybridization was used predominantly for the detection of viral genomes (Brahic and Haase, 1978; Haase *et al.*, 1981; Blum *et al.*, 1983). In more recent years, *in situ* hybridization has also been applied to the detection of RNA sequences, particularly in the fields of embryology and neurobiology (Cox *et al.*, 1984; Valentino *et al.*, 1987). For the histopathologist, detection of mRNA or viral genomes in human lesions is likely to be the major point of interest. Several improvements reported over the last 10 years made it possible to extend the range of applications for *in situ* hybridization from the visualization of highly abundant RNA transcripts to detecting mRNA species of low copy number.

In situ hybridization is now a widely used method in research. From 1983 to 1988 more than 2000 references using this technique are quoted in the data bank MEDLINE. Therefore, we feel that it is impossible to give a complete overview of the literature. The aim of this review is to discuss currently available *in situ* hybridization techniques for the demonstration of viral DNAs or RNAs and messenger RNAs at the light microscopy level. Based on the work done in the authors' laboratory, these methods and possible pitfalls will be discussed. Also, the significance of *in situ* hybridization in comparison to immunohistology will be considered. For detailed laboratory methods the reader is referred to comprehensive manuals (Hogan *et al.*, 1986; Pardue, 1985; Sambrook *et al.*, 1989). *In situ* hybridization techniques on the chromosomal level, using either metaphase spreads or interphase nuclei and ultrastructural *in situ* hybridization, are not within the scope of this review.

II. Methodology

DNA remains stable in tissues for a relatively long time. Therefore, it is possible to demonstrate DNA sequences even in poorly preserved or even autolytic autopsy tissues. In comparison to DNA–DNA hybridization, detection of RNA is technically more complicated and demanding with respect to the integrity of the cells. DNases are relatively labile enzymes that may be quickly denatured or inhibited by depletion of Mg^{2+} ions. Single-stranded RNA, on the other hand, is quickly degraded by RNases, which are ubiquitous and rather resistant to denaturation. Thus, the reliable detection of mRNA requires optimal procedures for tissue preparation and fixation. Furthermore, probe construction and labeling as well as hybridization and washing procedures differ in some aspects from DNA hybridization, whereas similar considerations apply to the choice of the method for signal detection.

A. Tissues, Fixatives, and Adhesives

DNA sequences can be detected *in situ* in almost any kind of cell or tissue preparation. Smears and cytocentrifuge preparations can be used as efficiently as sections of snap-frozen tissues. A variety of different fixatives have been used for *in situ* hybridization (Lawrence and Singer, 1985; Jilbert *et al.*, 1986; Mullink *et al.*, 1986b; Nuovo and Richart, 1989a). Precipitating fixatives such as methanol/acetic acid and Carnoy's fixative provide good probe penetration, whereas cross-linking fixatives such as paraformaldehyde and glutaraldehyde give better preservation of tissue morphology and nucleic acid retention. Most attractive, however, is the application of this technique to sections of formalin-fixed and paraffin-embedded tissues, because this opens the possibility of investigating tissue specimens that have been processed by routine histopathological techniques and stored for decades (e.g., Blum *et al.*, 1984a; Brigati *et al.*, 1983; Burns *et al.*, 1986; Jiwa *et al.*, 1989; McAllister and Rock, 1985; Niedobitek *et al.*, 1988b). Recently, the application of plastic-embedded tissues for *in situ* hybridization has also been described (Cao and Beckstead, 1989).

In comparison to DNA, the biological half-life of most RNA species is rather short. The function of some regulatory proteins is reflected by the short half-life of their specific mRNAs, e.g., approximately 10 minutes for c-*myc*. It is therefore mandatory to keep the time interval between removal of the tissue from the organism and fixation as short as possible. In this context, the period of hypoxemia prior to excision of surgical specimens also influences the content and integrity of intracellular RNA. On the other hand, it may be possible to detect certain highly abundant mRNA transcript species such as immunoglobulin (Ig) mRNA in plasma cells of autopsy material. Also, the detection of viral RNA in autopsy tissues has been reported (Brown et al., 1989). In such cases it is advisable to confirm the presence of relevant transcript levels with a highly expressed "indicator" gene transcript by *in situ* hybridization prior to prolonged autoradiographic procedures for the detection of other transcripts. Alternatively, hybridization to an appropriately labeled oligo-d(T) strand may indicate the presence of polyadenylated mRNA species (Pringle et al., 1989). The intensity of the autoradiographic signal obtained in a surgical specimen in comparison to an optimally fixed sample may indicate any loss of RNA due to delay in fixation. Examples for such indicator gene transcripts are albumin in liver specimens or Ig light chains in plasma cells. In our experience it is useless to try to detect a low-abundance gene transcript in a lymph node or mucosal tissue specimen if visualization of Ig light chain transcripts in plasma cells using ^{35}S-labeled RNA probes requires more than 12 hours of autoradiography.

Tissue for mRNA *in situ* hybridization or nucleic acid extraction should be snap frozen as quickly as possible and stored in liquid nitrogen or at least at −80°C. Storage in liquid nitrogen is required if extraction of cellular RNA for size determination by Northern blotting is intended. In most −80°C freezers, slight temperature fluctuations will result in mechanical disintegration of nucleic acid strands. The nucleic acids, however, will remain in the nuclei and cytoplasm of cells, and *in situ* hybridization for transcripts present in low copy numbers may still be possible after several years of storage.

Some protocols suggest fixation of tissue in 4% buffered paraformaldehyde followed by immersion in sucrose prior to freezing (Hogan et al., 1986). This will decrease artifacts, but is more time consuming and more expensive, and nucleic acid extraction from tissues fixed with cross-linking reagents will be impaired. Moreover, snap-frozen material is immediately available for immunohistological examination, but only a limited panel of antigens can be detected in paraformaldehyde-fixed tissues.

Paraffin sections may be used with varying success for demonstration of mRNA *in situ*, depending on the fixation conditions. If tissue specimens are processed within a short time after surgical excision and are subjected to fixation and paraffin embedding in thin slices, the loss of signal tends to be minimal in comparison to frozen sections prepared in parallel. However, the mRNA content of these tissues should be monitored using an indicator probe (see above).

Frozen sections are cut, mounted on pretreated slides, quickly dried on a hot plate, and fixed in 4% paraformaldehyde (Lawrence and Singer, 1985; Tournier et al., 1987). Whereas precipitating fixatives have been shown to reduce RNA retention in the tissue, other cross-linking fixatives inhibit probe penetration into cells, thus contributing to a reduced signal strength (Singer *et al.*, 1986). Pretreatment of slides is as for DNA target sequences, except that slides are subjected to baking for several hours at 250°C in order to eliminate possible RNase contamination.

To prevent loss of tissue sections from slides during the lengthy *in situ* hybridization and washing procedures, the use of adhesives is recommended. Several adhesives have been described in the literature, including poly(L-lysine), gelatin, and Elmer's glue. Poly(L-lysine) is commonly used in immunohistology but is not very efficient for *in situ* hybridization (Niedobitek *et al.*, 1989b). Good results are obtained with gelatin/chrome alum, in particular for mRNA detection (Pardue, 1985). Here, however, the preparation of slides is laborious and batches of gelatin have to be tested prior to use to obtain reproducible results. In our hands, aminopropyltriethoxysilane (APES) is the most efficient adhesive (Niedobitek *et al.*, 1989b). This adhesive provides the glass with aminoalkyl groups, which are believed to bind covalently to tissue sections (Rentrop *et al.*, 1986). Coating the slides with APES for DNA and RNA hybridization as well as for immunohistological applications is convenient and reproducible.

B. Probes

Probes for hybridization experiments are labeled nucleic acid molecules with a sequence complementary to the target nucleic acid. For the detection of specific DNA sequences *in situ*, double-stranded (ds) cDNA probes are usually employed. However, synthetic oligonucleotide probes have also occasionally been used for this purpose (Cubie and Norval, 1989).

Probe sequences may be amplified in bacteria, usually *Escherichia coli*, using plasmids or phages as vectors (Sambrook *et al.*, 1989). After extraction and purification, the total plasmid DNA and the specific insert, or the excised insert alone, are labeled. Several techniques are available for labeling cDNA probes. The most widely applied methods are "nick translation" and "random primer extension." In nick translation, DNase I is used to cut nicks in the DNA in a random fashion. These nicks are then repaired by DNA polymerase I, and in this way labeled deoxyribonucleoside triphosphates (dNTPs) present in the reaction are incorporated in the newly synthesized DNA (Rigby *et al.*, 1977). Random primer extension requires just one enzyme, DNA polymerase I. Denatured DNA is incubated with short oligonucleotides that hybridize randomly to the DNA strands. Starting from these oligonucleotides attached to the DNA, the DNA polymerase I synthesizes new complementary strands using labeled dNTPs present in the reaction mixture (Feinberg and Vogelstein, 1983). Both of these techniques are equally well-suited to obtain probes with high specific activity. Random primer extension is usually employed to label small amounts of inserts whereas nick translation can be utilized to label large amounts (up to 1 μg) of total plasmid DNA. Standardized kits from various suppliers are commercially available for both methods. Use of inserts alone may be helpful to reduce background staining because plasmid DNA may hybridize to bacterial contaminants (Ambinder et al., 1986). However, this is more a problem for the investigation of extracted DNAs. In contrast, use of total plasmid DNA may be advantageous for *in situ* hybridization because the formation of networks at the site of hybridization may contribute to an increased signal strength. Network formation is mediated by probe fragments consisting of both insert and plasmid sequences [junction pieces (Lawrence and Singer, 1985)]. As the plasmid sequences do not hybridize to the target, they remain available for hybridization with other plasmid sequences, thus increasing the number of reporter molecules at the site of hybridization. This effect is observed mainly with large probe fragments of about 1500 bases. As the effect produced by the network formation cannot be calculated, total plasmid DNA is not useful for quantitative *in situ* hybridization. The ratio of labeled to unlabeled strands within dsDNA probes can be considerably increased by use of a primer-directed polymerase chain reaction (PCR) in combination with the thermostable Taq DNA polymerase, which allows the amplification of sequences up to 3000 base pairs in length (Saiki et al., 1988).

Probes can be labeled with either radioactive or nonradioactive reporter molecules. Initially, mainly radioactively labeled probes were employed (Blum et al., 1983; Brahic and Haase, 1978). The most commonly used radionuclides in *in situ* hybridization are ^{3}H, ^{35}S, and ^{32}P. Tritium has a low energy resulting in a good autoradiographic resolution. However, due to the long half-life of this isotope and the low specific activity of tritiated nucleotides, exposure times are usually long. Phosphorus-labeled dNTPs, on the other hand, have a short half-life and a high specific activity, thus requiring only short exposure times. Due to its high energy, the resolution of ^{32}P-labeled probes is not adequate for many purposes. ^{35}S provides a good compromise with reasonable tissue resolution and exposure times and therefore is now the most widely used radionuclide in *in situ* hybridization (e.g., Crum et al., 1989; Fox et al., 1989; Milani et al., 1989a,b: Niedobitek et al., 1989a,c; Syrjanen et al., 1987a; Weiss et al., 1989a,b). ^{35}S has a half-life of about 87 days. Probes labeled with this nuclide can be used for *in situ* hybridization for up to 6 weeks. Probes should be stored at −20°C in aliquots to prevent repeated freezing and thawing, and dithiothreitol (DTT) should be added to the probe to a final concentration of 10 mM to inhibit oxidation.

For many reasons, the introduction of nonradioactive reporter molecules (Brigati et al., 1983) has promoted the use of *in situ* hybridization. Use of radiolabeled probes requires special facilities such as dark rooms and causes problems concerning personnel safety and handling of radioactive waste. The introduction of nonradioactive probes made it possible to avoid these problems. Also, the detection of these probes can be achieved by routine immunohistochemical techniques that are well within the scope of many laboratories. These techniques also enable a good signal resolution superior to autoradiographic techniques. The most widely applied nonradioactive reporter molecule is biotin (Brigati *et al.*, 1983). Biotin-labeled nucleotides are commercially available and are readily incorporated in DNA probes using either nick translation or random priming. Also, biotin labeling of probes can be achieved by the use of photobiotin and high-energy light (Forster *et al.*, 1985). While the stability of radiolabeled probes is limited by the half-life of the radionuclide, biotin-labeled probes are very stable and can be stored at 4°C for more than a year.

Meanwhile, many other nonisotopic techniques have been described. DNA probes have been labeled with bromodeoxyuridine (BrdU) using nick translation (Niedobitek *et al.*, 1988a; 1989a; Traincard *et al.*, 1983). Also, probes labeled with fluorochromes have been employed successfully (Bauman, 1985). Recently, digoxigenine-labeled DNA probes have been used for the detection of human papillomaviruses (Herrington *et al.*, 1989). Incorporation of these reporter molecules is usually achieved by enzymatic incorporation of modified nucleotides by means of DNA polymerase. DNA labeling with BrdU has been achieved also by growing bacteria in a BrdU-containing medium (Kitazawa *et al.*, 1989). In addition, several methods have been devised for chemical modification of DNA, including the incorporation of sulfone groups (Morimoto *et al.*, 1987; Perrot-Rechenmann *et al.*, 1989), mercury (Hopman *et al.*, 1986a), or aminoacetylfluorene groups (Cremers *et al.*, 1987), or the UV irradiation-induced introduction of T–T dimers (Lund *et al.*, 1989). These nonisotopic reporter molecules are usually employed to overcome some of the drawbacks of biotinylated probes or in double-labeling experiments (Hopman *et al.*, 1986b; Niedobitek *et al.*, 1989a; Mullink *et al.*, 1989b; Nederlof *et al.*, 1989; Herrington *et al.*, 1989).

Double-stranded cDNA probes may be employed also in *in situ* hybridization experiments for the detection of mRNA sequences. However, reannealing of double-stranded probes reduces the amount of labeled probe available for hybridization to the target sequence. This problem can be overcome by employing single-stranded DNA or RNA probes. Single-stranded DNA is either obtained by chemical synthesis (oligonucleotides) (Gait, 1984; Guitteny *et al.*, 1988; Hankin and Lloyd, 1989; Uhl *et al.*, 1985) or by oligonucleotide-primed second-strand synthesis with DNA polymerase on recombinant single-stranded bacteriophage genomes, such as M13 or plasmids containing an M13 origin of replication (Varndell *et al.*, 1984). The latter is not a very frequently used approach, however.

The development of *in vitro* run-off transcription systems led to the availability of another type of probe (Cox *et al.*, 1984; Melton *et al.*, 1984). *In situ* hybridization with single-stranded RNA probes results in highly thermostable, specific RNA–RNA hybrids. These hybrids are also resistant to attack by most ribonucleases and therefore allow a posthybridization RNase digestion that considerably reduces background signal by removing single-stranded RNA sequences that are not specifically bound. Plasmids containing a multiple cloning site flanked by two promoters allow the transcription of the insert in alternate directions. Promoter sequences employed for run-off transcription vectors are derived from the *Salmonella* bacteriophage SP6 and the *E. coli* bacteriophages T3 and T7. The corresponding polymerases and run-off transcription vectors are commercially available from a variety of companies. Using these plasmids it is not only possible to make "antisense" RNA with a sequence complementary to the target mRNA, but also to generate "sense" RNA with a sequence identical to the mRNA in the specimen. The latter should not hybridize to the target and therefore provides a good negative control, particularly for quantitative autoradiographic evaluation. For linearizing transcription plasmid vectors, use of restriction enzymes that produce 3'-protruding ends should be avoided, as some polymerases may bind nonspecifically to these ends, leading to extraneous transcription. The length of the insert should not exceed 800–1000 base pairs, as the polymerases may terminate transcription prior to arriving at the end of the insert. If large parts of the mRNA in the specimen are to be detected, it may be useful to construct several run-off transcription vectors with different fragments of the probe sequence. Alternatively, RNA transcripts can be prepared from synthetic oligonucleotides and plasmids carrying the SP6 or similar promoters, after annealing of the oligonucleotide and enzymatic second-strand synthesis (Wölfl *et al.*, 1986; Denny *et al.*, 1988).

After completion of the transcription, the vector DNA may be selectively removed by controlled DNase digestion. To increase penetration into tissue and cells, probes should have an average length between 50 and 150 bases (Cox *et al.*, 1984; Moench *et al.*, 1985). This is achieved by controlled nicking of DNA probes with DNase I during nick translation, or by a controlled alkaline hydrolysis in the case of RNA probes, using the equation

$$t = (L_0 - L_f)/kL_0L_f$$

where t is the time in minutes and L_0 and L_f are the initial and final fragment lengths in kilobases. The empirically determined rate constant for hydrolysis, k, is approximately $0.11 \text{ kb}^{-1} \text{ min}^{-1}$ (Cox *et al.*, 1984).

RNA probes are usually labeled with [^{35}S]UTP, but other nonisotopic reporter molecules can be incorporated as well. Biotinylation can be achieved using either biotinylated UTP or allyl-UTP and secondary biotinylation. Bromouridine is also efficiently incorporated in RNA probes (G. Niedobitek and H. Herbst, unpublished observations). The problem of probe reannealing can also be circumvented by employing single-stranded synthetic oligonucleotides. The automation of oligonucleotide synthesis in recent years has provided a convenient and inexpensive alternative to the use of cloned DNA probes (Gait, 1984). Oligonucleotides are rapidly and reliably synthesized using commercially available DNA synthesizers. After cleavage of the product from the column, the oligonucleotides can be directly labeled and used in *in situ* hybridization experiments. As with other probes, oligonucleotide probes can be labeled with either radioactive or nonisotopic reporter molecules. Usually, biotin- or digoxigenin-labeled nucleotides are added using terminal transferase (Larsson, 1989; Zischler *et al.*, 1989). Alternatively, oligonucleotides can be labeled to high specific activity with ^{32}P at the 5' end using polynucleotide kinase (Sambrook *et al.*, 1989). Nonisotopic labeling is also possible by including an amino linker during the automated DNA synthesis, with subsequent chemical incorporation of biotin or fluorochromes (Chu and Orgel, 1985).

Because of their nature as deoxyribonucleic acids, synthetic oligonucleotides are not sensitive to RNase digestion. This renders them more stable than RNA probes, thus making handling the probes more convenient. However, a reduction of nonspecific background by controlled RNase digestion after completion of *in situ* hybridization is not possible with oligonucleotide probes. Also, hybrids consisting of oligonucleotides and mRNA are less stable than are pure RNA–RNA hybrids. In addition, oligonucleotide probes are usually short (about 30 bases). As sensitivity of detection is proportional to the length of the probe (Berger, 1986), use of oligonucleotides for detection of low-abundance transcript sequences requires the preparation of oligonucleotide mixtures covering longer parts of the transcript. In such cases, use of oligonucleotides may be considerably more expensive than use of biologically propagated probes.

After completion of probe labeling, nonincorporated labeled nucleotides should be removed from the probe. This is usually achieved by gel filtration with Sephadex G50. This purification is of paramount importance for radiolabeled probes, whereas in our experience it is not necessary for nonisotopic probes. For RNA probes, gel filtration is not suitable because of possible RNase contamination of the gel columns. Therefore, in our laboratory RNA probes are separated from free labeled nucleotides by phenol extraction and subsequent ethanol precipitation. The first step also removes all enzymes from the probe.

Before using probes in hybridization experiments, the efficiency of the labeling reaction should be controlled. Nonradioactive probes can be spotted onto nitrocellulose membranes followed by immunoenzymatic detection of the reporter molecule. However, this allows at best a semiquantitative evaluation. Use of radioactive reporter molecules allows the calculation of the specific activity of DNA probes labeled by nick translation. This is usually not possible with probes labeled by random priming or with RNA probes, because the amount of newly synthesized probe in these reactions is unknown.

C. Pretreatment and Hybridization Conditions

Whole cell preparations and sections of frozen tissues exposed to mild, noncrosslinking fixatives usually can be hybridized to the probe without any special pretreatment. Paraformaldehyde-fixed and, in particular, formalin-fixed and paraffin-embedded tissues, however, require a pretreatment of the sections in order to make the DNA accessible to the probes. This pretreatment usually includes incubation with hydrochloric acid to remove basic proteins, treatment with the detergent Triton X-100, and a proteolytic digestion (Brigati *et al.*, 1983). Several proteolytic enzymes are recommended. In our laboratory, pronase is usually employed (Niedobitek *et al.*, 1988a,b); however, other authors have used other proteases successfully (Burns *et al.*, 1986; Lawrence and Singer, 1985; McQuaid *et al.*, 1990; Naoumov *et al.*, 1988; Pringle *et al.*, 1987). Optimal conditions have to be determined for every batch of enzyme. In our hands pronase concentrations as high as 10 mg/ml have to be used occasionally, depending on the temperature and the length of the incubation (Niedobitek *et al.*, 1988b).

In experiments using radiolabeled probes it is usually recommended to acetylate the slides with triethanolamine and acetic anhydride to reduce background signal due to nonspecific interaction of probe with glass and tissue (Hayashi *et al.*, 1978). Some protocols recommend a prehybridization of slides with a hybridization buffer containing sheared and denatured carrier DNA (e.g., herring sperm DNA) prior to the application of the probe (Pringle *et al.*, 1989). This procedure has proved useful in filter hybridization experiments to reduce unspecific probe binding. However, in *in situ* hybridization it has no significant effect (Lawrence and Singer, 1985).

To enable the probe to hybridize to the tissue, both probe and tissue DNA have to be denatured. Basically, denaturation of dsDNA can be achieved by thermal, alkaline, or acid treatment (Raap *et al.*, 1986). The most convenient method is to apply the probe to the tissue and then to denature both simultaneously by heat treatment (Brigati *et al.*, 1983). In our experience, heat treatment of slides in ovens or water baths is often insufficient to achieve DNA denaturation. Consistent results are obtained by placing the slides directly on heating blocks at temperatures between 90 and 100°C for 3 minutes (Niedobitek *et al.*, 1988a,b). This procedure does not lead to significant disruption of tissue morphology.

Hybridization and washing conditions vary, depending on the stringency required. The melting temperature (T_m) is an indicator of the hybrid stability. The T_m is the temperature at which half of the double-stranded molecules of a given DNA sequence are dissociated into single strands. Conditions of high stringency are close to T_m. The main parameters influencing T_m are summarized in the following equation:

$$T_m = 81.5 + 16.6 \lg[Na^+] + 0.41(\%GC) - 0.72(\%F) - 600/N$$

where [Na^+] is the sodium chloride concentration in moles/liter, %GC is the percentage G + C content, %F is the percentage formamide content (v/v), and N is the chain length in base pairs.

Increased concentration of positively charged sodium ions stabilizes DNA–DNA hybrids by neutralizing the negatively charged phosphate groups of DNA and by decreasing the solubility of the bases. As GC base pairs are stabilized by three hydrogen bonds, in contrast to the two hydrogen bonds of AT base pairs, an increased GC content contributes to the stability of hybrids. Formamide has the capacity of breaking up hydrogen bonds and therefore destabilizes double-stranded nucleic acids. Obviously, hybrid stability is also influenced by the probe length. The impact of mismatches on hybrid stability is higher with short oligonucleotide probes than with longer cDNA probes. Nick-translated cDNA probes usually have an average length of 500 base pairs, and therefore probe length does not affect hybrid stability significantly in this instance.

Temperatures close to the melting point of DNA prevent hybridization between DNA sequences of limited homology, e.g., different subtypes of human papillomaviruses, whereas lower temperatures allow some cross-hybridization between related but not identical sequences. Usually, washing conditions are chosen closer to the T_m than are hybridization conditions. For DNA–DNA hybridization, the hybridization mixture usually consists of formamide (up to 50% v/v), dextran sulfate (usually 10% w/v), 2× SSC (0.3 M sodium chloride/0.03 M sodium citrate, pH 7.6), a carrier DNA (e.g., sonicated herring sperm DNA), and the labeled probe. Dextran sulfate binds water and thus reduces the effective volume of the hybridization mixture, leading to an enhanced hybridization (Lawrence and Singer, 1985).

In liquid hybridization experiments the kinetics of hybridization can be easily calculated. In *in situ* hybridization experiments, however, other factors, such as probe penetration into the tissue, influence the hybridization kinetics and therefore optimal times and probe concentrations have to be determined empirically. It has been shown that hybridization is usually accomplished after approximately 3 hours (Lawrence and Singer, 1985; Bashir *et al.*, 1989). However, for convenience, overnight hybridization may be chosen. For non-radioactive probes, hybridization times as short as 30 minutes may be sufficient. However, this requires high probe concentrations of up to 2 µg/ml in the hybridization mixture. In general, the hybridization is driven by the probe concentration (Lawrence and Singer, 1985). Therefore, increasing the probe concentration allows reduction of hybridization time. However, high probe concentrations are also associated with high background signal, particularly when radiolabeled probes are used. Also, high probe concentrations lead to increased expenses of *in situ* hybridization. Using ^{35}S-labeled DNA probes of about $(3–5) \times 10^8$ dpm/µg specific activity, a probe concentration of 20–40 ng/ml [corresponding to $(2–5) \times 10^5$ dpm/slide] gives the best results in our hands (Niedobitek *et al.*, 1989c).

After DNA–DNA hybridization, slides are washed in a solution containing 50% formamide and $0.1 \times$ SSC. DTT should be added to the hybridization mixture and to all washing solutions to a final concentration of 10 mM when ^{35}S-labeled probes are employed. In general, washing has to be more extensive for *in situ* hybridization with radioactive probes than for experiments with nonisotopic probes.

In situ hybridization for the detection of mRNA sequences in paraformaldehyde-fixed tissue sections requires a pretreatment similar to DNA–DNA hybridization. However, care must be taken to avoid RNase contamination. Glassware is baked at 250°C prior to use to inactivate the enzyme. For the same reason, all aqueous solutions [except tris(hydroxymethyl)aminomethane (TRIS)-containing solutions] should be treated with the cross-linking agent diethyl pyrocarbonate (DEPC) and autoclaved. Heat treatment of probe and specimen is usually not required for RNA–RNA hybridization. Because RNA may form secondary structures, moderate heat treatment of RNA probes may be advantageous in some cases. Denaturation of tissue DNA, however, should be avoided, as this may result in hybridization of the probe to the gene rather than to its transcript and thus may lead to labeling of every nucleus. Hybridization with RNA probes is usually performed at higher temperatures than with DNA probes. After hybridization, a digestion with RNase A removes nonspecifically bound single-stranded RNA probe, thus reducing the background signal in autoradiography.

D. PROBE DETECTION

Bound radioactive probes are located by autoradiography. The most frequently used technique for *in situ* hybridization involves dipping slides into a nuclear track emulsion, whereby the sections are covered with a thin layer of the emulsion. Nuclear track emulsions are suspensions of silver bromide crystals in gelatin. Different emulsions are commercially available, providing different grain sizes. Large grains are recommended for photographic documentation of results and smaller grains are preferred for quantitative *in situ* hybridization requiring counting of grains. The emulsion has to be melted at 42°C and is diluted 1 : 1 using either water or 0.6 M ammonium acetate, which might better preserve stability of the hybrids. After drying for about 1 hour, slides are exposed in the dark at 4°C together with a desiccant. Decay of radionuclides leads to the formation of latent images in the emulsion layer. Latent images are converted into real images by photographic development and fixation (Rogers, 1979). Slides are then counterstained with hematoxylin and eosin. To avoid artifacts, slides should be allowed to warm up slowly after exposure at 4°C. Color microautoradiography for the simultaneous detection of different viral genomes using two radionuclides of different energy and two layers of emulsion separated by inert gelatin has been described (Haase *et al.*, 1985). Though repeated melting of nuclear track emulsions is usually not recommended, this can be done with the emulsion used in our laboratory (Ilford G5) without increasing the background signal. In our experience, rests of diluted emulsion can be stored in the dark at 4°C and reused once.

For the detection of biotinylated probes, several methods have been described (Brigati *et al.*, 1983; Burns *et al.*, 1985; Lewis *et al.*, 1987; Löning *et al.*, 1986; Niedobitek *et al.*, 1989b; Pringle *et al.*, 1987; Syrjanen *et al.*, 1988; Unger *et al.*, 1986). The principle of most of these techniques is the specific binding of biotin to avidin (or streptavidin). Unlike avidin, streptavidin is not glycosylated and therefore is less prone to unspecific interaction with the tissue. Avidin is either directly labeled with an enzyme or is made to form complexes with biotinylated enzymes. Alternatively, the use of gold-labeled avidins and secondary silver amplification has been described (P. Jackson *et al.*, 1989; Löning *et al.*, 1987). The introduction of polyclonal and monoclonal antibiotin antibodies has made it possible to use conventional immunoenzymatic techniques for the detection of biotinylated probes (Löning *et al.*, 1986; Niedobitek *et al.*, 1989b).

Many other nonradioactive tagging substances have been described, including bromodeoxyuridine, digoxigenine, and several fluorochromes. Also, several methods for chemical modification, wherein antigenic haptens are introduced into nucleic acids, have been described. Probes labeled with fluorochromes can be detected directly by fluorescence microscopy. Detection of the other reporter molecules is achieved by polyclonal or monoclonal antibodies and conventional immunohistochemical techniques. Monoclonal antibodies to bromodeoxyuridine cross-react with bromouridine (G. Niedobitek and H. Herbst, unpublished observations) and therefore should be useful also for the detection of bromouridine-labeled RNA probes.

Choice of appropriate enzymes and chromogens for the detection of nonradioactive probes is of importance. The most frequently used enzymes are peroxidase and alkaline phosphatase. These enzymes are then developed with appropriate substrates and chromogens, usually diaminobenzidine (DAB) or aminoethylcarbazole (AEC) for peroxidase and new fushsin, fast red, nitro blue tetrazolium (NBT), or fast blue for alkaline phosphatase. Peroxidase has been shown to be less sensitive than alkaline phosphatase. However, it provides better tissue resolution. Also, reflection contrast microscopy has been shown to ameliorate detection of small amounts of precipitated diaminobenzidine in peroxidase-stained tissue sections (Cornelese ten Velde *et al.*, 1989; Cremers *et al.*, 1987). In addition, DAB development of peroxidase allows secondary silver amplification and evaluation at the ultrastructural level (Przepiorka and Myerson, 1986). Several chromogens are available for the development of alkaline phosphatase. In our hands, nitro blue tetrazolium, which yields a blue precipitate, provides the best sensitivity (Niedobitek *et al.*, 1989b). However, NBT-developed sections cannot be counterstained with hematoxylin. Therefore, if counterstaining is required, a red chromogen, e.g., new fuchsin, is advantageous.

Some investigators have reported the high sensitivity of immunogold silver-staining systems for the detection of biotinylated DNA probes (Löning *et al.*, 1987; P. Jackson *et al.*, 1989).

E. Combined *in Situ* Hybridization and Immunohistology

The combination of *in situ* hybridization with immunohistochemistry allows the detection of nucleic acids and proteins in a single tissue section or cytological preparation. In virus research this approach can be used (1) to demonstrate viral genomes and virus-encoded proteins simultaneously and (2) to identify the phenotype of virus-infected cells. Concurrent detection of viral DNA and proteins associated with viral latency or replication may allow an assessment of the state of the virus in an infected cell (latent or replicative). The simultaneous demonstration of viral DNA and transforming viral proteins may allow an assessment of the potential significance of a virus in the pathogenesis of malignant tumor.

Combination of *in situ* hybridization with immunohistochemical demonstration of cell type-specific antigens such as intermediate filaments may be used for the identification of virus-infected cells. This technique may be helpful for the identification of the sites of viral latency.

Because *in situ* hybridization for the detection of DNA sequences requires heat denaturation of tissue and probe DNA, which might destroy antigens, it is usually recommended to perform immunohistology before *in situ* hybridization (van der Loos *et al.*, 1989; Roberts *et al.*, 1989; Porter *et al.*, 1990). However, methods wherein *in situ* hybridization is performed prior to immunohistology have been described for some stable antigens (Wolber and Lloyd, 1988). Immunohistochemistry can be readily combined with *in situ* hybridization employing either radioactive or nonradioactive probes. However, in some instances it may be more appropriate to use nonradioactive instead of radioactive *in situ* hybridization. The tissue resolution is usually better when enzymatic procedures are used for the demonstration of bound probe. Also, when radiolabeled probes are employed, an intense signal leading to saturation of the emulsion may hide the underlying immunohistochemical staining product.

Immunohistochemistry on frozen or paraffin sections as well as on cytological preparations is performed as usual (Mullink *et al.*, 1989a). After completion of immunohistology, including the enzymatic development of the reaction, a proteolytic treatment may be required to unmask the target DNA. This is necessary in particular for sections of formalin-fixed and paraffin-embedded tissues. In our hands, treatment of sections with a 3 M KCl solution in addition to proteolytic digestion has proved helpful. Attention has to be paid to the choice of enzymes and, most importantly, of the chromogen. If both immunohistology and *in situ* hybridization are developed by enzymatic procedures, the chromogens have to be chosen to give good contrast. Also, the chromogen used for immunohistology has to be resistant to organic solvents, in particular when *in situ* hybridization is performed with radioactive probes. Diaminobenzidine for peroxidase and new fuchsin for alkaline phosphatase result in stable precipitates still clearly visible even after photographic development of radioactive *in situ* hybridization. NBT results in a dark blue to brown precipitate that contrasts well with the red color of new fuchsin. NBT, however, is not resistant to organic solvents.

For the demonstration of a particular mRNA sequence and its polypeptide product within the same cell, immunohistology can be performed before *in situ* hybridization or vice versa. Performing *in situ* hybridization before immunohistology may not be suitable for every antigen because some antigens are damaged by protease digestion. Also, dextran sulfate, which is a constituent of hybridization mixtures in most published protocols, can bind to proteins and impair their antigenic properties. Therefore, dextran sulfate may have to be excluded from the mixture, at the expense of higher background labeling. When immunohistochemistry is conducted before *in situ* hybridization, RNase inhibitors must be added to the antibodies and other solutions to prevent RNA degradation. Heparin, placental RNase inhibitor (RNasin), and yeast tRNA or bacterial rRNA are useful to block RNase in monoclonal antibody culture supernatants and antisera (Höfler *et al.*, 1987). Also, low concentrations of diethyl pyrocarbonate may be used whereas high diethyl pyrocarbonate concentrations also degrade immunoglobulins and antigens. However, in spite of the application of RNase inhibitors, RNA degradation may occur during immunohistology. Therefore, control slides hybridized to the probe without prior immunohistology should be included in the experiment to assess RNA loss and avoid erroneous evaluation.

F. Pitfalls and Controls

A central reasoning of pathologists favoring nonradioactive *in situ* hybridization techniques is the high background attributed to radiolabeled probes (Syrjanen *et al.*, 1988; Seyda *et al.*, 1989). In radioactive *in situ* hybridization, background signal is influenced by two parameters: probe concentration and exposure time. Most investigators recommend a probe concentration of 100–900 μg/ml in the hybridization mixture whereas in our hands probe concentrations of as little as 20–40 ng/ml gave the best results. It seems advisable to use low concentrations of high-specific-activity probes [specific activities of $(3-5) \times 10^8$ dpm/μg are readily achieved with [^{35}S]dCTP and commercially available nick translation reagent kits] to overcome the problem of high background. Also, acetylation of slides is recommended to reduce unspecific binding of probes (Hayashi *et al.*, 1978). The second parameter influencing the intensity of background signal is the exposure time. Overexposure clearly leads to an increased radioactive background. However, this problem is also encountered in immunoenzymatic detection of nonradioactive probes, as overdevelopment of enzymes also leads to increased background staining. For nonradioactive techniques, microscopic control of the enzymatic reaction is suggested to prevent overstaining. As this is not a suitable procedure for radioactive probes, it is recommended to expose at least three sets of slides from every experiment and develop them after different exposure times.

Grain formation in nuclear track emulsions may be induced by factors other than radioactive decay. Light, heat, electrostatic discharges, inappropriately fast drying of the emulsion, and mechanical factors such as scratches, pressure, or uneven surface of the section may lead to a diffuse or focal aggregation of silver grains. Also, chemical factors in the tissues or solutions may have a negative or positive influence on the formation of silver grains (positive or negative chemography). A fading of latent images before development can be induced by heat or humidity (Rogers, 1979).

The introduction of biotin-labeled DNA probes (Brigati *et al.*, 1983) has greatly promoted the application of *in situ* hybridization, especially in virus research. Several authors have employed biotinylated probes for the study of hepatitis B virus-related liver disease (Brambilla *et al.*, 1986; Herrmann and Hübner, 1987; Negro *et al.*, 1985; Rijntjes et al., 1985). However, it is known that several tissues, including liver and kidney, contain endogenous biotin, mainly as a prosthetic group of various enzymes (Dakshinamurti and Mistry, 1963). This endogenous avidin-binding activity (EABA) has long been recognized as a potential cause of background staining in immunohistology on frozen tissue sections, and methods for blocking EABA employing incubation of sections with avidin and subsequent saturation of free biotin-binding sites have been described (Wood and Warnke, 1981). Recent studies have demonstrated that EABA may also cause unspecific staining in *in situ* hybridization experiments on paraffin sections (Naoumov *et al.*, 1988; Niedobitek *et al.*, 1989a). Incubation of tissue sections with avidin and biotin prior to the heat denaturation of DNA does not reduce background staining, whereas omitting the heat treatment or application of the blocking reagents after heat treatment led to a significant reduction of unspecific staining (Niedobitek *et al.*, 1989a). The latter procedures, however, are not suitable for DNA *in situ* hybridization because tissue DNA is usually denatured by heat treatment, and application of the blocking reagents after heat treatment would interfere with the detection of the bound probe. Recently, it has been suggested that the intensity of background staining due to endogenous biotin depends on the degree of the proteolytic pretreatment of tissue sections (Naoumov *et al.*, 1988).

Unspecific binding of DNA and RNA probes to eosinophilic granulocytes has been recognized by several authors (Fox *et al.*, 1989; Niedobitek *et al.*, 1989a; Patterson *et al.*, 1989) and methods for blocking this binding have been described (Fox *et al.*, 1989; Patterson *et al.*, 1989). This artifact is probably due to the presence in eosinophilic granulocytes of a major basic protein with the capacity to precipitate nucleic acids (Gleich *et al.*, 1974). In hematoxylin and eosin (HE)-counterstained tissue sections this artifact is easily identified by the intense cytoplasmic staining of eosinophilic granulocytes, and rare eosinophils usually do not interfere with the evaluation of *in situ* hybridization. However, in tissues infiltrated with numerous eosinophilic granulocytes, e.g., some cases of Hodgkin's disease or nasopharyngeal carcinoma, or in bone marrow sections it can impede evaluation of *in situ* hybridization. On the other hand, the presence of a few eosinophils can serve as an internal control for some parameters of the *in situ* hybridization procedure, e.g., the detection system. This can be useful particularly for *in situ* hybridization with radioactive probes because an accumulation of grains over eosinophilic granulocytes excludes the possibility that factors such as negative chemography or latent image fading have influenced the *in situ* hybridization results. Finally, lipofuscin has been reported to be a cause of misinterpretation of *in situ* hybridization results in neuronal tissues (Steiner *et al.*, 1989).

To ensure an unequivocal evaluation of DNA-DNA *in situ* hybridization experiments, several controls have to be performed. A positive control tissue known to harbor the nucleic acid of interest should be included to make sure that all of the many steps of the *in situ* hybridization protocol have been properly carried out. Southern blot hybridization of DNA extracted from the tissue may be used to confirm the specificity of *in situ* hybridization results. Other specificity controls include hybridization to another sequence of the same gene or virus and immunohistochemical detection of the gene product or viral antigens.

For a proper evaluation of *in situ* hybridization results several negative control experiments are mandatory. Tissues negative for the nucleic acid investigated should be included. After DNase predigestion, no signal should be seen upon *in situ* hybridization (Burns *et al.*, 1987; Gnann *et al.*, 1988). Most important is the hybridization of the tissue to an unrelated probe. Use of total plasmid DNA may give unspecific results due to hybridization to bacterial DNA (Ambinder *et al.*, 1986). Although this is mainly a problem in filter hybridization experiments, it is advisable to use labeled plasmid DNA without the specific insert as a control. In virus research, hybridization to unrelated viral DNA provides an additional negative control.

Similar considerations apply also to hybridization experiments for the detection of mRNAs. Additional specificity controls may be carried out, for example, to test the sensitivity of the signal to digestion with RNase. Cellular RNA will be easily digested by this enzyme. If RNA probes are to be used, however, micrococcal nuclease must be substituted for this enzyme (Williamson, 1988), as residual RNase may attack the probe RNA as well, leading to false results. Micrococcal nuclease is dependent on Ca^{2+} ions and is inhibited by high concentrations of sodium chloride.

Furthermore, it may be helpful to correlate *in situ* hybridization and previously obtained immunohistological results. Size determination by Northern blot analysis of the transcript to be detected by *in situ* hybridization should always be carried out if heterologous nucleic acid probes are used. When used as a negative control probe, the sense RNA must not produce a signal in *in situ* hybridization. Probing for different regions of a particular transcript in different reactions with nonoverlapping probes should result in identical expression patterns before unexpected *in situ* hybridization results are to be accepted.

G. Sensitivity of Radioactive and Nonradioactive Techniques

The introduction of nonradioactive probes has greatly stimulated the use of *in situ* hybridization. However, the question of the comparative sensitivity of radioactive *in situ* hybridization techniques versus nonradioactive ones is still a matter of controversy. This may be relatively unimportant for the diagnosis of acute viral infections, e.g., cytomegalovirus (CMV) infection in AIDS patients, which is usually accompanied by production of infectious virions. Thus, in such instances an abundance of viral DNA is regularly available for hybridization. The sensitivity of *in situ* hybridization techniques, however, is critical for studies aiming at the demonstration of low viral copy numbers in latent infections.

Several studies have evaluated the sensitivity of radioactive and nonradioactive *in situ* hybridization techniques (Burns *et al.*, 1987; Niedobitek *et al.*, 1989a; Nuovo and Richart, 1989b; Seyda *et al.*, 1989; Syrjanen *et al.*, 1987b, 1988; Walboomers *et al.*, 1988). Nuovo and Richart (1989b) have evaluated 80 epithelial lesions of the genital tract for the presence of human papillomavirus (HPV) DNA with biotin- and ^{35}S-labeled probes and have concluded that both techniques resulted in similar numbers of positive cases. Syrjanen *et al.* (1987b) demonstrated the detection of HPV DNA in suprabasal cells of cervical lesions with ^{35}S-labeled probes but not with biotin-labeled probes. However, using another detection system for biotinylated probes, the same authors reported a more frequent labeling of suprabasal cells with biotinylated than with ^{35}S-labeled probes (Syrjanen *et al.*, 1988). In a study comparing bromodeoxyuridine- and ^{35}S-labeled probes for the detection of hepatitis B virus (HBV) DNA in liver sections we demonstrated a high sensitivity of the radiolabeled probe. The sensitivity of the nonradioactive technique was insufficient for the detection of the HBV in infected liver, whereas CMV DNA was readily detected in infected hepatocytes with bromodeoxyuridine-labeled probes (Niedobitek *et al.*, 1989a).

Using ^{35}S-labeled DNA probes we have recently demonstrated the detection of the single copy of the EBV genome per cell in the AW Ramos cell line (Klein *et al.*, 1975; Andersson and Lindahl, 1976), an EBV-converted subline of the EBV-negative Burkitt lymphoma line, Ramos (Pahl *et al.*, 1991). In the B95.8 cell line, which has a small percentage of cells with virus replication (Miller *et al.*, 1972), the virus-producing cells showed a saturation of the emulsion after short exposure time whereas the other latently infected cells of this line displayed a strong nuclear signal of more than 100 grains per nucleus. In comparison, the sensitivity of *in situ* hybridization with biotin-labeled probes was limited to the detection of EBV-producing cells in the B95.8 cell line. Experiments with an RNase predigestion before probe application have demonstrated that hybridization to mRNA transcripts does not contribute significantly to the signal under our experimental conditions (Pahl *et al.*, 1991).

Our results confirm previous studies reporting a higher sensitivity of *in situ* hybridization techniques with radiolabeled probes than with nonradioactive techniques (Crum *et al.*, 1986; Höfler *et al.*, 1987; Syrjanen *et al.*, 1987b). Other reports, however, claim a high sensitivity of nonradioactive techniques, comparable or even superior to radioactive techniques (Allan *et al.*, 1989; Burns *et al.*, 1987; Nuovo and Richart, 1989b; Syrjanen *et al.*, 1988; Walboomers *et al.*, 1988). The difference between our results and these studies is difficult to explain. A central argument of authors favoring nonradioactive *in situ* hybridization is a high background signal ascribed to radioactive probes (Syrjanen *et al.*, 1988; Seyda *et al.*, 1989). This, however, may be due to inadequate technique. Whereas most other authors have used between 100 and 900 ng/ml of ^{35}S-labeled probe, our protocol requires a probe concentration of only 20-40 ng/ml. Use of inappropriately high probe concentrations may contribute to an unfavorable signal-to-noise ratio.

Also, it is well known that the sensitivity of *in situ* hybridization with nonradioactive probes depends on the detection system applied. An increased sensitivity of systems employing alkaline phosphatase as the marker enzyme has been demonstrated when compared to peroxidase-labeled reagents (Nuovo and Richart, 1989b; Niedobitek *et al.*, 1989b). Several reports concluded that the use of streptavidin and biotinylated alkaline phosphatase together with NBT as chromogen gives the best results (Bashir *et al.*, 1989; Burns *et al.*, 1987; Lewis *et al.*, 1987; Niedobitek *et al.*, 1989b). This system, which is also used in our laboratory, was introduced a couple of years ago and no major progress has since been made. Some authors recommend the application of an antibiotin antiserum and a biotinylated secondary antibody before incubation with a streptavidin– enzyme complex (Löning *et al.*, 1986; Naoumov *et al.*, 1988). However, this procedure may lead to an increased background staining (Niedobitek *et al.*, 1989b).

Concerning the question of sensitivity of nonradioactive techniques, it is interesting to note that most protocols for nonradioactive *in situ* hybridization employ much higher probe concentrations than recommended for radioactive *in situ* hybridization, ranging from 1 to 2 µg/ml (Borisch *et al.*, 1988; Brigati *et al.*, 1983; Burns *et al.*, 1987; Löning *et al.*, 1986; Mullink *et al.*, 1989b; Myerson *et al.*, 1984; Niedobitek *et al.*, 1989a,b; Walboomers *et al.*, 1988). In view of the stated high sensitivity of nonradioactive *in situ* hybridization, this difference is difficult to explain. The obvious necessity of a comparatively high probe concentration rather points to a lower sensitivity of ISH with biotinylated probes in comparison to ^{35}S-labeled probes.

The sensitivity of *in situ* hybridization is also determined by the size of the viral genome of interest and the choice of the probe. Human papillomaviruses and hepatitis B virus have comparatively small genomes of 9 and 3 kb, respectively. Therefore, the amount of DNA available for hybridization is limited in comparison to the larger herpesviruses, which have genomes of about 150–250 kb. Also, the size of the probe and the number of reiterations of the probe sequence in the viral genome is of importance. The *Bam*HI-W fragment used as a probe in our EBV *in situ* hybridization studies is 3.1 kb and is repeated between 10 and 15 times in the EBV genome. Thus, this probe covers about 30 to 35 kb of target DNA. Therefore, the copy number of viral genomes in a given cell necessary for detection by *in situ* hybridization is higher for smaller viruses, such as HPV or HBV, than for EBV. Similar considerations apply also for mRNA *in situ* hybridization. In particular, use of small synthetic oligonucleotide probes may lead to low sensitivity. This problem can be resolved by use of multiple oligonucleotides with different sequences covering different parts of the transcript.

Recently, integrated EBV genomes were demonstrated in a Burkitt lymphoma cell line (Namalwa) by means of biotin-labeled probes and fluoroscein isothiocyanate (FITC)-labeled streptavidin (Lawrence et al., 1988, 1989). These results, however, were obtained with isolated chromosomes and preparations of interphase nuclei and therefore probably cannot be compared to studies using whole cells or tissue sections.

Bashir et al. (1989) have demonstrated a staining of Namalwa cells with biotinylated probes and a streptavidin–alkaline phosphatase detection system. Their results, however, were mainly due to hybridization of the probe to RNA transcripts, and therefore an estimation of the sensitivity of their technique is not possible from their data. Because the presence of substantial amounts of mRNA in routinely processed tissues cannot be taken for granted, it would seem important to establish the threshold of detection of ISH techniques for DNA. In our experiments, predigestion with RNase demonstrated that hybridization with mRNA did not contribute significantly to the signal (Pahl et al., 1991).

In conclusion, though nonradioactive *in situ* hybridization techniques have been improved since their introduction, there is, to our best knowledge, currently no report that unequivocally demonstrates a sensitivity with nonradioactive probes that is similar or higher than that achieved with radioactive probes for the detection of viral DNA.

As detection of RNA and DNA probes is achieved virtually by the same techniques, the above considerations should apply also to RNA probes. Indeed, the superiority of ^{35}S-labeled RNA probes to biotinylated probes for the demonstration of HPV mRNA has been demonstrated (Crum et al., 1988).

III. Applications

A. *In Situ* Hybridization for the Detection of DNA

In situ hybridization can be used for the detection of specific DNA sequences in any kind of tissue or cell preparation. This technique has been applied to the demonstration of Y chromosomal DNA in tissue sections, allowing sex determination, for example (Burns et al., 1985; Handyside et al., 1989; West et al., 1987). Also, aneuploid cells have been demonstrated in cytological preparations (Giwercman et al., 1990) and human tissue xenografts in mice have been identified by *in situ* hybridization (Obara et al., 1986).

patic tissues also, e.g., pancreas and spleen, using *in situ* hybridization and Southern blot analysis (Jilbert *et al.*, 1987).

More recently, changes in the distribution of HBV DNA in the liver according to the stage of chronic hepatitis have been demonstrated by *in situ* hybridization (Michitaka *et al.*, 1988). Detection of HBV-encoded antigens, most notably the HBV surface (HBs) antigen and the HBV core (HBc) antigen by immunohistology is a valuable tool for the histopathological evaluation of liver diseases (Gerber and Thung, 1987). Simultaneous detection of HBV genomes and antigens in tissue sections by combined immunohistology and *in situ* hybridization has indicated the absence of the HBc antigen in hepatocytes with cytoplasmic virus replication (Blum *et al.*, 1984a). Thus, *in situ* hybridization may be more sensitive than immunohistology for the diagnosis of HBV infection. Also, this double-labeling technique may be used to study the pathogenesis of HBV-related hepatitis.

Involvement of HBV in the pathogenesis of inflammatory liver disease and of hepatocellular carcinoma and the potential high sensitivity of *in situ* hybridization for identification of the virus have stimulated many groups to apply *in situ* hybridization to HBV DNA in liver tissue in various diseases. Many of these studies were performed with biotinylated probes (Brambilla *et al.*, 1986; Herrmann and Hübner, 1987; Negro *et al.*, 1985; Rijntjes *et al.*, 1985). However, the presence of endogenous biotin in liver (Dakshinamurti and Mistry, 1963) may lead to background staining, making interpretation difficult or impossible (Niedobitek *et al.*, 1989a). Therefore, other nonradioactive reporter molecules have been used for labeling of DNA probes (Niedobitek *et al.*, 1989a). However, using bromodeoxyuridine-labeled HBV probes we did not obtain any signal in liver infected by HBV, whereas CMV-infected hepatocytes were readily detected by this technique (Niedobitek *et al.*, 1989a). Thus, *in situ* hybridization with isotopic probes currently provides the only reliable technique for the demonstration of the viral genome at the single-cell level.

B. *In Situ* Hybridization for the Detection of RNA

Almost any kind of intracellular RNA may be detected by *in situ* hybridization, and its sensitivity has been greatly increased by the introduction of complementary RNA probes. Most publications deal with detection of gene transcripts, i.e., messenger RNA (mRNA) and its precursors, heterogeneous nuclear RNA (hnRNA), but *in situ* hybridization for genomes of RNA viruses and ribosomal RNA (rRNA) has been carried out as well (Buongiorno-Nardelli and Amaldi, 1970). The purpose of the following paragraphs is not to provide a complete list of the abundance of genes and cellular targets analyzed by *in situ* hybridization during recent years. Rather, the following paragraphs will focus on some applications to human tissues, which illustrate the value of *in situ* hybridization as an additional technique in histopathology, in particular by comparison to immunohistology. The application of *in situ* hybridization to problems in some specialized fields, such as neurobiology, embryology, and endocrinology, is not included here, as it has been extensively reviewed by others (e.g., DeLellis and Wolfe, 1987; Höfler, 1987; Valentino *et al.*, 1987).

1. *Transcripts of Oncogenes, Growth Factor Genes, and Homeotic Genes*

If the polypeptide product of a particular gene cannot be localized in histological or cytological specimens by histochemical or immunohistological techniques, *in situ* hybridization represents the only method for the assessment of gene expression at the single-cell level. This applies to the products of many newly identified genes, in particular to those isolated by nucleic acid hybridization with heterologous gene probes. Examples for such genes are cellular oncogenes (c-*onc*), genes encoding growth factors and growth factor receptors, and homeobox genes. Cellular oncogenes were initially identified by their homology to viral oncogenes (v-*onc*) included in the genome of acutely transforming retroviruses, or were identified by their transforming properties in certain fibroblastoid cell lines. Other cellular oncogenes were isolated by homology to other c-*onc* genes such as N-*myc* (Schwab *et al.*, 1983). Consequently, nucleic acid probes were available earlier than were antisera or antibodies of immunohistological quality. Furthermore, some immunological reagents, in particular antibodies directed against short peptide sequences, may exhibit cross-reactivity with unrelated proteins. In this context, cross-reactivities of antibodies raised against cytoskeletal proteins with oncogene and viral gene products were described (Crabbe, 1985).

In situ hybridization techniques have been employed in the study of the expression patterns of various oncogenes in chick and murine fetal tissues, as well as for the analysis of human malignancies. To understand of the contribution of c-*onc* gene expression to carcinogenesis, morphological criteria must be considered as well, because many c-*onc* genes may be expressed at high levels not only in the tumor cell population but in reactive stromal or inflammatory cells within the tumor tissue as well.

The expression of different c-*onc* genes has been investigated for a number of human malignancies. Hamatani *et al.* (1989a) studied the expression of several oncogenes in non-Hodgkin lymphomas using biotinylated probes. Their experiments showed high levels of nuclear oncogene expression in the tumor cell population in the majority of lymphomas regardless of histology and phenotype. Similarly, bone marrow cells (Emilia *et al.*, 1986), hydatiform mole (Sarkar *et al.*, 1986), medullary thyroid tumors (Klimpfinger *et al.*, 1988), gliomas (Bigner *et al.*, 1988), and sarcomas (Fahrer *et al.*, 1989) were investigated for expression of several oncogenes by *in situ* hybridization. Among the oncogenes subjected to detailed expression studies by *in situ* hybridization is the c-*fms* gene, which encodes the receptor for colony-stimulating factor 1. The c-*fms* gene was thus found to be expressed in myelomonocytic precursor cells (Wakamiya *et al.*, 1987; Bicknell *et al.*, 1988) and in cases of acute myeloblastic leukemias (Rambaldi *et al.*, 1988), but not in Reed–Sternberg cells of Hodgkin's disease (Farhi, 1989). The c-*fms* mRNA was also detected at high levels during placental development (Arceci *et al.*, 1989) and in uterine epithelium; consequently, c-*fms* transcripts were also present in endometrial adenocarcinomas at particularly high levels in clinically aggressive forms (Kacinski *et al.*, 1988). In a study of c-*abl* expression in leukemic and lymphoma cells by Greil *et al.* (1989), it was emphasized that *in situ* hybridization detected few copies of the transcript in small subpopulations of the malignant cell clones, signals that were otherwise not detectable by extractive methods. The c-*fos* gene, which encodes a nuclear oncogene, is expressed during monocytoid cell differentiation and in neutrophilic, but not eosinophilic, granulocytes (Kreipe *et al.*, 1987), and in erythroblasts (Caubet *et al.*, 1989). The c-*fos* gene is also expressed during bone, cartilage, and tooth development (Caubet and Bernaudin, 1988). It was studied in more detail in growth plates of long bones and calvarial bones (Sandberg *et al.*, 1988a,b). The *ras* genes are expressed in many cell types and malignancies, such as pancreatic carcinomas (Parsa *et al.*, 1986), lymphomas (Hamatani *et al.*, 1989b), oral squamous carcinomas (Hoellering and Shuler, 1989), or stomach carcinomas (Ohuchi *et al.*, 1987). Although high levels of expression have been occasionally detected, no strict correlation to differentiation and histological type or to point mutations in *ras* genes were seen. The *int-2* gene, a member of the basic fibroblast growth factor (FGF) gene family, was found to be expressed in human breast carcinomas with amplification at the *int-2* locus (Liscia *et al.*, 1989). Mammary carcinomas were also studied by *in situ* hybridization for expression of the c-*erbB-2* (Walker *et al.*, 1989), the c-*erbB-1* (EGF receptor), and the estrogen receptor genes (Barrett-Lee *et al.*, 1987; Kacinski *et al.*, 1988), which are all homologues of the oncogenes v-*erbB* and v-*erbA*, respectively, of the chicken erythroblastosis virus. The c-*myc* gene was found to be expressed in mitogen-activated B lymphocytes (Lacy *et al.*, 1986) during human placental development (Pfeifer-Ohlsson *et al.*, 1984; Rydnert *et al.*, 1987), in spermatogonia (but not in spermatocytes and spermatids) (Koji *et al.*, 1988), in normal human intestinal mucosa (ten Kate *et al.*, 1989), as well as in a variety of malignancies such as lung cancer (Lee *et al.*, 1988), colonic adenomas, and adenocarcinomas (Mariani-Costantini et al., 1989), and acute myelogenous leukemias (Evinger-Hodges et al., 1988). The N-*myc* gene, which is amplified in some neuroblastomas (Schwab et al., 1983), shows high homology to c-*myc* and also encodes a nuclear protein. Its amplification and expression were studied by *in situ* hybridization in fetal human brain and kidney (Grady et al., 1987; Hirvonen et al., 1989), as well as in related malignancies, such as neuroblastoma (Schwab et al., 1984; Grady-Leopardi et al., 1986; Noguchi et al., 1988) and Wilm's tumor (Shaw et al., 1988). The c-*sis* gene, encoding the B chain of the platelet-derived growth factor (PDGF), was seen in sarcomas (Fahrer et al., 1989), in breast lesions with marked desmoplasia (pointing to paracrine action) (Ro et al., 1989), and in acute myelogenous leukemias (Evinger-Hodges et al., 1988). The c-*src* gene is expressed in fetal human liver and brain (Grady et al., 1987), and c-*yes* is expressed at high levels in Purkinje cells (Sudol et al., 1989).

In the authors' laboratory, the spatial and temporal expression patterns of several oncogenes were investigated in acute toxic rat liver injury and in human liver biopsies (Herbst et al., 1991b). Previously, characteristic kinetics of c-*onc* transcript levels have been observed following partial hepatectomy (PH) or administration of hepatotoxins. After partial hepatectomy, compensatory growth is initiated within minutes, resulting in sequential activation of c-*ets* and c-*fos* genes, followed by increasing c-*myc* transcript levels within the first 4 hours, while c-K-*ras* and c-H-*ras* mRNA levels reach peak values 24–48 hours after surgery (Thompson et al., 1986; Fausto, 1986; Bhat et al., 1987). All these studies employed dot blot and Northern blot hybridization techniques and were thus not suitable for defining the cell types responsible for the alterations in gene expression. We have analyzed by *in situ* hybridization with single-stranded, ^{35}S-labeled cRNA probes the cellular distribution of c-*fos*, c-*jun*, c-*myc*, c-H-*ras*, c-K-*ras*, and c-*fms* transcripts in adult rat liver at various time points following intraperitoneal administration of carbon tetrachloride. Administration of CCl_4 results in hepatocellular necrosis predominantly of centrilobular (zone III) hepatocytes and severe fibrosis with architectural remodeling of the liver after chronic intoxication.

Very low levels of c-*fos*, c-*jun*, c-*myc*, and c-*ras* transcripts were observed in the cytoplasm of a large proportion of hepatocytes and, in the case of c-*myc* and c-*fms*, of some nonparenchymal cells. As early as 30 minutes after administration of CCl_4, strong expression of c-*fos* and c-*jun* was visible in hepatocytes of the lobular zone III, which showed centrifugal progression through zones II and I within the next 3 hours. Similarly, expression of c-*myc* becomes visible in zone III hepatocytes 1 hour after intoxication, and progresses within the next 6 hours through the lobule. The c-*myc* transcripts are then seen for up to 48 hours in nonparenchymal cells of zone III and in hepatocytes of zones I and II. The c-H-*ras* and c-K-*ras* expression was slightly delayed as compared to c-*myc*; hepatocytes of zone III showed a stronger signal as compared to zone I and II parenchymal cells; in general, hepatocellular c-H-*ras* transcripts were localized over cytoplasm and nucleus, whereas c-H-*ras* transcripts were found only on scattered nonparenchymal cells. The c-*myc* transcripts were found mainly in the cytoplasm of most hepatocytes and in some portal tract and lobular nonparenchymal cells. The expression of c-*myc* and c-H-*ras* decreased after 48 and 72 hours, respectively, concomitantly with the development of liver cell necrosis in zone III of the lobule. The c-*fms* gene, which was expressed in many Kupffer cells of normal liver, showed a considerable increase in the number of labeled cells per lobule 48–72 hours after intoxication, particularly in areas of necrosis.

These experiments demonstrate that sequential oncogene activation in hepatocytes is initiated at the site of toxic injury, then spreads over the whole parenchymal compartment, resulting in vigorous mitotic activity within the following days. Delayed expression of oncogenes in nonparenchymal cells points to mechanisms of activation different from hepatocytes, perhaps via stimulation of Kupffer cells by necrotic material and subsequent activation of other mesenchymal cells. Even if immunohistologic reagents had been available for this study, the differences in oncogene activation observed in this model were unlikely to be resolved by methods other than *in situ* hybridization with autoradiographic development, allowing semiquantitative evaluation.

Recently, *in situ* hybridization has also been successfully applied to the identification of the cellular sources of various cytokines (such as interleukins and other lymphokines), transforming growth factors, tumor necrosis factors, interferons, insulin-like growth factors, and platelet-derived growth factor. Despite the development of a large number of highly specific immunological reagents and of sensitive immunohistological techniques, immunohistology may fail to provide information about the cellular source of a protein. This failure may be the result of uptake of peptides by specific receptors, providing false positive information, or a lack of signal may be influenced by the rate of polypeptide synthesis, degradation, and secretion. Several studies dealt with the expression of interleukin 1 (IL-1) in different forms of human monocytes (Bernaudin *et al.*, 1988; Roy *et al.*, 1988; Tron *et al.*, 1988), or with expression of IL-2 in fetal thymocytes (Carding *et al.*, 1989), HTLV-I-infected T cells (Goebels *et al.*, 1988), or placental syncytiotrophoblast cells (Boehm *et al.*, 1989). IL-3 gene transcripts were shown in blood mononuclear cells (Wimperis *et al.*, 1989), as well as in astrocytes and neuronal cell bodies of mouse brain (Farrar *et al.*, 1989); IL-4 gene transcripts were shown in developing thymus and peripheral lymphocytes (Sideras *et al.*, 1988), and IL-6 mRNA was shown in psoriatic skin and isolated keratinocytes (Grossman *et al.*, 1989) and human monocytes (Navarro *et al.*, 1989). Using an oligonucleotide probe, IL-5 expression was studied in Hodgkin's disease by *in situ* hybridization and was found in the tumor cell population in some cases that also displayed a marked eosinophilia (Samoszuk and Nansen, 1990). Tumor necrosis factor-α (TNF-α) expression was detected in basophils (Steffen et al., 1989) and cells of the monocytoid lineage in peripheral blood and lung tissue (Strieter et al., 1989), in acute myeloid leukemias (Wakamiya et al., 1989), and in macrophages infiltrating colorectal adenocarcinomas (Beissert et al., 1989). Peripheral blood mononuclear leukocytes producing interferon-α (IFN-α) were characterized by Gobl et al. (1988) and by Sandberg et al. (1989b). Because of the lack of antibodies that can discriminate between insulin-like growth factors I and II (IGF-I and IGF-II; somatomedins C and A), in situ hybridization has been employed primarily for morphologic studies in this field, demonstrating these factors in placenta (Wang et al., 1988; Ohlsson et al., 1989), fetal tissues (Han et al., 1987a,b; Hirvonen et al., 1989), cardiomyocytes (Engelmann et al., 1989), striated muscle cells (Edwall et al., 1989), and Wilm's tumors (Paik et al., 1989). In mammary carcinoma, the in situ hybridization pattern showed evidence of a paracrine role for IGF-I (Yee et al., 1989). TGF-α synthesis occurs in a variety of neoplastic cells and during early fetal development (Han et al., 1988), and has also been demonstrated by in situ hybridization in normal human keratinocytes (Coffey et al., 1987). TGF-β appears to be implicated in bone development (Sandberg et al., 1988a,b). PDGF was found to be expressed in fibroblasts, smooth muscle cells (Terracio et al., 1988), and glioblastomas (Hermannsson et al., 1988), and is related to the development of atherosclerotic plaques (Wilcox et al., 1988).

Another example of gene families primarily identified by homology to other nucleic acid sequences are homeotic genes. Many of the genes controlling segmentation and pattern formation in *Drosophila* contain a conserved 183-base pair sequence known as the homeobox. Homeobox sequences have also been found in mouse and man. This striking conservation suggests a fundamental role for homeotic genes in developmental processes. To test this hypothesis, in situ hybridization has been used by several authors for the analysis of the spatial and temporal patterns of homeobox gene expression during embryogenesis in correlation to major morphogenetic events. Most homeotic genes have been found to be expressed in a region-specific manner during the formation and differentiation of the embryonic axis, and striking gene transcript patterns were seen in segmented structures of the embryo (i.e., somites, neural tube, or dorsal spinal ganglia) as well as in tissues with no obvious segmental origin (Dony and Gruss, 1987, 1988; Davis and Joyner, 1988; Gaunt, 1988; Graham et al., 1988; Hogan et al., 1988; Le Mouellic et al., 1988; Bogarad et al., 1989; Murphy et al., 1989; Robert et al., 1989). In situ hybridization may well be suited to reveal the potential role of homeotic genes not only for human morphogenesis, but also for differentiation and metastatic properties of human tumors.

2. Transcripts of Extracellular Matrix Protein Genes

The immunohistological analysis of the intracellular precursors of extracellular matrix proteins in tissue sections is complicated by the low concentration of intracellular antigenic determinants as compared to their concentration in the extracellular space. This results either in the absence of any detectable signal in the cytoplasm of a potential producer cell, or in difficulty in discriminating a positive signal from background, or "spill-over" of reaction product from the extracellular space, particularly in the case of fibroblast-like cells with little cytoplasm.

Eukaryotic cells are surrounded by a complex assembly of macromolecules termed the extracellular matrix (ECM). This specialized tissue compartment consists of the interstitium, which may separate cells from each other over long distances; the pericellular matrix components, which interact with structures of the cell membrane; and the basement membrane, which supports epithelial, endothelial, and certain mesenchymal cells. It was once assumed that only few species of molecules were involved in ECM formation. During the last 20 years, however, more than 30 polypeptides contributing to the ECM have been characterized. The ECM not only provides support and cohesiveness, but also plays an important role in the regulation of gene expression because of the interaction of certain ECM molecules with specific receptors on cell membranes. It is thus of particular interest to analyze the patterns of ECM component gene expression and to determine the cellular sources of the ECM.

In situ hybridization has been employed by several authors studying the differential localization of the most frequently occurring types of collagens in injured and normal skin (Scharffetter *et al.*, 1989a,b), in fractured and developing bone and cartilage (Sandberg *et al.*, 1989a,b), or in conditions such as scleroderma (Kahari *et al.*, 1988), neurofibromatosis (Peltonen *et al.*, 1988a; Jaakkola *et al.*, 1989), periodontal inflammation (Larjava *et al.*, 1989, 1990), or mammary cancer (Clavel *et al.*, 1989), as well as in adult and fetal human (Sandberg *et al.*, 1989c,d) or animal tissues (Hayashi *et al.*, 1986, 1988; Nah *et al.*, 1988; Devlin *et al.*, 1988). For myocardium, it was determined by *in situ* hybridization that fibroblasts are capable of producing types I, III, and IV collagen, whereas myocytes express only the type IV basement membrane collagen (Eghbali *et al.*, 1989). Elevated levels of type I collagen were found in distinct cells of arterial walls of hypertensive calves as compared to normotensive animals (Prosser *et al.*, 1989). *In situ* hybridization was also employed to study the origin of basement membrane components in developing kidney and in a murine model of polycystic kidney disease (Ebihara *et al.*, 1988; Laurie *et al.*, 1989). Other ECM components studied by *in situ* hybridization constitute cartilage proteoglycan core protein, amelogenin, or fibronectin (Mallein-Gerin *et al.*, 1988; Snead *et al.*, 1988; Peltonen *et al.*, 1988b).

The usefulness of *in situ* hybridization for the discrimination of ECM-producing or nonproducing cells is best illustrated by its application to the problem of liver fibrosis. Similar to other tissues and organs, fibrosis of the liver is associated with an increased deposition of ECM proteins. The bulk of these proteins is formed of the interstitial collagen types I and III, whereas type IV (basement membrane) collagen, other types of collagens, and ECM proteins (such as laminin) are quantitatively minor components. Because in progressive stages excessive deposition of ECM results in severely impaired organ function, it may be desirable to inhibit the formation of ECM deposits for therapeutic purposes. Some of the suggested therapeutic approaches to the prevention of liver fibrosis aim at inhibiting secretion and deposition of the newly synthesized procollagen, and most of these approaches consider the hepatocyte as the primary target (Chojkier and Brenner, 1988). The cellular source of hepatic collagens, however, has remained controversial, because biochemical, immunohistological, and other methods have yielded, in part, contradictory results when applied to *in vivo* and *in vitro* models, ranging from negligible amounts to a contribution of up to 75% to the hepatic collagen pool (Friedman *et al.*, 1985; Chojkier *et al.*, 1988). Immunohistological approaches have suffered from the shortcomings mentioned above, and *in vitro* cultivation methods were complicated by the fact that other cells with similar biophysical properties, such as Ito (fat-storing) cells, may contaminate primary hepatocyte cultures (Maher *et al.*, 1988). Furthermore, it is possible that disintegration prior to cultivation of the organ may alter the gene expression patterns of hepatocytes. Similarly, immunohistological methods had not been able to unequivocally establish the cell type producing laminin.

To rule out problems related to fixation procedures, to the specificity of immunological reagents, to phagocytosis, or to *in vitro* cultivation, *in situ* hybridization was chosen to localize ECM protein gene transcripts at the single-cell level in rat and human liver. The first experimental rat model examined was CCl_4-induced liver fibrosis (Milani *et al.*, 1989a). CCl_4 is toxic to hepatocytes and, as stated above, may induce liver cell necrosis predominantly in zone III of the lobule in a dose-dependent manner. Continuous application (1 ml/kg body weight) induces architectural changes progressing to cirrhosis within 4–5 weeks. However, administration of CCl_4 results in a severely distorted lobular architecture with steatosis and extensive necrosis of hepatocytes impairing the morphological discrimination of the various cell types, and technical problems in the preparation of frozen sections of good quality. Our studies were therefore extended to another experimental model, liver fibrosis secondary to common bile duct ligation and scission (Milani *et al.*, 1990a). This type of fibrosis is morphologically characterized by a progressive enlargement of portal tracts due to vigorous bile duct proliferation and massive deposition of collagens in portal tracts and periportal areas associated with only modest signs of inflammation and necrosis. Chemical irritation and mechanical compression due to cholestasis are considered to be the major triggers for the fibrosis that begins at zone I and progresses to zone III of the lobule. In addition, it should theoretically be possible to detect differences between zone I and zone III hepatocytes in this model, if hepatocytes contributed significantly to the hepatic collagen production. As it remained to be shown that the conclusions drawn from the rat models also apply to human subjects, a total of 20 biopsies were studied, including those with normal histology and those with fibrosis or cirrhosis of varying degree and of heterogeneous etiology (Milani et al., 1990b).

All tissues were hybridized with α-2(I), α-1(III), and α-1(IV) procollagen gene probes. An α-1(I) procollagen probe was additionally applied to human tissues to test whether the two genes encoding the type I collagen polypeptide chains are expressed in similar anatomical locations. A serum albumin probe served the purpose of quickly providing information about the mRNA content of the sample.

In normal liver, procollagen type I, III, and IV transcripts were detected in stromal and vascular mesenchymal cells of portal tracts and central veins as well as in some perisinusoidal cells of the lobule. In fibrotic liver, increased levels of these procollagen mRNAs were observed in the same locations, and were particularly enhanced in stromal cells of fibrotic septa and portal tracts, as well as in perisinusoidal cells. Expression of α-1(IV) procollagen RNA was also found in some vascular endothelial and bile duct epithelial cells. Despite the limited sequence homology among the four procollagen gene cDNA probes employed in our study, a common pattern of cellular transcript localization emerged in both normal and fibrotic liver: interstitial procollagen (type I and III) gene transcripts were distributed in regions occupied by mesenchymal cells, such as portal tracts, central veins, sinusoids, and fibrotic septa. Even in the presence of dense pericellular fibrosis around groups of hepatocytes, procollagen mRNA expression was confined to cells with a fibroblast-like morphology rather than to hepatocytes. The α-1(IV) procollagen gene transcripts showed a similar cellular distribution and were additionally observed in some epithelial cells of newly formed bile ducts with a distinct, although less intense, signal.

In sinusoids of rat liver, collagen-expressing cells and desmin-positive cells are colocalized. In the rat, desmin is a marker of myofibroblasts or modified Ito cells (Yokoi et al., 1984). Thus the intralobular formation of collagen can in part be attributed to this cell type. Recently, fat-storing cells have been identified as the collagen-producing cells in primary hepatocyte cultures (Maher et al., 1988). The fact that essentially identical cellular patterns of procollagen gene expression were observed, regardless of the etiology of the fibrosis or cirrhosis, points to a common final pathway of procollagen synthesis in rat and human liver.

Although previously suggested as the major source of liver collagens, hepatocytes showed no significant procollagen transcript levels in any of our samples. Thus procollagen synthesis does not appear to be a function of hepatocytes, but rather of mesenchymal, endothelial, and bile duct epithelial cells in adult human liver. Saber *et al.* (1983a,b) performed *in situ* hybridization for α-2(I) procollagen transcripts in both isolated hepatocytes and hepatic tissue from normal and *Schistosoma mansoni*-infected mice. Although in their model abundant procollagen expression was localized in the nonparenchymal cells of the fibrotic tissue, thus supporting our data, a weak positive hybridization signal was also observed in the hepatocytes of normal and fibrotic liver. This signal on hepatocytes is likely to be related to the characteristics of the cell type and the heterologous cDNA probe employed, because a similar picture can be seen with cRNA probes prior to removal of nonspecifically bound probe by RNase. On the basis of our data, however, a minimal expression of procollagen genes in hepatocytes cannot be excluded; its extent, however, then seems to be insignificant for the development of fibrosis as compared to the strong transcriptional activity in nonparenchymal cells.

The cellular localization of laminin B1 transcripts in adult human (Milani *et al.*, 1989b) and fetal mouse liver (Senior *et al.*, 1988) was almost identical to the distribution of collagen type IV mRNA, i.e., both hepatic cell populations capable of interstitial collagen synthesis as well as bile duct epithelial cells showed an *in situ* hybridization signal. Thus, the same considerations as for collagen synthesis apply to laminin as well; laminin synthesis does not appear to be a function of hepatocytes, but rather of mesenchymal, endothelial, and bile duct epithelial cells in the liver.

These examples illustrate that *in situ* hybridization on tissue sections is unsurpassed as a powerful morphological method for the analysis of the cellular origin of different ECM components and the temporal and spatial patterns of ECM gene expression.

3. *Cellular Origin of Serum Proteins*

The intracellular demonstration of serum proteins may not necessarily correlate with protein synthesis at these locations, but may instead reflect specific or nonspecific active uptake by the cell due to membrane receptors or phagocytosis, or may be related to nonspecific influx of serum protein as a supravital or fixation artifact, depending on their quantity in the extracellular space. It is possible to resolve such problems at the ultrastructural level by immunoelectron microscopy, but this technique is restricted to specialized laboratories. In such cases, *in situ* hybridization can provide information at a semiquantitative level, because the mRNA detected is unlikely to be subject to diffusion processes from one cell to another. The application of *in situ* hybridization for the detection of serum albumin, α-fetoprotein, macrophage proteins, and immunoglobulin gene transcripts convincingly illustrates its usefulness in problems for which immunohistology proved to be less helpful.

Immunohistological techniques have yielded conflicting results concerning the percentage of hepatocytes engaged in albumin production in normal adult liver. A homogeneous distribution of albumin message in hepatocytes in all locations in the lobule is not necessarily to be expected. Marked differences were shown by *in situ* hybridization in the expression of transcripts of the enzyme glutamine synthetase in different parts of liver lobules. Expression was predominant in hepatocytes in centrilobular areas (Kuo *et al.*, 1988; Gebhardt *et al.*, 1988). Using a probe for serum albumin, Bernuau *et al.* (1985) and Poliard *et al.* (1986) were able to analyze the contribution of individual hepatocytes to the serum albumin pool in adult and fetal rat liver and found little variation of the hepatocytic albumin transcript content. Similar observations were made by Milani *et al.* (1989a,b, 1990a,b) for rat and human liver.

Konttinen *et al.* (1989) applied *in situ* hybridization to the analysis of type A synovial cells. These cells have been shown to contain in their lysosomes the protein lysozyme, which might have originated in other cells because synovial fluid contains elevated levels of this enzyme, particularly under conditions of acute inflammation. The presence of lysozyme RNA allowed the attribution of these synovial cells to the mononuclear phagocytic lineage.

Occasionally immunoglobulin (Ig) of polyclonal origin may be detected by immunohistology in normal squamous epithelial cells or in giant cells of varied histogenetic origin, such as anaplastic carcinomas, glioblastomas, sarcomas, or some immunoblastic or anaplastic large cell lymphomas. Such immunostaining results are often seen following suboptimal fixation prior to paraffin embedding or following delayed freezing of fresh biopsy material. Frequently such reactivity can be seen on paraffin-embedded material stained for immunoglobulin, but not in corresponding frozen sections, and this fact strongly suggests influx of serum proteins. This is particularly the case if the staining is detected in cells that must be considered Ig nonproducers, such as carcinomas or squamous epithelial cells. The problem is more complex in the case of cells expressing certain types of receptors for constant domains of Ig (Fc receptors), such as macrophages or B lymphocytes.

Use of *in situ* hybridization for the detection of immunoglobulin gene transcripts, however, may not only be valuable for such situations, but— within limits—also allows analysis of the clonal composition, isotype usage, and Ig heavy chain class switching on the single-cell level. Berger (1986) investigated the increase of μ heavy chain (HC)-specific mRNA and the appearance of switched μ heavy chain-expressing cells after mitogenic activation. Analyzing the functional repertoires by examining κ variable (v) gene family expression in mitogen-activated adult and fetal B cells, Teale and Morris (1989) demonstrated considerable variation in the V gene usage. Similarly, Kastner et al. (1989) studied the immunoglobulin heavy chain variable gene utilization in murine lupus erythematosus, with emphasis on the relative contribution of 3' and 5' gene families. Seibel and Kirsch (1989) and Mar et al. (1989) studied human lymphatic B lymphoid malignancies on the single-cell level in relation to the Ig gene rearrangement status. Such analysis of gene segment family utilization can also be achieved by means of immunohistology, using idiotype-specific reagents. Such reagents, however, are available for only a few, mainly murine, V_H gene families. *In situ* hybridization allows application to all gene segments and may be particularly useful in the clonal analysis *in situ* of human B lymphomas.

In situ hybridization has been used in the authors' laboratory to address the question of whether Hodgkin and Reed–Sternberg cells of Hodgkin's disease may have the potential to express immunoglobulin light chain (IgLC) genes and whether such expression would be restricted to only one type of IgLC, κ or λ (Herbst et al., 1991a). Using *in situ* hybridization with single-stranded RNA probes specific for IgLC constant gene segments, 22 Hodgkin's disease biopsies were studied. Plasma cells and reactive B lymphocytes provided internal positive controls, showing within 2 and 4 days of autoradiography a mosaic-like arrangement of positive cells congruent with the immunohistologically assessed pattern. Hybridization with an IL-2-receptor gene probe verified the presence and integrity of the RNA within the malignant cell population and ruled out the possibility of a preferential depletion of mRNA in Hodgkin and Reed–Sternberg cells. IgLC transcripts could be demonstrated in Hodgkin and Reed–Sternberg cells in 3 out of 22 cases of Hodgkin's disease, with restriction to either κ or λ IgLC type, whereas such transcripts were absent in the tumor cells in the other cases, despite polyclonal Ig immunoreactivity in paraffin sections in some instances. One biopsy, which showed an Ig λ gene rearrangement in Southern blot hybridization of DNA extracts, also contained λ IgLC gene transcripts in the tumor cells.

These findings provide direct evidence for the monoclonal B lymphoid origin of Hodgkin and Reed–Sternberg cells in some cases and support previous investigations that attributed such gene rearrangements to the Hodgkin and Reed–Sternberg cells rather than to reactive clonal B cell expansions. In other cases, most of which displayed a B cell phenotype, IgLC transcripts were undetectable in the tumor cell population even after prolonged autoradiography. This strongly suggests that in most HD cases with the B cell phenotype, Hodgkin and Reed–Sternberg cells correspond to early B cell differentiation stages. In seven Hodgkin's disease biopsies the tumor cells displayed immunolabeling for both Ig κ and Ig λ in paraffin sections.

Because of the absence of any IgLC transcripts in these cases, this polyclonal IgLC-specific immunostaining cannot reflect synthesis of IgLC proteins by the cells, but rather uptake of serum immunoglobulin either via specific Ig receptors or by nonspecific mechanisms. These results emphasize the usefulness of *in situ* hybridization for areas that are difficult to assess by immunohistology alone.

4. RNA Virus Genomes

In parallel to its use for detecting DNA viruses and DNA viral gene transcripts (Stevens *et al.*, 1987; Croen *et al.*, 1987; Wolber *et al.*, 1989), *in situ* hybridization proved useful for the demonstration of RNA viral genomes. Among the viruses investigated with this technique are measles virus in human brain (Dowling *et al.*, 1986; Moench *et al.*, 1988) and Paget's bone disease tissue (Basle *et al.*, 1986), rubella virus (Filipenko *et al.*, 1988), enteroviruses (Kandolf *et al.*, 1987; Rotbart *et al.*, 1988), poliovirus type 1 (Couderc *et al.*, 1989), rabies virus (A. C. Jackson *et al.*, 1989), and hepatitis A virus (Harmon *et al.*, 1989; Xi *et al.*, 1989).

In situ hybridization has been used occasionally for detecting complex RNA sequences of retroviruses (e.g., Godard, 1983). With the identification of AIDS as a new clinical entity and the discovery of the human immunodeficiency virus (HIV) as the causative agent, *in situ* hybridization became a major tool of retroviral research. Harper and Marselle (1986), Biberfeld *et al.* (1986), Baroni *et al.* (1988), and Tenner-Racz *et al.* (1988) studied lymph nodes of HIV-I-seropositive individuals, detecting rare cells with lymphoid morphology containing HIV-I RNA at levels consistent with viral replication (20–300 copies per cell); these cells were clustered in germinal centers. These authors also described fine granular patterns superimposable on the meshwork of follicular dendritic cells. This was interpreted as trapping of viral particles in immune complexes or active replication of the virus in these cells, an explanation also suggested by Prevot *et al.* (1989). The finding of HIV in high endothelial venules with sulfonated HIV probes (Baroni *et al.*, 1988) is likely to represent a staining artifact, as HIV genomes were not detected in this cell type using ^{35}S-labeled RNA probes in a large number of cases (Tenner-Racz *et al.*, 1988; Spiegel *et al.*, 1991). Presence and replication of HIV genomes was demonstrable, however, in other cell types, such as macrophages in brain tissue from AIDS patients with encephalopathy (Koenig *et al.*, 1986; Wiley *et al.*, 1986), or in spinal cord (Eilbott *et al.*, 1989), in mononuclear cells of esophageal ulcers (Kotler *et al.*, 1989), and in the lamina propria of AIDS patients with gastrointestinal disease (Fox *et al.*, 1989; Levy *et al.*, 1989). Although many aspects of HIV infection are far from being understood, it has to be expected that *in situ* hybridization, in particular in combination with immunohistological techniques, will play a pivotal role in resolving the uncertainties regarding the site of latent viral infection, i.e., the cellular virus reservoir.

IV. Practical Value for Histopathology

Classical histological techniques identify tissue components either by their specific binding of certain dyes or by their function in enzyme histochemistry. The advent of immunohistology has revolutionized histology and histopathology because it allows the demonstration of cellular and extracellular tissue constituents by their antigenic properties, thus expanding the range of detectable molecules. Immunohistology using either polyclonal or monoclonal antibodies has provided great advances of our understanding of normal and malignant cell growth and differentiation, and concepts based entirely on morphological grounds have been challenged by immunohistological results. Also, though the examination of conventionally stained slides still is the basis of histopathology, immunohistochemical detection of antigens has replaced many classical histochemical techniques. However, the specificity of monoclonal antibodies, and even more so of polyclonal antibodies, is often ill-defined, and precise definition of the immunohistological reactivity pattern of an antibody is laborious. For example, leukocyte differentiation antigens defined by monoclonal antibodies are clustered during workshops held at regular intervals (Knapp *et al.*, 1989). Also, monoclonal antibodies detect only short peptide sequences or carbohydrate residues of an antigen. That unrelated proteins may share the same epitopes is, however, not an uncommon phenomenon and may lead to unexpected results open to misinterpretation. Molecular biological techniques, on the other hand, employ nucleic acid probes of defined specificity and sequence. This allows one to chose appropriate hybridization conditions that exclude cross-hybridization with unrelated sequences. *In situ* hybridization is the molecular biological technique of choice for the pathologist. Unlike methods based on the extraction of nucleic acids from tissues, it allows the attribution of signal to a particular cell type and the simultaneous evaluation of the underlying pathology. *In situ* hybridization has become a valuable tool in various areas of research. This technique is a useful complement to immunohistology; it may be used to verify immunohistological results and vice versa. Also, this technique is particularly helpful when antibodies against a gene product are not available. In the study of extracellular proteins of uncertain cellular origin, *in situ* hybridization has proved useful. The introduction of nonisotopic reporter molecules has promoted the widespread application of the method in several areas.

Coffey, R. J., Jr., Derynck, R., Wilcox, J. N., Bringman, T. S., Goustin, A. S., Moses, H. L., and Pittelkow, M. R. (1987). *Nature (London)* **328,** 817–820.
Condere, T., Guinguene, B., Hourand, F., Aubert-Combiescu, A., and Crainic, R. (1989). *Eur. J. Epidemiol.* **5,** 270–274.
Cornelese ten Velde, I., Wiegant, J., Tanke, H. J., and Ploem, J. S. (1989). *Histochemistry* **92,** 153–160.
Cox, K. H., DeLeon, D. V., Angerer, L. M., and Angerer, R. C. (1984). *Dev. Biol.* **101,** 485–502.
Crabbe, M. I. (1985). *Biosci. Rep.* **5,** 167–174.
Cremers, A. F. M., Jansen in de Wal, N., Wiegant, J., Dirks, R. W., Weisbeek, P., van der Ploeg, M., and Landegent, J. (1987). *Histochemistry* **86,** 609–615.
Croen, K. D., Ostrove, J. M., Dragovic, L. J., Smialek, J. E., and Straus, S. E. (1987). *N. Engl. J. Med.* **317,** 1427–1432.
Crum, C. P., Nagai, N., Levine, R. U., and Silverstein, S. (1986). *Am. J. Pathol.* **123,** 174–182.
Crum, C. P., Nuovo, G., Friedman, D., and Silverstein, S. (1988). *Lab. Invest.* **58,** 354–359.
Crum, C. P., Symbula, M., and Ward, B. E. (1989). *Am. J. Pathol.* **134,** 1183–1188.
Cubie, H. A., and Norval, M. (1989). *J. Clin. Pathol.* **42,** 988–991.
Dakshinamurti, K., and Mistry, S. P. (1963). *J. Biol. Chem.* **238,** 294–296.
Davis, C. A., and Joyner, A. L. (1988). *Genes Dev.* **2,** 1736–1744.
Dawson, C. W., Rickinson, A. B., and Young, L. S. (1990). *Nature (London)* **344,** 777–780.
Deacon, E. M., Matthews, J. B., Potts, A. J. C., Hamburger, J., Bevans, I. S., and Young, L. S. (1990). *J. Pathol.*, in press.
DeLellis, R. A., and Wolfe, H. J. (1987). *J. Histochem. Cytochem.* **35,** 1347–1351.
Denny, P., Hamid, Q., Krause, J. E., Polak, J. M., and Legon, S. (1988). *Histochemistry* **89,** 481–483.
de Souza, Y. G., Greenspan, D., Felton, J. R., Hartzog, G. A., Hammer, M., and Greenspan, J. S. (1989). *N. Engl. J. Med.* **320,** 1559–1560.
Devlin, C. J., Brickell, P. M., Taylor, E. R., Hornbruch, A., Craig, R. K., and Wolpert, L. (1988). *Development* **103,** 111–118.
Dimery, I. W., Lee, J. S., Blick, M., Pearson, G., Spitzer, G., and Hong, W. K. (1988). *Cancer* **61,** 2475–2480.
Dony, C., and Gruss, P. (1987). *EMBO J.* **6,** 2965–2975.
Dony, C., and Gruss, P. (1988). *Differentiation (Berlin)* **37,** 115–122.
Dowling, P. C., Blumberg, B. M., Kolakofsky, D., Cook, P., Jotkowitz, A., Prineas, J. W., and Cook, S. D. (1986). *Virus Res.* **5,** 97–107.
Dürst, M., Gissmann, L., Ikenberg, H., and zur Hausen, H. (1983). *Proc. Natl. Acad. Sci. U.S.A.* **80,** 3812–3815.
Ebihara, I., Killen, P. D., Laurie, G. W., Huang, T., Yamada, Y., Martin, G. R., and Brown, K. S. (1988). *Lab. Invest.* **58,** 262–269.
Edwall, D., Schalling, M., Jennische, E., and Norstedt, G. (1989). *Endocrinology (Baltimore)* **124,** 820–825.
Eghbali, M., Blumenfeld, O. O., Seifter, S., Buttrick, P. M., Leinwand, L. A., Robinson, T. F., Zern, M. A., and Giambrone, M. A. (1989). *J. Mol. Cell. Cardiol.* **21,** 103–113.
Eilbott, D. J., Peress, N., Burger, H., LaNeve, D., Orenstein, J., Gendelman, H. E., Seidman, R., and Weiser, B. (1989). *Proc. Natl. Acad. Sci. U.S.A.* **86,** 3337–3341.
Emilia, G., Donelli, A., Ferrari, S., Torelli, U., Selleri, L., Zucchini, P., Moretti, L., Venturelli, D., Ceccherelli, G., and Torelli, G. (1986). *Br. J. Haematol.* **62,** 287–292.
Engelmann, G. L., Boehm, K. D., Haskell, J. F., Khairallah, P. A., and Ilan, J. (1989). *Mol. Cell. Endocrinol.* **63,** 1–14.
Ernberg, I., and Altiok, E. (1989). *Acta Pathol. Microbiol. Scand.* **8,** 58–61.
Evinger-Hodges, M. J., Bresser, J., Brouwer, R., Cox, I., Spitzer, G., and Dicke, K. (1988). *Leukemia* **2,** 45–49.

Fahraeus, R., Li Fu, H., Ernberg, I., Finke, J., Rowe, M., Klein, G., Falk, K., Nilsson, E., Yadar, M., Busson, P., Tursz, T., and Kallin, B. (1988). *Int. J. Cancer* **42**, 329–338.
Fahraeus, R., Rymo, L., Rhim, J. S., and Klein, G. (1990). *Nature (London)* **345**, 447–449.
Fahrer, C., Brachmann, R., and von der Helm, K. (1989). *Int. J. Cancer* **44**, 652–657.
Farhi, D. C. (1989). *Hematol. Pathol.* **3**, 85–90.
Farnsworth, A., Laverty, C., and Stoler, M. H. (1989). *Int. J. Gynecol. Pathol.* **8**, 321–330.
Farrar, W. L., Vinocour, M., and Hill, J. M. (1989). *Blood* **73**, 137–140.
Fausto, N. (1986). *Cancer Res.* **46**, 3111–3117.
Feinberg, A. P., and Vogelstein, B. (1983). *Anal. Biochem.* **132**, 6–13.
Filipenko, D., Hobman, T., MacDonald, I., and Gillam, S. (1988). *J. Virol. Methods* **22**, 109–118.
Forster, A. C., McInnes, J. L., Skingle, D. C., and Symons, R. H. (1985). *Nucleic Acids Res.* **13**, 745–761.
Fox, C. H., Kotler, D., Tierney, A., Wilson, C. S., and Fauci, A. S. (1989). *J. Infect. Dis.* **159**, 467–471.
Fox, R. I., Pearson, G., and Vaughan, J. H. (1986). *J. Immunol.* **137**, 3162–3168.
Francis, N. D., Boylston, A. W., Roberts, A. H. G., and Parkin, J. M. (1989). *J. Clin. Pathol.* **42**, 1055–1064.
Friedmann, S. L., Roll, F. J., Boyles, J., and Bissell, D. M. (1985). *Proc. Natl. Acad. Sci. U.S.A.* **82**, 8681–8685.
Gait, M. J. (1984). "Oligonucleotide Synthesis—A Practical Approach." IRL Press, Oxford, England.
Gall, J. G., and Pardue, M. L. (1969). *Proc. Natl. Acad. Sci. U.S.A.* **63**, 378–383.
Gaunt, S. J. (1988). *Development* **103**, 135–144.
Gebhardt, R., Ebert, A., and Bauer, G. (1988). *FEBS Lett.* **241**, 89–93.
Gerber, M. A., and Thung, S. N. (1987). *Hum. Pathol.* **18**, 771–774.
Gissmann, L., Boshart, M., Dürst, M., Ikenberg, H., Wagner, D., and zur Hausen, H. (1984). *J. Invest. Dermatol.* **83**, 26s–28s.
Giwercman, A., Hopman, A. H. N., Ramaekers, F. C. S., and Skakkebaek, N. E. (1990). *Am. J. Pathol.* **136**, 497–502.
Gleich, G. J., Loegering, D. A., and Kueppers, F. (1974). *J. Exp. Med.* **139**, 313–332.
Gnann, J. W., Ahlmen, J., Svalander, C., Olding, L., Oldstone, M. B., and Nelson, J. A. (1988). *Am. J. Pathol.* **132**, 239–248.
Gobl, A. E., Funa, K., and Alm, G. V. (1988). *J. Immunol.* **140**, 3605–3609.
Godard, C. M. (1983). *Histochemistry* **77**, 123–131.
Goebels, N., Waase, I., Pfizenmaier, K., and Krönke, M. (1988). *J. Immunol.* **141**, 1231–1235.
Grady, E. F., Schwab, M., and Rosenau, W. (1987). *Cancer Res.* **47**, 2931–2936.
Grady-Leopardi, E. F., Schwab, M., Ablin, A. R., and Rosenau, W. (1986). *Cancer Res.* **46**, 3196–3199.
Graham, A., Papalopulu, N., Lorimer, L., McVey, J. H., Tuddenham, E. G., and Krumlauf, R. (1988). *Genes Dev.* **2**, 1424–1438.
Granelli-Piperno, A. (1988). *J. Exp. Med.* **168**, 1649–1658.
Gratama, J. W., Oosterveer, M. A. P., Zwaan, F. E., Lepoutre, J., Klein, G., and Ernberg, I. (1988). *Proc. Natl. Acad. Sci. U.S.A.* **85**, 8693–8699.
Greenspan, D., Greenspan, J. S., Conant, M., Petersen, V., and Silverman, S. (1984). *Lancet* **2**, 831–834.
Greenspan, J. S., Greenspan, D., Lennette, E. T., Abrams, D. I., Conant, M. A., Petersen, V., and Freese, U. K. (1985). *N. Engl. J. Med.* **313**, 1564–1571.
Greil, R., Fasching, B., and Huber, H. (1989). *Lab. Invest.* **60**, 574–582.
Grossman, M., Krueger, J., Yourish, D., Granelli-Piperno, A., Murphy, D. P., May, L. T., Kupper, T. S., Sehgal, P. B., and Gottlieb, A. B. (1989). *Proc. Natl. Acad. Sci. U.S.A.* **86**, 6367–6371.

Grussendorf-Conen, E. I. (1987). *In* "Papillomaviruses and Human Disease" (K. Syrjanen, L. Gissmann, and L. G. Koss, eds.), pp. 158–181. Springer-Verlag, Berlin.
Grussendorf-Conen, E. I., Deutz, F. J., and De Villiers, E. M. (1987). *Cancer* **60,** 1832–1835.
Guitteny, A. F., Fouque, B., Mougin, C., Teoule, R., and Bloch, B. (1988). *J. Histochem. Cytochem.* **36,** 563–571.
Haase, A. T., Ventura, P., Gibbs, C. J., and Tourtelotte, W. W. (1981). *Science* **212,** 672–675.
Haase, A. T., Walker, D., Stowring, L., Ventura, P., Geballe, A., Blum, H., Brahic, M., Goldberg, R., and O'Brien, K. (1985). *Science* **227,** 189–192.
Hamatani, K., Yoshida, K., Kondo, H., Toki, H., Okabe, K., Motoi, M., Ikeda, S., Mori, S., Shimaoka, K., and Akiyama, M. (1989a). *Blood* **74,** 423–429.
Hamatani, K., Nagata, Y., Abe, M., Abe, K., Toki, H., Ikeda, S., Nakayama, E., and Shiku, H. (1989b). *Gann* **80,** 706–710.
Hamilton-Dutoit, S. J., Pallesen, G., Karkov, J., Skinhoj, P., Franzmann, M. B., and Pedersen, C. (1989). *Lancet* **1,** 554–555.
Han, V. K., d'Ercole, A. J., and Lund, P. K. (1987a). *Science* **236,** 193–197.
Han, V. K., Hill, D. J., Strain, A. J., Towle, A. C., Lauder, J. M., Underwood, L. E., and d'Ercole, A. J. (1987b). *Pediatr. Res.* **22,** 245–249.
Han, V. K., d'Ercole, A. J., and Lee, D. C. (1988). *Can. J. Physiol. Pharmacol.* **66,** 1113–1121.
Handyside, A. H., Pattinson, J. K., Penketh, R. J., Delhanty, J. D., Winston, R. M., and Tuddenham, E. G. (1989). *Lancet* **1,** 347–349.
Hankin, R. C., and Lloyd, R. V. (1989). *Am. J. Clin. Pathol.* **92,** 166–171.
Hanto, D. W., Sakamoto, K., Purtilo, D. T., Simmons, R. L., and Najarian, J. S. (1981). *Surgery* **90,** 204–213.
Harmon, S. A., Summers, D. F., and Ehrenfeld, E. (1989). *Virus Res.* **12,** 361–369.
Harper, M. E., and Marselle, L. M. (1986). *Cancer. Genet. Cytogenet.* **19,** 73–80.
Harper, M. E., Marselle, L. M., Gallo, R. C., and Wong-Staal, F. (1986). *Proc. Natl. Acad. Sci. U.S.A.* **83,** 772–776.
Hayashi, M., Ninomiya, Y., Parsons, J., Hayashi, K., Olsen, B. R., and Trelstad, R. L. (1986). *J. Cell Biol.* **102,** 2302–2309.
Hayashi, M., Ninomiya, Y., Hayashi, K., Linsenmayer, T. F., Olsen, B. R., and Trelstad, R. L. (1988). *Development* **103,** 27–36.
Hayashi, S., Gillam, I. C., Delaney, A. D., and Tener, G. M. (1978). *J. Histochem. Cytochem.* **26,** 677–679.
Henle, G., Henle, W., and Diehl, V. (1968). *Proc. Natl. Acad. Sci. U.S.A.* **59,** 94–101.
Herbst, H., Niedobitek, G., Kneba, M., Hummel, M., Finn, T., Anagnostopoulos, I., Bergholz, M., Krieger, G., and Stein, H. (1990). *Am. J. Pathol.* **137,** 13–18.
Herbst, H., Kratzsch, H. C., Niedobitek, G., Anagnostopoulos, I., Dienemann, D., Falini, B., and Stein, H. (1991a). Submitted for publication.
Herbst, H., Milani, S., Schuppau, D., and Stein, H. (1991b). Submitted for publication.
Hermansson, M., Nister, M., Betsholtz, C., Heldin, C. H., Westermark, B., and Funa, K. (1988). *Proc. Natl. Acad. Sci. U.S.A.* **85,** 7748–7752.
Herrington, C. S., Burns, J., Graham, A. K., Bhatt, B., and McGee, J. O. D. (1989). *J. Clin. Pathol.* **42,** 601–606.
Herrmann, G., and Hübner, K. (1987). *Hepato-gastroenterology* **34,** 148–151.
Hesse, J., Andersen, E., Levine, P. H., Ebbesen, P., Halberg, P., and Reisher, J. I. (1973). *Int. J. Cancer* **11,** 237–243.
Hirvonen, H., Sandberg, M., Kalimo, H., Hukkanen, V., Vuorio, E., Salmi, T. T., and Alitalo, K. (1989). *J. Cell Biol.* **108,** 1093–1104.
Hoellering, J., and Shuler, C. F. (1989). *J. Oral Pathol. Med.* **18,** 74–78.
Höfler, H. (1987). *Pathol., Res. Pract.* **182,** 421–430.

Höfler, H., Pütz, B., Ruhri, C., Wirnsberger, G., Klimpfinger, M., and Smolle, J. (1987). *Virchows Arch. B* **54,** 144–151.
Hogan, B., Costantini, F., and Lacy, E. (1986). "Manipulating the Mouse Embryo: A Laboratory Manual." Cold Spring Harbor Lab., Cold Spring Harbor, New York.
Hogan, B. L., Holland, P. W., and Lumsden, A. (1988). *Cell. Differ. Dev.* **25,** 39–44.
Hogg, J. C., Irving, W. L., Porter, H., Evans, M., Dunnill, M. S., and Fleming, K. (1989). *Am. Rev. Respir. Dis.* **139,** 1531–1535.
Hopman, A. H., Wiegant, J., and van Duijn, P. (1986a). *Histochemistry* **84,** 169–178.
Hopman, A. H., Wiegant, J., Raap, A. K., Landegent, J. E., van der Ploeg, M., and van Duijn, P. (1986b). *Histochemistry* **85,** 1–4.
Jaakkola, S., Peltonen, J., and Uitto, J. J. (1989a). *J. Cell Biol.* **108,** 1157–1163.
Jackson, A. C., Reimer, D. L., and Wunner, W. H. (1989). *J. Virol. Methods* **25,** 1–11.
Jackson, P., Lewis, F. A., and Wells, M. (1989). *Histochem. J.* **21,** 425–428.
Jilbert, A. R., Burrell, C. J., Gowans, E. J., and Rowland, R. (1986). *Histochemistry* **85,** 505–514.
Jilbert, A. R., Freiman, J. S., Gowans, E. J., Holmes, M., Cossart, Y. E., and Burrell, C. J. (1987). *Virology* **158,** 330–338.
Jiwa, N. M., Raap, A. K., van de Rijke, F. M., Mulder, A., Weening, J. J., Zwaan, F. E., The, T. H., and van der Ploeg, M. (1989). *J. Clin. Pathol.* **42,** 749–754.
Johansson, B., Klein, G., Henle, W., and Henle, G. (1970). *Int. J. Cancer* **6,** 450–462.
John, H. A., Birnstil, M. L., and Jones, K. W. (1969). *Nature (London)* **223,** 582–587.
Kacinski, B. M., Carter, D., Mittal, K., Kohorn, E. I., Bloodgood, R. S., Donahue, J., Donofrio, L., Edwards, R., Schwartz, P. E., and Chambers, J. T. (1988). *Int. J. Radiat. Oncol., Biol. Phys.* **15,** 823–829.
Kahari, V. M., Sandberg, M., Kalimo, H., Vuorio, T., and Vuorio, E. (1988). *J. Invest. Dermatol.* **90,** 664–670.
Kandolf, R., Ameis, D., Kirschner, P., Canu, A., and Hofschneider, P. H. (1987). *Proc. Natl. Acad. Sci. U.S.A.* **84,** 6272–6276.
Kastner, D. L., McIntyre, T. M., Mallett, C. P., Hartman, A. B., and Steinberg, A. D. (1989). *J. Immunol.* **143,** 2761–2767.
Keh, W. C., and Gerber, M. A. (1988). *Am. J. Pathol.* **131,** 490–496.
Kitazawa, S., Takenaka, A., Abe, N., Maeda, S., Horio, M., and Sugiyama, T. (1989). *Histochemistry* **92,** 195–199.
Klein, G. (1979). *In* "The Epstein–Barr Virus" (M. A. Epstein and B. G. Achong, eds.), pp. 339–350. Springer-Verlag, Berlin.
Klein, G., Giovanella, B. C., Lindahl, T., Fialkow, P. J., Singh, S., and Stehlin, J. S. (1974). *Proc. Natl. Acad. Sci. U.S.A.* **71,** 4737–4741.
Klein, G., Giovanella, B., Westman, A., Stehlin, J. S., and Mumford, D. (1975). *Intervirology* **5,** 319–334.
Klimpfinger, M., Ruhri, C., Pütz, B., Pfragner, R., Wirnsberger, G., and Höfler, H. (1988). *Virchows Arch. B* **54,** 256–259.
Knapp, W., Dörken, B., Gilks, W. R., Rieber, E. P., Schmidt, R. E., Stein, H., and von dem Borne, A. E. G. K. (1989). "Leukocyte Typing IV." Oxford Univ. Press, Oxford, England.
Koenig, S., Gendelman, H. E., Orenstein, J. M., Dal-Canto, M. C., Pezeshkpour, G. H., Yungbluth, M., Janotta, F., Aksamit, A., Martin, M. A., and Fauci, A. S. (1986). *Science* **233,** 1089–1093.
Koji, T., Izumi, S., Tanno, M., Moriuchi, T., and Nakane, P. K. (1988). *Histochem. J.* **20,** 551–557.
Konttinen, Y. T., Bergroth, V., Kulomaa, M., Nordstrom, D., Segerberg-Konttinen, M., Keinanen, R., Kemppinen, P., Hukkanen, M., and Gronblad, M. (1989). *Ann. Rheum. Dis.* **48,** 912–917.
Koropchak, C. M., Solem, S. M., Diaz, P. S., and Arvin, A. M. (1989). *J. Virol.* **63,** 2392–2395.
Kotler, D. P., Wilson, C. S., Haroutiounian, G., and Fox, C. H. (1989). *Am. J. Gastroenterol.* **84,** 313–317.

Kreipe, H., Radzun, H. J., Heidorn, K., Mader, C., and Parwaresch, M. R. (1987). *J. Histochem. Cytochem.* **35,** 837–842.
Kulski, J., Demeter, T., Sterrett, G. F., and Shilkin, K. B. (1986). *Lancet* **2,** 683–684.
Kuo, C. F., Paulson, K. E., and Darnell, J. E. (1988). *Mol. Cell. Biol.* **8,** 4966–4971.
Lacy, J., Sarkar, S. N., and Summers, W. C. (1986). *Proc. Natl. Acad. Sci. U.S.A.* **83,** 1458–1462.
Larjava, H., Sandberg, M., and Vuorio, E. (1989). *J. Periodontal Res.* **24,** 171–177.
Larjava, H., Sandberg, M., Happonen, R. P., and Vuorio, E. (1990). *Lab. Invest.* **62,** 96–103.
Larsson, L. I. (1989). *Arch. Histol. Cytol.* **52,** 55–62.
Laurie, G. W., Horikoshi, S., Killen, P. D., Segui-Real, B., and Yamada, Y. (1989). *J. Cell Biol.* **109,** 1351–1362.
Lawrence, J. B., and Singer, R. H. (1985). *Nucleic Acids Res.* **13,** 1777–1799.
Lawrence, J. B., Villnave, C. A., and Singer, R. H. (1988). *Cell* **52,** 51–61.
Lawrence, J. B., Singer, R. H., and Marselle, L. M. (1989). *Cell* **57,** 493–502.
Lee, J. H., Lee, D. H., Park, S. S., Seok, S. E., and Lee, J. D. (1988). *Chest* **94,** 1046–1049.
Lemon, S. M., Hutt, L. M., Shaw, J. E., Li, J. L. H., and Pagano, J. S. (1977). *Nature (London)* **268,** 268–270.
Le-Mouellic, H., Condamine, H., and Brulet, P. (1988). *Genes Dev.* **2,** 125–135.
Levy, J. A., Margaretten, W., and Nelson, J. (1989). *Am. J. Gastroenterol.* **84,** 787–789.
Lewis, F. A., Griffiths, S., Dunnicliff, R., Wells, M., Dudding, N., and Bird, C. C. (1987). *J. Clin. Pathol.* **40,** 163–166.
Leyvraz, S., Henle, W., Cahinian, A. P., Perlmann, C., Klein, G., Gordon, R. E., Rosenblum, M., and Holland, J. F. (1985). *N. Engl. J. Med.* **312,** 1296–1299.
Liscia, D. S., Merlo, G. R., Garrett, C., French, D., Mariani-Costantini, R., and Callahan, R. (1989). *Oncogene* **4,** 1219–1224.
Löning, T., Ikenberg, H., Becker, J., Gissmann, L., Hoepfer, I., and zur Hausen, H. (1985). *J. Invest. Dermatol.* **84,** 417–420.
Löning, T., Milde, K., and Foss, H. D. (1986). *Virchows Arch. A: Pathol. Anat. Histol.* **409,** 777–790.
Löning, T., Henke, R. P., Reichart, P., and Becker, J. (1987). *Virchows Arch. A: Pathol. Anat. Histol.* **412,** 127–133.
Lund, V., Lindqvist, B. H., and Eggset, G. (1989). *Nucleic Acids Res.* **17,** 539–551.
Maher, J. J., Bissell, D. M., Friedman, S. L., and Roll, F. J. (1988). *J. Clin. Invest.* **82,** 450–459.
Mallein-Gerin, F., Kosher, R. A., Upholt, W. B., and Tanzer, M. L. (1988). *Dev. Biol.* **126,** 337–345.
Mar, P., Pachmann, K., Reinecke, K., Emmerich, B., and Thiel, E. (1989). *Blood* **74,** 638–644.
Mariani-Costantini, R., Theillet, C., Hutzell, P., Merlo, G., Schlom, J., and Callahan, R. (1989). *J. Histochem. Cytochem.* **37,** 293–298.
McAllister, H. A., and Rock, D. L. (1985). *J. Histochem. Cytochem.* **33,** 1026–1032.
McGuire, L. J., Huang, D. P., Teoh, R., Arnold, M., Wong, K., and Lee, J. C. K. (1988). *Am. J. Pathol.* **131,** 385–390.
McQuaid, S., Isserte, S., Allan, G. M., Taylor, M. J., Allen, I. V., and Cosby, S. L. (1990). *J. Clin. Pathol.* **43,** 329–333.
Melton, D. A., Krieg, P. A., and Rebagliati, M. R. (1984). Nucleic Acids Res. **12,** 7035–7056.
Michitaka, K., Horiike, N., Nadano, S., Onji, M., and Ohta, Y. (1988). *Liver* **8,** 247–253.
Milani, S., Herbst, H., Schuppan, D., Hahn, E. C., and Stein, H. (1989a). *Hepatology* **10,** 84–92.
Milani, S., Herbst, H., Schuppan, D., Surrenti, C., Riecken, E. O., and Stein, H. (1989b). *Am. J. Pathol.* **134,** 1175–1182.
Milani, S., Herbst, H., Schuppan, D., Kim, K. Y., Riecken, E. O., and Stein, H. (1990a). *Gastroenterology* **98,** 175–184.
Milani, S., Herbst, H., Schuppan, D., Surrenti, C., Riecken, E. O., and Stein, H. (1990b). *Am. J. Pathol.* **137,** 59–70.

Miller, G., Shope, T., Liscoe, H., Stitt, D., and Lipman, M. (1972). *Proc. Natl. Acad. Sci. U.S.A.* **69,** 383–387.
Moench, T. R., Gendelman, H. E., Clements, J. E., Narayan, O., and Griffin, D. E. (1985). *J. Virol. Methods* **11,** 119–130.
Moench, T. R., Griffin, D. E., Obriecht, C. R., Vaisberg, A. J., and Johnson, R. T. (1988). *J. Infect. Dis.* **158,** 433–442.
Morimoto, H., Monden, T., Shimano, T., Higashiyma, M., Tomita, N., Murotani, M., Matsuura, N., Okuda, H., and Mori, T. (1987). *Lab. Invest.* **57,** 737–741.
Mueller, N., Evans, A., Harris, N. L., Comstock, G. W., Jellum, E., Magnus, K., Orentreich, N., Polk, F., and Vogelman, J. (1989). *N. Engl. J. Med.* **320,** 689–695.
Mullink, H., Walboomers, J. M. M., Raap, A. K., and Meyer, C. J. L. M. (1989a). *Histochemistry* **91,** 195–198.
Mullink, H., Walboomers, J. M., Tadema, T. M., Jansen, D. J., and Meijer, C. J. (1989b). *J. Histochem. Cytochem.* **37,** 603–609.
Munoz, N., Davidson, R. J. L., Witthoff, B., Ericsson, J. E., and De-The, G. (1978). *Int. J. Cancer* **22,** 10–13.
Murphy, P., Davidson, D. R., and Hill, R. E. (1989). *Nature (London)* **341,** 156–159.
Myerson, D., Hackman, R. C., Nelson, J. A., Ward, D. C., and McDougall, J. K. (1984). *Hum. Pathol.* **15,** 430–439.
Nah, H. D., Rodgers, B. J., Kulyk, W. M., Kream, B. E., Kosher, R. A., and Upholt, W. B. (1988). *Collagen Relat. Res.* **8,** 277–294.
Naoumov, N. V., Alexander, G. J. M., Eddleston, A. L. W. F., and Williams, R. (1988). *J. Clin. Pathol.* **41,** 793–798.
Navarro, S., Debili, N., Bernaudin, J. F., Vainchenker, W., and Doly, S. (1989). *J. Immunol.* **142,** 4339–4345.
Nederlof, P. M., Robinson, D., Abuknesha, R., Wiegant, J., Hopman, A. H., Tanke, H. J., and Raap, A. K. (1989). Cytometry **10,** 20–27.
Negro, F., Berninger, M., Chiaberge, E., Gugliotta, P., Bussolati, G., Actis, G. C., Rizzetto, M., and Bonino, F. (1985). *J. Med. Virol.* **15,** 373–382.
Niederman, J. C., Miller, G., Pearson, H. A., Pagano, J. S., and Dowaliby, J. M. (1976). *N. Engl. J. Med.* **294,** 1355–1359.
Niedobitek, G., Finn, T., Herbst, H., Bornhöft, G., Gerdes, J., and Stein, H. (1988a). *Am. J. Pathol.* **131,** 1–4.
Niedobitek, G., Finn, T., Herbst, H., Gerdes, J., Grillner, L., Landqvist, M., Zweygberg Wirgart, B., and Stein, H. (1988b). *J. Clin. Pathol.* **41,** 1005–1009.
Niedobitek, G., Finn, T., Herbst, H., and Stein, H. (1989a). *Am. J. Pathol.* **134,** 633–639.
Niedobitek, G., Finn, T., Herbst, H., and Stein, H. (1989b). *Pathol. Res. Pract.* **184,** 343–348.
Niedobitek, G., Hamilton-Dutoit, S., Herbst, H., Finn, T., Vetner, M., Pallesen, G., and Stein, H. (1989c). *Hum. Pathol.* **20,** 796–799.
Niedobitek, G., Pitteroff, S., Herbst, H., Shepherd, P., Finn, T., Anagnostopoulos, I., and Stein, H. (1990). *J. Clin. Pathol.* **43,**
Niedobitek, G., Fietze, E., Herbst, H., Reinke, P., Schöne, J., Offermann, G., Kaden, J., Ditscherlein, G., Volk, H.-D., and Stein, H. (1991a). Submitted for publication.
Niedobitek, G., Hansmann, M. L., Herbst, H., Young, L. S., Dienemann, D., Hartmann, C. A., Finn, T., Pitteroff, S., Welt, A., Anagnostopoulos, I., Friedrich, R., Lobeck, H., Sam, C. K., Aranjo, I., Rickinson, A. B., and Stein, H. (1991b). Submitted for publication.
Noguchi, M., Hirohashi, S., Tsuda, H., Nakajima, T., Hara, F., and Shimosato, Y. (1988). *Mod. Pathol.* **1,** 428–432.
Nonoyama, M., Huang, C. H., Pagano, J. S., and Singh, S. (1973). *Proc. Natl. Acad. Sci. U.S.A.* **70,** 3265–3268.

Nuovo, G. J., and Richart, R. M. (1989a). *Am. J. Pathol.* **134**, 837–842.
Nuovo, G. J., and Richart, R. M. (1989b). *Lab. Invest.* **61**, 471–476.
Obara, T., Conti, C. J., Baba, M., Resau, J. H., Trifillis, A. L., Trump, B. F., and Klein-Szanto, A. J. P. (1986). *Am. J. Pathol.* **122**, 386–391.
Ohlsson, R., Holmgren, L., Glaser, A., Szpecht, A., and Pfeifer-Ohlsson, S. (1989). *EMBO J.* **8**, 1993–1999.
Ohuchi, N., Hand, P. H., Merlo, G., Fujita, J., Mariani-Costantini, R., Thor, A., Nose, M., Callahan, R., and Schlom, J. (1987). *Cancer Res.* **47**, 1413–1420.
Ostrow, R. S., Manias, D. A., Clark, B. A., Okagaki, T., Twiggs, L. B., and Faras, A. J. (1987). *Cancer Res.* **47**, 649–653.
Pahl, C., Niedobitek, G., Finn, T., Herbst, H., Klein, G., and Stein, H. (1991). Submitted for publication.
Paik, S., Rosen, N., Jung, W., You, J. M., Lippman, M. E., Perdue, J. F., and Yee, D. (1989). *Lab. Invest.* **61**, 522–526.
Pardue, M. L. (1985). *In* "Nucleic Acid Hybridisation—A Practical Approach" (B. D. Hames and S. J. Higgins, eds.), pp. 179–202. IRL Press. Oxford, England.
Parsa, I., Cleary, C. M., Marsh, W. H., Butt, K. M. and Foye, C. A. (1986). *Int. J. Pancreatol.* **1**, 299–308.
Patel, D., Shepherd, P. S., Naylor, J. A., and McCance, D. J. (1989). *J. Gen. Virol.* **70**, 69–77.
Patterson, S., Gross, J., and Webster, A. D. (1989). *J. Virol. Methods* **23**, 105–109.
Peltonen, J., Jaakkola, S., Lask, G., Virtanen, I., and Uitto, J. (1988a). *J. Invest. Dermatol.* **91**, 289–293.
Peltonen, J., Jaakola, S., Lebwohl, M., Renvall, S., Risteli, L., Virtanen, I., and Uitto, J. (1988b). *Lab Invest.* **59**, 760–771.
Perrot-Rechenmann, C., Joannes, M., Squalli, D., and Lebacq, P. (1989). *J. Histochem. Cytochem.* **37**, 423–428.
Pfeifer-Ohlsson, S., Goustin, A. S., Rydnert, J., Wahlstrom, T., Bjersing, L., Stehelin, D., and Ohlsson, R. (1984). *Cell* **38**, 585–596.
Poliard, A. M., Bernuau, D., Tournier, I., Legres, L. G., Schoevaert, D., Feldmann, G., and Sala-Trepat, J. M. (1986). *J. Cell Biol.* **103**, 777–786.
Poppema, S., van Imhoff, G., Torensma, R., and Smit, J. (1985). *Am. J. Clin. Pathol.* **84**, 385–390.
Porter, H. J., Khong, T. Y., Evans, M. F., Chan, V. T. W., and Fleming, K. A. (1988). *J. Clin. Pathol.* **41**, 381–383.
Porter, H. J., Heryet, A., Quantrill, A. M., and Fleming, K. A. (1990). *J. Clin. Pathol.* **43**, 129–132.
Portnoy, J., Ahronheim, G. A., Ghibu, F., Clecner, B., and Joncas, J. H. (1984). *N. Engl. J. Med.* **311**, 966–968.
Prevot, S., Fournier, J. G., Tardivel, I., Audouin, J., and Diebold, J. (1989). *Pathol. Res. Pract.* **185**, 187–193.
Pringle, J. H., Homer, C. E., Warford, A., Kendall, C. H., and Lauder, I. (1987). *Histochem. J.* **19**, 488–496.
Pringle, J. H., Primrose, L., Kind, C. N., Talbot, I. C., and Lauder, I. (1989). *J. Pathol.* **158**, 279–286.
Prosser, I. W., Stenmark, K. R., Suthar, M., Crouch, E. C., Mecham, R. P., and Parks, W. C. (1989). *Am. J. Pathol.* **135**, 1073–1088.
Przepiorka, D., and Myerson, D. (1986). *J. Histochem. Cytochem.* **34**, 1731–1734.
Raab-Traub, N., and Flynn, K. (1986). *Cell* **47**, 883–889.
Raab-Traub, N., Flynn, K., Pearson, G., Huang, A., Levine, P., Lanier, A., and Pagano, J. (1987). *Int. J. Cancer* **39**, 25–29.
Raap, A. K., Marijnen, J. G., Vrolijk, J., and van der Ploeg, M. (1986). *Cytometry* **7**, 235–242.
Rambaldi, A., Wakamiya, N., Vellenga, E. Horiguchi, J., Warren, M. K., and Kufe, D. (1988). *J. Clin. Invest.* **81**, 1030–1035.

Rentrop, M., Knapp, B., Winter, H., and Schweizer, J. (1986). *Histochem. J.* **18**, 271–276.
Resnick, R. M., Cornelissen, M. T. E., Wright, D. K., Eichinger, G. H., Fox, H. S., ter Schegget, J., and Manos, M. M. (1990). *J. Natl. Cancer Inst.* **82**, 1477–1484.
Rigby, P. B., Dieckmann, M., Rhodes, C., and Berg, P. (1977). *J. Mol. Biol.* **113**, 237–251.
Rijntjes, P. J. M., Van Ditzhuijsen, T. J. M., Van Loon, A. M., Van Haelst, U. J. G. M., Bronkhorst, F. B., and Yap, S. H. (1985). *Am. J. Pathol.* **120**, 411–418.
Ro, J., Bresser, J., Ro, J. Y., Brasfield, F., Hortobagyi, G., and Blick, M. (1989). *Oncogene* **4**, 351–354.
Robert, B., Sassoon, D., Jacq, B., Gehring, W., and Buckingham, M. (1989). *EMBO J.* **8**, 91–100.
Roberts, W. H., Sneddon, J. M., Waldman, J. M., and Stephens, R. E. (1989). *Arch. Pathol. Lab. Med.* **113**, 461–464.
Rogers, A. W. (1979). "Techniques in Autoradiography." Elsevier, Amsterdam.
Rotbart, H. A., Abzug, M. J., Murray, R. S., Murphy, N. L., and Levin, M. J. (1988). *J. Virol. Methods* **22**, 295–301.
Roy, S., Fitz-Gibbon, L., Poulin, L., and Wainberg, M. A. (1988). *Immunology* **64**, 233–239.
Rydnert, J., Pfeifer-Ohlsson, S., Goustin, A. S., and Ohlsson, R. (1987). *Placenta* **8**, 339–345.
Saber, M. A., Zern, M. A., and Shafritz, D. A. (1983a). *Proc. Natl. Acad. Sci. U.S.A.* **80**, 4017–4020.
Saber, M. A., Shafritz, D. A., and Zern, M. A. (1983b). *J. Cell Biol.* **97**, 986–992.
Saemundsen, A. K., Albeck, H., Hansen, J. P. H., Nielsen, N. H., Anvret, M., Henle, W., Henle, G., Thomsen, K. A., Kristensen, H. K., and Klein, G. (1982). *Br. J. Cancer* **46**, 721–727.
Saglie, R., Cheng, L., and Sadighi, R. (1988). *J. Periodontol.* **59**, 121–123.
Saiki, R. K., Gelfand, D. H., Stoffel, S., Scharf, S. J., Higuchi, R., Horn, G. T., Mullis, K. B., and Erlich, H. A. (1988). *Science* **239**, 487–491.
Saito, I., Servenius, B., Compton, T., and Fox, R. I. (1989). *J. Exp. Med.* **169**, 2191–2198.
Sambrook, J., Fritsch, E. F., and Maniatis, T. (1989). "Molecular Cloning: A Laboratory Manual." Cold Spring Harbor Lab. Cold Spring Harbor, New York.
Samoszuk, M., and Nansen, L. (1990). *Blood* **75**, 13–16.
Sandberg, M., Autio-Harmainen, H., and Vuorio, E. (1989a). *Dev. Biol.* **130**, 324–334.
Sandberg, M., Vuorio, T., Hirvonen, H., Alitalo, K., and Vuorio, E. (1988b). *Development* **102**, 461–470.
Sandberg, M., Aro, H., Multimaki, P., Aho, H., and Vuorio, E. (1989a). *J. Bone Jt. Surg., Am. Vol.* **71**, 69–77.
Sandberg, K., Gobl, E., Funa, K., and Alm, G. V. (1989b). *Scand. J. Immunol.* **29**, 651–658.
Sandberg, M., Makela, J. K., Multimaki, P., Vuorio, T., and Vuorio, E. (1989c). *Matrix* **9**, 82–91.
Sandberg, M., Tamminen, M., Hirvonen, H., Vuorio, E., and Pihlajaniemi, T. (1989d). *J. Cell Biol.* **109**, 1371–1379.
Sarkar, S., Kacinski, B. M., Kohorn, E. I., Merino, M. J., Carter, D., and Blakemore, K. K. (1986). *Am. J. Obstet. Gynecol.* **154**, 390–393.
Scharffetter, K., Stolz, W., Lankat-Buttgereit, B., Mauch, C., Kulozik, M., and Krieg, T. (1989a). *Virchows Arch. B* **56**, 299–306.
Scharffetter, K., Kulozik, M., Stolz, W., Lankat-Buttgereit, B., Hatamochi, A., Sohnchen, R., and Krieg, T. (1989b). *J. Invest. Dermatol.* **93**, 405–412.
Schrier, R. D., Nelson, J. A., and Oldstone, M. B. A. (1985). *Science* **230**, 1048–1051.
Schuurman, H. J., Schemmann, M. H. G., De Weger, R. A., Aanstoot, H., and Hene, R. (1989). *Am. J. Clin. Pathol.* **91**, 461–463.
Schwab, M., Alitalo, K., Klempnauer, K. H., Varmus, H. E., Bishop, J. M., Gilbert, F., Brodeur, G., Goldstein, M., and Trent, J. (1983). *Nature (London)* **305**, 245–248.
Schwab, M., Ellison, J., Busch, M., Rosenau, W., Varmus, H. E., and Bishop, J. M. (1984). *Proc. Natl. Acad. Sci. U.S.A.* **81**, 4940–4944.
Seibel, N. L., and Kirsch, I. R. (1989). *Blood* **74**, 1791–1795.

and macrophages can be induced to produce tissue factor (TF) (also known as factor III, or tissue thromboplastin) in response to a variety of immunological mediators, cytokines, and microorganismal products (reviewed by Ryan and Geczy, 1987). TF must be present for the extrinsic pathway of coagulation to function (reviewed by Stern et al., 1988). However, under normal conditions, TF is not present in the circulation and is not in contact with the circulation. Instead, TF appears to be sequestered away from the bloodstream, being undetectable by immunohistochemical staining with TF-specific monoclonal antibodies (MAbs) in vascular ECs and peripheral blood cells, but present in vascular adventitia, organ capsules, epidermis, and mucosal epithelium (Drake et al., 1989). These observations led to the suggestion that this distribution of TF evolved to facilitate coagulation whenever vascular integrity was disrupted (Drake et al., 1989). However, Dvorak et al. (1985) have argued that increased vascular permeability alone, which also occurs in DTH lesions (reviewed by Dvorak et al., 1986), is sufficient to induce extravascular coagulation, suggesting that saturating levels of TF (or other procoagulants) are present in normal tissues. This more conservative view does not rule out the involvement of cytokines, however, because various cytokines have been shown to increase the permeability of confluent EC monolayers *in vitro* (Brett et al., 1989) and to increase vascular permeability when injected *in vivo* (Martin et al., 1988).

Several groups have reported that cytokines can stimulate the conversion of the normally anticoagulant EC surface into a procoagulant one, at least *in vitro*. In 1983, Lyberg et al. showed that human umbilical vein ECs (HUVECs) are induced to express TF when incubated with peripheral blood lymphocytes, granulocytes, or various cell lines or, in some cases, with cell-free supernatants from cultures of those cells. The induction of TF was blocked by the presence of either actinomycin D or cycloheximide, demonstrating that induction required *de novo* RNA and protein synthesis. Bevilacqua et al. (1984, 1986a) then reported that the recombinant cytokines interleukin 1 (IL-1) and tumor necrosis factor α (TNF-α) could also induce the synthesis and cell-surface expression of TF by cultured human ECs. Again, the induction was shown to be dependent on *de novo* RNA and protein synthesis. IL-1 and TNF induced TF with similar kinetics—TF activity peaked at 4 hours and then declined to near baseline levels by 24 hours. Interestingly, the effects of the two cytokines were additive, even when apparently maximal doses of each were tested (Bevilacqua et al., 1986a). The latter two observations argue against the possibility that TNF acts indirectly to induce TF by stimulating the production of IL-1 by the ECs (Nawroth et al., 1986a; Libby et al., 1986; Kurt-Jones et al., 1987; Locksley et al., 1987). Gerlach et al. (1989) have observed that subconfluent EC monolayers express higher affinity TNF receptors than do confluent monolayers, and are therefore more susceptible to the procoagulant-inducing effects of TNF. These results suggest that ECs at sites of neovascularization *in vivo* could be more easily induced to express TF, and therefore would tend to stimulate coagulation.

Other studies have shown that antibodies can also induce TF on ECs. Because patients with systemic lupus erythematosus (SLE) have an increased risk for thrombosis and often produce antibodies that react with ECs, sera from such patients were tested for their ability to induce TF activity on cultured HUVECs (Tannenbaum *et al.*, 1986). Unfractioned sera, fractions containing only monomeric IgG, and fractions containing immune complexes were all effective in inducing TF. It was concluded that ECs are stimulated to produce TF when exposed to either anti-EC antibodies or immune complexes (Tannenbaum *et al.*, 1986). It is also of interest to note that Carlsen *et al.* (1988) have reported that cyclosporine significantly augmented the level of TF induced on cultured ECs by IL-1 or TNF. This result suggests that one potential risk of cyclosporine therapy in transplant recipients is the development of thromboses.

IL-1 and TNF have other effects on ECs that would also tend to favor a procoagulant state. Thus, incubation of *in vitro* cultures of ECs with either IL-1 or TNF resulted in increased production and/or release of plasminogen activator inhibitor (PAI) and von Willebrand factor (vWF). The increase in PAI activity was shown to be dependent on *de novo* RNA and protein synthesis (Schleef *et al.*, 1988; Emeis and Kooistra, 1986; van Hinsbergh *et al.*, 1988). In contrast, the IL-1 mediated increase in release of vWF was not blocked by cycloheximide, and a corresponding decrease in intracellular vWF was noted (Schorer *et al.*, 1987), suggesting that IL-1 stimulated the release of preformed vWF. The TNF-mediated increase in PAI was not blocked by anti-IL-1 antibodies (van Hinsbergh *et al.*, 1988), again suggesting that the effect of TNF was not mediated via EC-derived IL-1. Importantly, it has been shown that intravenous injection of either IL-1 (Emeis and Kooistra, 1986) or TNF (van Hinsbergh *et al.*, 1988) into rats increased the concentration of PAI in the blood. Because TNF did not increase production of PAI by cultured hepatocytes, it was concluded that the increase in PAI induced in the plasma of the TNF-injected rats was due to an effect of TNF on the vascular ECs and not due to an effect in the liver (van Hinsbergh *et al.*, 1988).

TNF and IL-1 have also been shown to inhibit EC production of tissue plasminogen activator (tPA) and thrombomodulin (Bevilacqua *et al.*, 1986b; Nawroth *et al.*, 1986b; Schleef *et al.*, 1988; Moore *et al.*, 1989; Schorer *et al.*, 1987). The decreased expression of TM on the cell surface of TNF-treated ECs was reported to be due to the internalization and degradation of the TM molecule (Moore *et al.*, 1989). There were at least two notable differences in the effects of IL-1/TNF on TF activity compared to their effects on PAI and tPA. First, the effects of the cytokines on tPA and PAI were relatively slow compared to their effects on TF, at least 18–24 hours being necessary for maximal effects (Emeis and Kooistra, 1986; van Hinsbergh et al., 1988; Bevilacqua et al., 1986b). Second, the effects of the two cytokines were additive on TF activity but were much less than additive on tPA and PAI activity (Schleef et al., 1988). Based on the above in vitro experiments, it would be predicated that ECs exposed in vivo to either IL-1 or TNF would be induced to activate the extrinsic clotting pathway. Direct in vivo evidence for this comes from the observation that intravenous infusion of IL-1 into rabbits resulted in the deposition of fibrin strands onto the luminal surface of ECs lining major arteries (Nawroth et al., 1986b).

Interestingly, thrombin has important effects on the balance of EC procoagulant and anticoagulant properties. Thrombin treatment of microvascular ECs in vitro stimulated both tPA and PAI production (van Hinsbergh et al., 1987). In addition, thrombin stimulated the release of factor VIII antigen from cultured HUVECs (Levine et al., 1982). It has also been reported that thrombin induced IL-1 production by ECs (Stern et al., 1985), which, by inducing TF activity on nearby cells, could stimulate an even stronger procoagulant response. Other possible roles for thrombin in the development of a chronic inflammatory lesion are (1) its chemotactic effect on monocytes (Bar-Shavit et al., 1983) and (2) its ability to increase EC adhesiveness for mononuclear cells (Saegusa et al., 1988).

In addition to the involvement of the clotting system in the pathophysiology of DTH reactions, several reports of the importance of the clotting system in immunologically mediated diseases have appeared. For example, when MAbs were used to study the possible role of cell-mediated immunity and clotting factors in human patients with proliferative glomerulonephritis (GN), it was observed that fibrin-positive biopsies showed significantly more mononuclear cell infiltration and TF reactivity than did fibrin-negative biopsies (Neale et al., 1988). Although the importance of cell-mediated immunity in GN is still controversial, the above results are consistent with the hypothesis that activated immune system cells can indirectly cause tissue damage at local sites by their ability to induce TF expression and, subsequently, coagulation. Second, it has been reported that injection of an inhibitor of plasminogen activator prevented the development of experimental autoimmune encephalomyelitis in rats (Koh and Paterson, 1987). Normally, clinical disease in this model is associated with the deposition of fibrin in the vasculature of the central nervous system and an increase in the permeability of the blood–brain barrier (BBB), presumably following fibrinolysis and the generation of vasoactive peptides. Consistent with this hypothesis was the observation that inhibition of disease following injection of the PA inhibitor correlated with an inhibition of the increase in BBB permeability.

It is also relevant to note that damage to ECs at sites of inflammation may stimulate the expression of receptors for the Fc portion of IgG (FcR) as well as receptors for complement components (C'R) (reviewed by Ryan, 1986). Subsequent binding of IgG and immune complexes to the vascular EC surface may lead to increased adhesion of other receptor-positive cells, including polymorphonuclear leukocytes (PMNs); activation of bound PMNs would then increase the release of vasoactive products, causing additional damage to the endothelium. As a result, vascular permeability would be increased and coagulation would be favored. In addition, as noted above, the binding of immune complexes or anti-EC antibodies induces ECs to synthesize TF (Tannenbaum *et al.*, 1986), thereby favoring the formation of a thrombus.

Finally, as reviewed by others (Cines, 1989), antibodies with reactivity to ECs have been reported in patients with diverse forms of thrombosis and/or vasculitis. In some cases, the antibodies bind only to ECs treated with particular cytokines (Leung *et al.*, 1986a,b). Some of these antibodies are capable of directly damaging ECs, at least *in vitro*, following complement fixation. Even the non-complement-fixing antibodies could damage ECs *in vivo* by stimulating adherence of platelets or PMNs or, as noted above, by stimulating the production of TF (Cines, 1989).

III. Lymphocyte/Endothelial Cell Interactions in Lymphocyte Recirculation

A. Organ-Specific Interactions

The classic morphological and electron microscopic studies by Gowans, Knight, and Marchesi (Gowans and Knight, 1964; Marchesi and Gowans, 1964) demonstrated that recirculating lymphocytes preferentially leave the bloodstream to enter lymph nodes and Peyer's patches by passing through the walls of specialized postcapillary venules (PCVs) referred to as high endothelial venules (HEVs). The term HEV is based on the morphological observation that the ECs of such PCVs are much more columnar and/or cuboidal than are the relatively flat ECs lining other PCVs in the body. In addition to their atypical morphology, the ECs of HEVs have distinctive histochemical and ultrastructural features. Thus, light microscopic examinations have shown that the ECs of HEVs in both experimental animals (Anderson *et al.*, 1976; Wenk *et al.*, 1974) and man (Freemont and Jones, 1983a) are not only "taller" than the relatively flat endothelium found in most PCVs, they also exhibit increased cytoplasmic pyroninophilia, ribonuclease-labile metachromasia, and anabolic enzymatic activities. Electron microscopic studies have further demonstrated that such ECs have increased numbers of polyribosomes, relatively dispersed chromatin, one or more prominent nucleoli, and a well-developed Golgi apparatus (Anderson et al., 1976; Wenk et al., 1974; Freemont and Jones, 1983a). Thus, both light and electron microscopic observations suggest that the ECs of HEVs are metabolically activated. The possible role of cytokines in the development of HEVs will be discussed in a subsequent section.

In vivo experiments in laboratory rodents and other animals have demonstrated that lymphocyte recirculation is not random and that lymphocytes vary in their abilities to enter different lymphoid organs through the HEVs (reviewed by Stoolman, 1989). Thus, lymphocytes from intestinal lymph tend to recirculate through the gut-associated lymphoid tissue (GALT), whereas lymphocytes isolated from peripheral lymph nodes (LNs) tend to recirculate through those organs. In addition, B cells, regardless of their tissue of origin, tend to home to GALT, in comparison to T cells, which tend to recirculate to peripheral lymph nodes. These preferences are not absolute and most lymphocytes appear capable of entering all lymphoid organs.

The molecular bases for these recirculatory pathways remained obscure until an *in vitro* assay was developed to study lymphocyte adhesion to HEV. In 1976, Stamper and Woodruff showed that rat lymphocytes would preferentially adhere to the ECs of HEVs when overlaid on frozen tissue sections of various lymphoid organs. The relevance of this assay to normal lymphocyte recirculation was demonstrated when it was shown that lymphocyte subsets vary in their levels of binding to HEVs from different lymphoid organs, and that those differences corresponded to their abilities to migrate into the various secondary lymphoid organs *in vivo* (reviewed by Woodruff et al., 1987). It was concluded from these studies (1) that ECs may express organ-specific molecules on their surface, and (2) that lymphocytes may vary in their expression of the corresponding surface molecules that bind to those tissue-specific EC ligands. The term lymphocyte-homing receptors has been commonly used to describe the lymphocyte cell surface molecules. The term vascular addressins has been suggested for the corresponding organ-specific EC molecules (Streeter et al., 1988).

Several groups of investigators, using monoclonal antibodies directed against the putative organ-specific lymphocyte cell surface molecules, have provided strong support for the above concept. The most well-characterized lymphocyte and EC molecules involved in these interactions are listed in Table II. The first such MAb to be described was MEL-14, which almost totally blocked the adhesion of murine lymphocytes to peripheral LN HEVs in a modified version of the Stamper–Woodruff assay (Gallatin et al., 1983). MEL-14 also partially inhibited the adhesion of murine lymphocytes to mesenteric LN HEVs but did not block lymphocyte binding to Peyer's patch HEVs. Impor-

TABLE II

WELL-CHARACTERIZED LYMPHOCYTE/EC ADHESION MOLECULES

Lymphocyte adhesion molecules
  1. Experimental animals: MEL-14, LPAM-1, LPAM-2, LFA-1
  2. Human: LFA-1, CD44, VLA-4, CD4
EC ligands
  1. Experimental animals: None
  2. Human: ICAM-1, ICAM-2(?), HLA-DR, VCAM-1/INCAM-110

tantly, it was demonstrated that MEL-14 also specifically inhibited the migration of lymphocytes into peripheral LNs during *in vivo* lymphocyte trafficking studies (Gallatin *et al.*, 1983; Mountz *et al.*, 1988). These observations were interpreted to suggest that MEL-14 recognizes a lymphocyte cell surface molecule that specifically binds to a ligand found on ECs in peripheral LNs and mesenteric LN HEVs, but not on Peyer's patch HEVs (Gallatin *et al.*, 1983). In addition, it was concluded that peripheral LN ECs and PP ECs express distinct, nonoverlapping ligands for lymphocyte homing receptors, whereas mesenteric LN ECs may express both peripheral LN and PP ligands (reviewed by Gallatin *et al.*, 1986). Chin, Rasmussen, Woodruff, and colleagues have published similar data in rats, in which MAbs were produced that selectively inhibited lymphocyte binding to either peripheral LN or PP HEVs (Rasmussen *et al.*, 1985; Chin *et al.*, 1986). Biochemical characterization and molecular cloning of the homing receptors on rodent lymphocytes (described below) have supported the hypothesis that the lymphocyte receptors for peripheral LN and PP HEVs are distinct.

When Gallatin *et al.* (1983) used SDS–PAGE to examine the cell surface molecules on murine lymphocytes and lymphomas that could be immunoprecipitated by MEL-14, a single band of 80–95 kDa was observed, the apparent size depending on the particular cell population examined. Based on inhibition studies with various mono- and polysaccharides, it was suggested that the molecule defined by MAb MEL-14 may be lectinlike, and the corresponding EC ligand may be carbohydrate in nature (Stoolman *et al.*, 1984; Rosen *et al.*, 1985; Rosen and Yednock, 1986; Yednock *et al.*, 1987). Thus, mannose-6-phosphate, and polymers of that molecule, but not various other mono- and polysaccharides or their derivatives, inhibited the binding of both rat and mouse lymphocytes to HEVs in peripheral LN tissue sections. Geoffroy and Rosen (1989) have recently shown that the lymphocyte cell surface molecule which can be purified by affinity chromatography on MEL-14-coated columns blocked lymphocyte adhesion to lymph node HEVs when it was preincubated with the tissue sections prior to the addition of the lymphocytes. Moreover, mannose-6-phosphate and related monosaccharides could inhibit this activity of the isolated receptor. Further evidence for the lectinlike nature of the lymphocyte homing receptors has come from molecular cloning studies.

Two groups have now isolated, cloned, and sequenced the gene encoding the MEL-14 core polypeptide (Lasky *et al.*, 1989; Siegelman *et al.*, 1989). The mature polypeptide is approximately 330 amino acids long and is estimated to be 37 kDa. The amino acid sequence suggested the molecule has 10 potential sites of N-glycosylation. The N-terminal sequence of 118 amino acids is 20–30% homologous to various animal lectins, again consistent with the evidence that the MEL-14 molecule may recognize a carbohydrate determinant on ECs. However, the orientation of the lectin binding domain is reversed with respect to its homologous lectins, which are oriented with their amino termini in the plasma membrane and the carboxyl termini facing extracellularly (reviewed by Drickamer, 1988). The next 33–37 amino acids consist of an epidermal growth factor (EGF)-like domain. Siegelman *et al.* (1989) noted that a 12-amino acid sequence of this domain is 58% identical and 83% homologous to a sequence found in the CD18 molecule [the common β chain of the lymphocyte function-associated antigen 1 (LFA-1) family of leukocyte glycoproteins]. This is of interest in view of the evidence discussed below that (1) LFA-1 seems to be involved in lymphocyte trafficking in a non-organ-specific manner, possibly by strengthening interactions between organ-specific receptor–ligand pairs, and (2) the higher molecular weight chain of the murine PP homing receptor is homologous to the α chain of the human VLA-4 molecule, which, like LFA-1, is a member of the integrin superfamily (Hemler, 1990) of adhesion molecules. The remaining extracellular portion of the MEL-14 molecule includes two identical repeats of a 62-amino acid sequence that is homologous to a number of "complement regulatory" proteins, which primarily bind to either C3b or C4b. These repeats presumably resulted from a recent gene duplication event, as they are identical not only at the protein level, but also at the DNA level. The DNA sequence suggests a hydrophobic transmembrane region of 23-amino acids, followed by a hydrophilic cytoplasmic tail of 18-amino acids. Interestingly, as will be discussed in more detail below, a similar domain structure has been found for the ELAM-1 molecule, a cell surface glycoprotein that is upregulated by cytokines on *in vitro* cultures of human ECs, and which appears to be an EC ligand for polymorphonuclear leukocytes.

In contrast to MAb MEL-14, MAb R1-2 blocked binding of murine lymphocytes to PP HEVs, but not to peripheral LN HEVs (Holzmann *et al.*, 1989). R1-2 reacted with two distinct heterodimeric proteins, named LPAM-1 and LPAM-2, which shared a common α subunit. This α subunit was shown to be homologous to the human VLA-4α chain because it could be precipitated with a monospecific rabbit antiserum to the human molecule. However, the α chain, unlike other known integrin molecules, was demonstrated to be capable of forming heterodimers with either of two β chains, the common β_1 chain of the VLA family or a novel β chain (Holzmann and Wiessman, 1989). Interestingly, MAb R1-2 inhibited the binding of lymphoma cell lines expressing either LPAM-1 or LPAM-2 to PP HEVs. However, LPAM-2 was expressed on some nonbinding lymphomas and LPAM-1 was not expressed on a LPAM-2+ line capable of binding to HEVs (Holzmann and Wiessman, 1989), suggesting that the expression of either molecule alone was not sufficient for binding to occur. Although LFA-1 has been shown to be involved in the binding of murine and human lymphocytes to HEVs *in vitro* (Pals *et al.*, 1988; Hamann *et al.*, 1988), some of the nonbinding LPAM+ murine lymphomas coexpressed LFA-1 (Holzmann and Weissman, 1989). It was concluded that multiple adhesion molecules may be involved in lymphocyte adhesion to HEVs.

MAbs that specifically inhibit the adhesion of human lymphocytes to LN or PP HEVs have also been reported. Although human lymphocytes stained very weakly with the MEL-14 antibody (Jalkanen *et al.*, 1987), that MAb almost totally inhibited binding of human cells to peripheral LN HEVs and immunoprecipitated a 90-kDa molecule (Jalkanen *et al.*, 1987); this mass is similar to that of the murine peripheral lymph node homing receptor described above (Gallatin *et al.*, 1983). As will be described later, a gene for a MEL-14-like molecule in humans has now been cloned and sequenced but it has not yet been formally shown that the human MEL-14-like molecule functions as an adhesion molecule. Butcher and colleagues have produced another MAb, Hermes-3, which specifically blocked the adhesion of human lymphocytes to mucosal HEVs and immunoprecipitated a molecule on human lymphocytes with a similar molecular weight (Jalkanen *et al.*, 1987). As reviewed recently (Haynes *et al.*, 1989), it is now clear that the molecule recognized by the Hermes-3 MAb is identical to both the human homologue of the murine Pgp-1 molecule and the CD44 molecule (Picker *et al.*, 1989). Pgp-1 and CD44 were originally described as a polymorphic antigen of mesenchymal cells (Hughes *et al.*, 1981), and as a marker of thymocyte maturation (Haynes *et al.*, 1983), respectively. A very similar molecule, identified by the Hutch-1 MAb, has been found on the lymphocytes of baboons (Idzerda *et al.*, 1989). Two different groups have now cloned and sequenced the relevant gene in humans (Goldstein *et al.*, 1989; Stamenkovic *et al.*, 1989). Both groups noted that the amino-terminal portion of this transmembrane molecule was approximately 30% homologous with chicken and rat cartilage link proteins and with rat cartilage proteoglycan core protein. Surprisingly, the molecule shared no homology with either MEL-14 or members of the CD11/CD18 (LFA-1, Mac-1, and p150,95) family. Because cartilage link and proteoglycan core proteins interact with ECM molecules, it is of interest to note that CD44 appears to be very similar, if not identical, to a previously described collagen receptor (see later). The relationship between receptors for ECM proteins and lymphocyte homing receptors has already been noted with regard to the apparent homology between the murine PP homing receptor and the human VLA-4 molecule. Because VLA molecules are known to function as receptors for extracellular matrix (ECM) proteins, it is intriguing to consider the possibility that lymphocyte homing receptors and receptors for ECM proteins may be related. In fact, because ECs are known to secrete various components of the ECM, it is possible that the PP HEV receptor on lymphocytes may be recognizing a tissue-specific ECM component expressed on the cell surface of the ECs of PP HEVs.

The existence of apparently identical mRNAs for the Hermes antigen in lymphoma cell lines with specificities for HEVs from different lymphoid organs (Goldstein et al., 1989) suggests, as pointed out by Stamenkovic et al. (1989), that Hermes may be a non-organ-specific adhesion molecule that, like LFA-1 (Pals et al., 1988; Hamann et al., 1988), may facilitate organ-specific interaction with MEL-14-like molecules. This conclusion would be consistent with the earlier observations (1) that Hermes-3 stained both mucosal HEV-specific lymphomas as well as lymphomas that bound only to LN HEVs, even though it selectively inhibited the binding to mucosal HEVs, and (2) that a polyclonal anti-Hermes antiserum blocked adhesion to HEVs from all organs examined (Jalkanen et al., 1987).

The human equivalent of the murine MEL-14 molecule has now been cloned by several groups and was shown to be the molecule recognized by the MAb Leu-8 (Tedder et al., 1989; Bowen et al., 1989; Camerini et al., 1989; Siegelman and Weissman, 1989). The overall amino acid sequence homology between the murine and human molecules is 77%. Although the proteins are nearly identical in the transmembrane and immediately surrounding regions, suggesting that this is a functionally important region, Camerini et al. (1989) provided evidence that the human molecule could be expressed in both transmembrane and phospholipid-anchored forms. The gene for this human molecule, called lymphocyte-associated cell surface molecule 1 (LAM-1) by one group (Tedder et al., 1989), was localized to chromosome 1. It has not yet been formally shown that the human molecule mediates adhesion to either HEVs in tissue sections or to cultured ECs.

It is of interest that Bevilacqua et al. (1989) have recently cloned an adhesion molecule expressed by human ECs that is similar in structure to MEL-14. This molecule, named endothelial leukocyte adhesion molecule 1 (ELAM-1), appears to be an EC ligand for an unknown receptor on PMNs. The mRNA for this protein was induced within 1–2 hours in *in vitro* cultures by ECs by IL-1, TNF, or LT (but not by IFN-γ) and then declined to near basal levels by 24 hours. Surface expression of this molecule closely paralleled the expression of the mRNA. The rapid induction and decline of ELAM-1 expression *in vitro* is consistent with its postulated importance in promoting PMN adhesion and migration into sites of acute inflammation. The involvement of this molecule in the *in vitro* adhesion of PMNs to ECs was demonstrated by showing that COS cells transfected with the ELAM-1 cDNA supported PMN adhesion, whereas control COS monolayers did not. In addition, treatment of the transfected COS cells with the anti-ELAM-1 MAb H18/7 almost totally blocked that adhesion. Others have shown that lymphoid cell lines do not recognize this molecule (Osborn *et al.*, 1989). The extracellular portion of the molecule is strikingly similar to the structure of the murine LN homing receptor detected by MAb MEL-14. The N-terminal region of ~120 amino acids, like the N-terminal part of the MEL-14 molecule, is homologous to the family of lectinlike proteins. The following 34 or so amino acids contain the EGF motif. In these two portions of the molecule, MEL-14 and ELAM-1 were found to be 61% identical. Unlike MEL-14, however, ELAM-1 contains six tandem repeats of a sequence that is homologous to the complement regulatory proteins (Bevilacqua *et al.*, 1989). It has recently been shown that degranulation of mast cells by substance P or other secretagogues in organ cultures of human skin induces the release of a TNF-like molecule from the mast cells, and also induces the expression of ELAM-1 on the surface of the ECs of nearby PCVs (Klein *et al.*, 1989; Matis *et al.*, 1990). Thus, it was hypothesized that the release of substance P by stimulated dermal nerve fibers may be important in the regulation of EC/leukocyte interactions *in vivo*.

In addition to the apparent presence of organ-specific EC ligands on the ECs of HEVs in the different secondary lymphoid organs, recent studies have suggested that ECs of HEV-like PCVs in various inflammatory lesions may also possess organ-specific ligands that are recognized by specific lymphocyte receptors. Thus, Jalkanen *et al.* (1987) reported that MEL-14 and Hermes-3 inhibited human lymphocyte binding to peripheral LN HEVs and mucosal HEVs, respectively, but neither MAb had any effect on binding to ECs of HEV-like PCVs in synovial membranes from rheumatoid arthritis patients. Similarly, Sackstein *et al.* (1988) observed that the binding of rat thoracic duct lymphocytes to HEV-like PCVs in tissue sections of psoriatic human skin could not be blocked by MAbs that were capable of inhibiting their binding to either peripheral LN HEVs or to PP HEVs.

B. NON-ORGAN-SPECIFIC INTERACTIONS

Two groups have recently reported that MAbs to the lymphocyte function-associated antigen 1 (LFA-1) molecule significantly, but incompletely, inhibited *in vitro* adhesion of murine and human lymphocytes to both peripheral and mucosal HEV (Pals *et al.*, 1988; Hamann *et al.*, 1988). It was also shown that anti-LFA-1 MAb partially inhibited lymphocyte migration into peripheral LN and PP *in vivo* in the mouse (Hamann *et al.*, 1988). As will be discussed below, several groups have shown that anti-LFA-1 MAbs also decrease the adhesion of lymphocytes to monolayers of viable ECs *in vitro*. Thus, LFA-1 has been definitively established as an important, albeit probably non-organ specific, lymphocyte cell surface adhesion molecule for ECs.

LFA-1 is one member of a family of three heterodimeric leukocyte cell surface adhesive glycoproteins that share a common β chain but have distinct α chains (reviewed by Kishimoto *et al.*, 1989). The other two members of this family are Mac-1 and p150,95. Mac-1 is also known as the CR3 receptor, and binds C3bi; p150,95 also is capable of binding C3bi. The LFA-1 family of molecules is one of three families of molecules comprising the integrin superfamily of adhesion molecules (reviewed by Hemler, 1990). The other two families, which are also cell surface heterodimeric structures, are known as the VLA family and the cytoadhesion family. Like the LFA-1 family, the individual members of the VLA and cytoadhesion families share a family-specific common β chain and are distinguished by their α chains. The name VLA arose because the first members of this family were originally described as "very late activation" antigens on T cells (Hemler *et al.*, 1986). It is now known, however, that these molecules serve as receptors for ECM proteins (Hemler, 1990). The cytoadhesion molecules, which have been best characterized on platelets, also bind to ECM proteins as well as to other proteins.

As noted above, various lines of evidence suggest that the Hermes molecule(s) on human lymphocytes may be a non-organ-specific lymphocyte receptor for vascular ECs. Further support for that hypothesis comes from the observation that the CD44/Hermes/Pgp-1 molecule is similar, if not identical, to extracellular matrix receptor type III (ECMRIII), originally defined by Carter and Wayner. Using a human fibrosarcoma cell line, these investigators characterized a transmembrane, phosphorylated glycoprotein that bound to collagen types I and VI in affinity chromatography experiments and that appeared to be associated with the cytoskeletal protein vimentin (Carter and Wayner, 1988). The biochemical similarities of this molecule to those of the Hermes and Hutch-1 molecules led to an investigation of the possible relationship between the three. When the molecules immunoprecipitated by MAbs, Hutch-1, Hermes-1, and P1G12 (anti-ECMRIII) were digested with proteases, identical peptides were obtained (Gallatin *et al.*, 1989). However, sequential immunoprecipitation experiments showed that preclearing with the anti-ECMRIII MAb removed reactivity to all three MAbs, whereas preclearing with the Hermes or Hutch MAb removed most but not all reactivity to the ECMRIII MAb. Thus, the lymphocyte homing receptors defined by the Hermes and Hutch MAbs may be a subset of the molecules immunoprecipitated with P1G12. Alternatively, all three MAbs may recognize the same molecule(s), but vary in their efficiencies in immunoprecipitation. Although this molecule has been referred to as a homing receptor, many groups have commented on its widespread tissue distribution, which includes fibroblasts, lymphocytes, monocytes, granulocytes, some but not all epithelial cells, endothelial cells, and keratinocytes (Kansas *et al.*, 1989; Pals *et al.*, 1989; Picker *et al.*, 1989; Carter and Wayner, 1988). These observations are consistent with its possible function as a receptor for ECM proteins.

Recently, the expression of Pgp-1 (CD44) on murine lymphocytes has been suggested to be a marker of previously activated, memory cells (Budd *et al.*, 1987). Thus, it was demonstrated that activation of murine Pgp-1− lymphocytes with alloantigens or mitogens led to cell surface expression of Pgp-1. In addition, the frequency of antigen-specific cells was greatly enriched in the Pgp-1+ subset in comparison to the Pgp-1− subset. Similar experiments with human neonatal and adult lymphocytes reached the same conclusion, although the differential expression of Pgp-1 on naive and memory cells was not as definitive as the expression of the LFA-3 or CD45RO antigens (Sanders *et al.*, 1988a). The activation-induced increase in expression of a cell surface molecule (CD44/Hermes/Pgp-1) that may act as a receptor for ECM proteins is consistent with earlier reports that activation of human T cells also induces expression of certain VLA proteins, now known to also have ECM receptor function (Hemler, 1990).

IV. Interactions between Endothelial Cells and Immune System Cells in the Regulation of Mononuclear Cell Migration into Inflammatory Lesions

Since the original discovery by Gowans and Knight (1964), it has been accepted that lymphocytes preferentially migrate from the bloodstream into lymph nodes and Peyer's patches from unique postcapillary venules, the high endothelial venules. Interestingly, HEV-like PCVs are found not only in lymph nodes and Peyer's patches, but also at sites of chronic inflammation in both man and experimental animals (Freemont and Jones, 1983b; Graham and Shannon, 1972; Chin *et al.*, 1990; Kabel *et al.*, 1989; Freemont and Ford, 1985; Nightingale and Hurley, 1978; Heng *et al.*, 1988; Iguchi and Ziff, 1986). In many of these studies, it was observed that the HEV-like PCVs were usually adjacent to densely aggregated lymphocytic infiltrates (Freemont and Jones, 1983b; Freemont and Ford, 1985; NIghtingale and Hurley, 1978; Iguchi and Ziff, 1986), suggesting that they were sites of active lymphocyte migration. Studies of lymphocyte migration into inflammatory lesions in experimental animals have clearly shown that such HEV-like PCVs are, in fact, the major sites of lymphocyte migration into those lesions (Freemont and Ford, 1985; Nightingale and Hurley, 1978), just as they are in lymph nodes and Peyer's patches.

It appears that the HEV phenotype is inducible, reversible, and regulated by the cells of the immune system. As noted above, HEVs have been repeatedly observed at sites of chronic inflammation. Second, HEVs are uncommon in T-cell-deficient experimental animals (Wright *et al.*, 1983; Parrott *et al.*, 1966). Moreover, HEVs in lymph nodes disappear over a period of a few weeks when the afferent lymphatics are ligated, but then reappear when the lymph node is stimulated by antigen (Hendriks and Estermans, 1983). It is of interest to note that a decrease in the adhesiveness of the HEV for lymphocytes appears to precede the loss of the HEV morphology (Hendriks *et al.*, 1987), suggesting, as might have been expected, that the concentration of adhesion molecules on the cell surface can be altered more rapidly than the overall metabolic status of the cell.

Because HEV-like PCVs are prominent at sites of chronic inflammation, as well as in lymph nodes, and because such PCVs appear to be the major site of lymphocyte migration in both cases, my collaborators and I hypothesized that cytokines produced by immune system cells might stimulate lymphocyte–EC adhesion and/or the development of HEV-like properties in cultured ECs. To test this hypothesis, a system was needed in which viable ECs could be incubated with cytokines prior to the performance of relevant assays. *In vitro* cultures of ECs derived from human umbilical cords provided a reliable, convenient source of viable ECs for these experiments. As a first test of the hypothesis that cytokines might affect T cell adhesion to ECs, Yu *et al.* examined the effects of crude supernatants from mixed lymphocyte reactions and mitogen-stimulated cultures on the adhesion of human lymphocytes to confluent monolayers of HUVECs. They reported that such supernatants, when preincubated with the ECs, increased the proportions of both B and T cells that adhered to the ECs, but had no effect on red blood cell adhesion (Yu *et al.*, 1985). The supernatants did not stimulate adhesion when preincubated with the lymphocytes. Subsequent experiments with recombinant cytokines and other molecules have been reviewed previously (Cavender, 1989) and will not be discussed in detail here. Briefly, it was demonstrated that preincubation of monolayers of either HUVEC monolayers or dermal microvascular ECs with recombinant human IFN-γ, IL-1α, IL-1β, lymphotoxin (LT; also known as TNF-β), or TNF (Cavender *et al.*, 1986, 1987b, 1989; Haskard *et al.*, 1987) led to a significant increase in the ability of the ECs to bind lymphocytes. Evidence suggesting that IL-1 and TNF may upregulate EC adhesiveness by the same mechanism will be presented below. Maximal adhesiveness of ECs following preincubation with either TNF or IL-1 was observed at a concentration of only 0.1 ng/ml (approximately 6 pM). In addition, those cytokines stimulated maximal adhesion after only 4–8 hours of incubation. Of all the cytokines, IFN-γ had, by far, the weakest effect (peak effect at 3 ng/ml and only about a 5–10% increase in the number of cells that bound) and required a longer incubation period (24 hours) to cause a maximal effect compared to the other cytokines. However, it should be noted that IL-1 and TNF, but not IFN-γ, have also been reported to up-regulate EC adhesiveness for PMNs, monocytes, natural killer cells, basophils, and/or eosinophils (Bevilacqua et al., 1985; Dunn and Fleming, 1984; Schleimer and Rutledge, 1986; Bender et al., 1987; Thornhill et al., 1990b; Gamble and Vadas, 1988; Bochner et al., 1988; Lamas et al., 1988). On the basis of those observations, it appeared that IFN-γ may be the only cytokine that specifically enhances lymphocyte adhesion. Recently, however, it has been reported that IL-4 also stimulates EC adhesiveness for T cells without an effect on PMN adhesion (Thornhill et al., 1990a). As yet, no data exist on the adhesion of other leukocyte types to IL-4-treated ECs. It is also of interest to note that preincubation of ECs with either lipopolysaccharide (LPS) or thrombin stimulated EC adhesiveness for T cells (Yu et al., 1986; Saegusa et al., 1988). The effects of these agents may be of particular importance at sites of infection and inflammation. Finally, it has been demonstrated that pretreatment of EC monolayers *in vitro* with IFN-γ not only increased T cell–EC adhesion, but also stimulated T cell migration through the EC monolayer (Oppenheimer-Marks and Ziff, 1988).

The above results clearly supported the hypothesis that immune system cytokines secreted at sites of inflammation or other immune activity may act on the ECs of nearby PCVs to increase their adhesiveness for circulating lymphocytes. Thus, these results provide a rational explanation for the development of lymphocytic infiltrates at sites of chronic inflammation. Unlike the homing receptor-type binding described above, the cytokine-induced increase in lymphocyte–EC adhesion is presumably not tissue specific. This view was supported by the results of additional studies performed by ourselves and others that showed that ECs isolated from various organs and different species all responded to the same cytokines with increased adhesiveness for lymphocytes (Haskard et al., 1987; Bender et al., 1987; Issekutz, 1990; Hughes et al., 1988).

Results of MAb inhibition studies have suggested that several ligand–receptor pairs may be involved in the adhesion of lymphocytes to cultured EC monolayers. Several groups have reported that antibodies to the LFA-1 molecule nearly completely inhibited T cell adhesion to non-cytokine-treated ECs (Dustin and Springer, 1988; Haskard et al., 1986). Thus, MAbs to either the α or β chain of LFA-1 almost totally blocked the adhesion of either resting or phorbol ester-stimulated T cells to untreated ECs (Haskard et al., 1986). Others have shown that anti-LFA-1 MAbs also inhibit the binding of both CD4+ and CD8+ human T cell clones to ECs (Mentzer et al., 1986). Using

MAbs against intracellular adhesion molecule 1 (ICAM-1) (Rothlein et al., 1986), Dustin and Springer (1988) have suggested that this LFA-1-dependent adhesion may actually involve two different ligand–receptor pairs: (1) LFA-1 on the T cell recognizing ICAM-1 on the EC (LFA-1 dependent, ICAM-1 dependent), and (2) LFA-1 on the T cell binding to a second, unknown ligand on the EC (LFA-1 dependent, ICAM-1 independent). As will be discussed below, this unknown ligand may be the recently described (Staunton et al., 1989) ICAM-2 molecule. In contrast to the inhibitory effects of anti-LFA-1 MAbs on the binding of untreated and phorbol ester-treated T cells to unstimulated ECs (Haskard et al., 1986), we and others have shown that such MAbs had almost no inhibitory effect on the increase in adhesion observed when the ECs were pretreated with TNF, LPS, IL-1, IL-4, or thrombin (Saegusa et al., 1988; Cavender et al., 1987a; Haskard et al., 1986; Thornhill et al., 1990b), suggesting that the ECs synthesized another receptor for lymphocytes following incubation with those stimulants. The inability of anti-LFA-1 MAbs to inhibit T cell adhesion to cytokine-treated ECs has been confirmed by other laboratories, using normal lymphocytes (Dustin and Springer, 1988) as well as lymphoblastoid cell lines from LFA-1-deficient patients (Haskard et al., 1989). The apparent induction of an alternative EC receptor for lymphocytes following incubation with cytokines is consistent with the observation that cycloheximide, when used at appropriate doses, inhibited the adhesion-promoting effects of the cytokines (Cavender et al., 1987a). A large number of other MAbs, including anti-HLA class I or II, anti-CD2, anti-CD3, anti-LFA-3, anti-Mac-1, and anti-p150,95 had no effect on either unstimulated or cytokine-stimulated lymphocyte–EC adhesion (Haskard et al., 1986).

Cytokine treatment of ECs has also been reported to enhance the binding of monocytes (Bevilacqua et al., 1985; Downs et al., 1987). Although there is general agreement that members of the CD11/CD18 family are involved in monocyte adhesion to ECs *in vitro*, there is some disagreement concerning which of the three molecules (LFA-1, Mac-1, and p150,95) is of prime importance (Wallis et al., 1985; TeVelde et al., 1987; Prieto et al., 1988; Mentzer et al., 1987).

The inhibitory effects of anti-LFA-1 MAbs on the adhesion of T cells to untreated ECs are consistent with the results obtained in our separate experiments designed to determine whether specific subsets of T cells could be identified based on varying degrees of adhesiveness for ECs (Cavender et al., 1988). In these experiments, human peripheral blood T cells were separated into weakly and strongly adherent subsets by consecutive incubations on untreated and cytokine-activated ECs, and then were stained with various MAbs. Thus, the weakly adherent subpopulation was empirically defined as those cells that failed to adhere to either untreated or cytokine-stimulated ECs, whereas the strongly adherent subset was defined as those cells that bound to untreated ECs. Although there was no detectable difference between CD4+ and CD8+ T cells in their abilities to bind to ECs, the strongly adherent subpopulation was enriched for cells that stained brightly with anti-LFA-1 MAbs and the weakly adherent subpopulation contained mostly LFA-1-dull cells (Cavender et al., 1988). It was also observed that panning T cells on IL-1, LPS, or TNF-treated EC monolayers resulted in a marked depletion of cells capable of binding to either IL-1, LPS, or TNF-treated ECs in rebinding experiments (Cavender et al., 1988). These results suggested that IL-1, LPS, and TNF up-regulated EC adhesiveness by the same mechanism. The conclusion that IL-1, LPS, and TNF all stimulate EC adhesiveness for T cells by the same mechanism is consistent with (1) the similarity in the kinetics of the increases in adhesion induced by these agents, and (2) the lack of effect of anti-LFA-1 MAb on the increases in adhesion. Because both LPS and TNF are known to stimulate ECs to produce IL-1 (Nawroth et al., 1986a; Libby et al., 1986; Kurt-Jones et al., 1987; Miossec et al., 1986), one possible explanation of the above results was that IL-1 is the final common mediator of the stimulatory effect of all three agents on EC adhesiveness. However, when neutralizing amounts of monospecific anti-IL-1α and/or anti-IL-1β antisera were added to EC cultures in the presence of either LPS or TNF, no inhibitory effects of the antisera on the increases in EC adhesiveness were observed (Cavender et al., 1987b; D. E. Cavender, Y. Saegusa, and M. Ziff, unpublished observations). These results suggest that LPS and TNF do not increase EC adhesiveness by stimulating EC production of IL-1, which then acts in an autocrine fashion to stimulate EC adhesiveness. However, it has been reported that EC-derived IL-1 does increase the adhesiveness of fresh EC monolayers for T cells, suggesting that an autocrine, positive-feedback loop is theoretically possible and may be important *in vivo* (Miossec et al., 1988).

Recent studies on the lymphocytes present in chronic inflammatory lesions support the importance of LFA-1 in lymphocytic infiltration, and suggest that the monolayer adhesion assay is physiologically relevant to the understanding of lymphocyte migration at sites of inflammation. Human peripheral blood CD4+ T cells can be roughly divided into two approximately equal-sized, almost nonoverlapping groups based on reactivities with MAbs 4B4 and 2H4—a 4B4+, 2H4− group and a 4B4−, 2H4+ group (reviewed by Sanders et al., 1988b). Interestingly, most CD4+ T cells present in various chronic inflammatory lesions react positively with MAb 4B4 and very few react with MAb 2H4 (Pitzalis et al., 1988; Morimoto et al., 1988; Modlin et al., 1988). Pitzalis et al. (1988) demonstrated, using the panning procedure described above, that 4B4+ cells had a greater ability to bind to ECs, at least *in vitro*, compared to the 2H4+ cells. Moreover, isolated 4B4+ cells were shown to contain a higher proportion of cells staining strongly with anti-LFA-1 MAb than did the 2H4+ cells. However, when the adhesion of 4B4+ and 2H4+ T cells was tested in the presence of anti-LFA-1 MAb, the differences between the subsets were not completely abolished, suggesting that non-LFA-1-dependent mechanisms are also of importance in lymphocyte adhesion to EC monolayers *in vitro* (Pitzalis *et al.*, 1988).

It has recently been shown that the 4B4+ subpopulation of human peripheral blood T cells also adheres significantly better than the 2H4+ subset to HEV-like PCVs in frozen sections of human psoriatic lesions (Chin *et al.*, 1990). As was observed for the binding of 4B4+ cells to cultured ECs (Pitzalis *et al.*, 1988), the binding to psoriatic HEVs appeared to involve both LFA-1-dependent and -independent mechanisms, because the anti-CD18 MAb 60.3 only partially inhibited binding (~40%) (Chin *et al.*, 1990). Sanders *et al.* (1988a,b) have recently provided strong evidence that the subpopulation of human CD4+ T cells that is 4B4+ and expresses relatively high levels of LFA-1 is the *in vivo*-primed, memory helper T cell subset. Thus, this subset of cells contains almost all of the cells capable of proliferating in response to recall antigens *in vitro*. In addition, almost all neonatal T cells were 2H4+, 4B4−, but could be converted to the opposite phenotype following stimulation with polyclonal mitogens. It is now known that the 4B4 MAb reacts with the common β chain of the VLA family of markers (Knapp *et al.*, 1989), consistent with the knowledge that a subset of peripheral blood T cells expresses VLA-4, a receptor for fibronectin (FN) (Wayner *et al.*, 1989). Also, as noted above, VLA-4 appears to function as a lymphocyte homing receptor for PP HEVs in the mouse. Sanders *et al.* (1988a) also showed that these memory cells have an increased expression of other molecules, including CD2, LFA-3 (CD58), UCHL1 (CD45O), and Pgp-1 (CD44; the Hermes lymphocyte homing receptor molecule; see earlier). Thus, memory T cells in the human express increased levels of at least three molecules that have been implicated in adhesion to ECs: LFA-1, VLA-4, and CD44. In addition, their expression of VLA and Hermes antigens may enable them to interact with ECM proteins in the connective tissue. Therefore, as might have been predicted, it appears that many memory T cells have a greater capacity to bind to ECs than do naive T cells and, therefore, may have a greater ability to recirculate *in vivo*. Finally, Damle and Doyle (1990) have confirmed the greater adherence of the memory subset of T cells and also demonstrated that this subset, upon activation, significantly increased the permeability of endothelial monolayers to macromolecules. It was suggested that this capability may facilitate their transendothelial migration into extravascular connective tissue *in vivo*.

Recently, using a novel functional cloning method, Staunton *et al.* (1989) cloned the gene for a second ligand for LFA-1, which they refer to as ICAM-2. ICAM-2, like ICAM-1 (Rothlein *et al.*, 1986), is an integral membrane protein. However, ICAM-2 has only two immunoglobulin-like domains, unlike ICAM-1, which has five. It seems likely that ICAM-2 is the relevant EC ligand involved in the "LFA-1-dependent, ICAM-1-independent" type of binding, although this question has not yet been directly addressed. Because neither ICAM-1 nor ICAM-2 contains an Arg-Gly-Asp (RGD) sequence, common to a variety of ligands for integrin molecules (reviewed by Ruoslahti and Pierschbacher, 1987), LFA-1 does not apparently recognize the RGD sequence in its ligands. In contrast to the situation with ICAM-1, ICAM-2 mRNA was present at high levels in untreated ECs and did not increase upon exposure of the ECs to lipopolysaccharide (LPS). Therefore, the increase in T cell binding that is observed following treatment of ECs with LPS (Yu *et al.*, 1986), which was demonstrated to be almost completely independent of LFA-1 (Haskard *et al.*, 1986), also appears to be independent of ICAM-2. However, LFA-1-dependent, ICAM-1-independent binding to untreated ECs may involve ICAM-2.

Recent *in vivo* experiments in the rat have provided further evidence for the concept that memory T cells have a greater affinity for cultured ECs and may therefore have a greater ability to recirculate *in vivo*. Issekutz (1990) has demonstrated that lymph node lymphocytes, which migrate poorly to inflammatory sites *in vivo*, are poor binders to unstimulated and cytokine-treated microvascular ECs, whereas small, resting, peritoneal exudate lymphocytes, which actively migrate into inflammatory sites, bind relatively well to microvascular ECs *in vitro*. Most importantly, it was shown that the subpopulation of peritoneal exudate lymphocytes that did not adhere to cytokine-treated EC monolayers *in vitro* did not migrate efficiently into inflammatory sites.

Major histocompatibility complex (MHC) antigens on the surface of cultured ECs may also function as adhesion molecules for lymphocytes. Masuyama *et al.* (1986) reported that the stimulatory effect of IFN-γ on the adhesiveness of ECs for T cells required 72 hours of incubation to reach a maximum. The kinetics of the increased adhesion closely paralleled the kinetics of the induction of endothelial cell surface expression of HLA-DR antigens, which were induced much more strongly than were DP or DQ antigens. T cell subset analyses indicated that Leu-3+ (CD4+) T cells preferentially bound to the IFN-γ–EC. In addition, it was reported that MAbs to the T cell CD4 molecule or to the EC DR antigens significantly, but incompletely, inhibited T cell adhesion to IFN-γ–EC. The increased adhesion of CD4+ T cells to IFN-γ–EC was observed in both syngeneic and allogeneic combinations of cells, suggesting that the increased binding could not be explained on the basis of T cell recognition of foreign class II antigens (Masuyama *et al.*, 1986). Similar results have been reported by others (Thornhill *et al.*, 1989), and are consistent with the observation that interaction of the CD4 molecule with MHC class II antigens can mediate cell adhesion (Doyle and Strominger, 1987).

At least one other ligand–receptor pair may be involved in the adhesion of T cells to *in vitro* cultures of ECs. Osborn, Elices, and colleagues (Osborn *et* al., 1989; Elices et al., 1990) have cloned an EC adhesion molecule for lymphocytes, which they named vascular cell adhesion molecule 1 (VCAM-1). VCAM-1, like ICAM-1 and ICAM-2, belongs to the immunoglobulin superfamily; its amino acid sequence is 26% identical to that of ICAM-1. VCAM-1 mRNA was barely detectable in untreated HUVECs but increased greatly within 2 hours after exposure of the cells to either IL-1 or TNF, and remained high for at least 72 hours. Transfection experiments with the VCAM-1 cDNA and VLA-4 cDNA demonstrated that VLA-4 on lymphoid cells bound specifically to VCAM-1-transfected cells (Elices et al., 1990). PMNs showed no specific adhesion to COS cells transfected with VCAM-1 cDNA, whereas lymphoid cell lines failed to recognize COS cells transfected with ELAM-1 cDNA. These results confirm that cytokine-treated ECs express distinct adhesion molecules for PMNs and lymphocytes. Interestingly, inhibition experiments with MAbs and fibronectin fragments showed that the binding site on VLA-4 for fibronectin was distinct from its binding site for VCAM-1 (Elices et al., 1990). Rice and colleagues, in independent experiments (Rice and Bevilacqua, 1989; Rice et al., 1990), produced a MAb, E1/6, that appears to recognize VCAM-1. These investigators, who called this molecule inducible cell adhesion molecule 110 (INCAM-110), reported that E1/6 markedly inhibited the adhesion of melanoma cell lines to IL-1- or TNF-treated HUVECs (Rice and Bevilacqua, 1989). Moreover, additional MAb inhibition studies, which used combinations of E1/6 with either anti-LFA-1 or anti-ICAM-1 MAbs, suggested that lymphocytes and monocytes may recognize both INCAM-110 and ICAM-1 on ECs (Rice et al., 1990). Preliminary immunohistochemical experiments on tissue sections suggested that INCAM-110 was present on ECs at sites of immune reactions *in vivo* (Rice et al., 1990). Thus, at least four gene families appear to be involved in lymphocyte–EC interactions: (1) members of the integrin superfamily, including both the CD11/CD18 family (particularly LFA-1), and the VLA/ECM receptor family (particularly VLA-4/LPAM-1/LPAM-2); (2) members of the immunoglobulin superfamily (ICAM-1, ICAM-2, VCAM-1, CD4, and HLA-DR); (3) members of the family with homology to C-type lectins, EGF, and complement regulatory proteins (the MEL-14 antigen and ELAM-1); and (4) CD44 (Hermes, Pgp-1, Hutch-1, and ECMRIII).

It is obvious that much has been learned concerning the cytokines and receptors that may be involved in the stimulation of lymphocyte adhesion to vascular ECs. Equally important, particularly from a therapeutic point of view, are the factors that may inhibit or down-regulate this interaction. In this regard, it is important to note that Gamble and Vadas (1988) have demonstrated that preincubation of EC monolayers *in vitro* with transforming growth factor β (TGF-β) inhibited the subsequent binding of PMNs. Moreover, when the ECs were incubated with both TGF-β and TNF, TGF-β totally inhibited the expected TNF-mediated increase in adhesion. As will be discussed in more detail below, we have reported that IL-1 totally inhibited the TNF-induced increases in EC metabolism (RNA and protein synthesis) and cell volume, although IL-1 did not inhibit the increase in EC adhesiveness for T cells induced by TNF (Cavender and Edelbaum, 1988). Finally, Gimbrone and colleagues have shown that cytokine-treated ECs secrete a soluble inhibitor of PMN adhesion (Wheeler et al., 1988), which they subsequently identified as an amino-terminal-extended form of IL-8 (Gimbrone et al., 1989). Importantly, the EC-derived IL-8 was also shown to prevent PMN-mediated damage to EC monolayers *in vitro*. If similar inhibitors of mononuclear cell adhesion could be found, it might be possible to block selectively the development of chronic inflammatory lesions.

V. The Role of Cytokines in the Activation of Endothelial Cells at Sites of Inflammation

Several characteristics common to HEVs in secondary lymphoid organs and HEV-like PCVs at sites of chronic inflammation suggest that the ECs of these vessels are metabolically activated. First, the ECs of HEVs have been reported to be cuboidal or columnar, in contrast to the relatively flat ECs lining the other PCVs in the body. Second, electron microscopic studies have documented increases in biosynthetic organelles (increased amounts of rough endoplasmic reticulum and Golgi apparatus) and a relatively great ability to incorporate radioactive sulfate. Third, the ECs exhibit an increase in ribonuclease-sensitive metachromasia. In an attempt to model this process *in vitro*, my colleagues and I measured the effects of various cytokines on RNA synthesis, protein synthesis, and cell volume of cultured ECs. Although IL-1α, IL-1β, IFN-γ, LT, and TNF all stimulated EC adhesiveness for T cells, only TNF and LT stimulated EC RNA and protein synthesis and cell volume (Cavender et al., 1989). To our surprise, IL-1 was a potent inhibitor of those actions of TNF and LT (Cavender and Edelbaum, 1988). Therefore, we suggested that TNF and LT, but not IL-1 or IFN-γ, may be important in the induction of HEV-like PCVs at sites of inflammation *in vivo*, whereas EC-derived IL-1 may function to downregulate EC activation.

Other evidence suggests that cytokines are important in the regulation of EC activation at inflammatory sites. As will be discussed in more detail below, class II+ ECs have been observed in various diseased organs, suggesting the local production of IFN-γ by activated T cells. Other studies have demonstrated that MAbs produced against cytokine-treated ECs *in vitro* selectively bind to ECs at sites of inflammation *in vivo* (Munro et al., 1989; Cotran et al., 1986; Rice et al., 1990; Lewis et al., 1989). In some cases, injection of impure (Dumonde et al., 1982) or recombinant (Munro et al., 1989; Issekutz et al.,

1988; Rosenbaum et al., 1988; Kaplan et al., 1987) cytokines into human (Dumonde et al., 1982; Kaplan et al., 1987) or animals (Munro et al., 1989; Issekutz et al., 1988; Rosenbaum et al., 1988) has induced a mononuclear cell infiltrate and/or evidence of EC activation.

A recent study comparing the effects of intradermally injected IFN-γ and TNF in baboons (Munro et al., 1989) is of particular interest. IFN-γ alone induced a modest migration of mononuclear cells but little or no increase in EC expression of ICAM-1 or ELAM-1 molecules. TNF, however, induced a more intense mononuclear cell infiltrate, which was apparent by 9 hours after injection and which consisted of approximately equal numbers of T cells and monocytes. ICAM-1 and ELAM-1 expression were markedly increased on ECs, and hypertrophy of venular ECs was observed starting at about 24 hours (Munro et al., 1989). At the electron microscopic level, it could be seen that ECs near TNF-injected sites possessed dilated rough endoplasmic reticulum and increased numbers of intracellular organelles. Combining IFN-γ with TNF produced results similar to those obtained with TNF alone, although slightly increased staining of ECs for ELAM-1 and ICAM-1 was noted. These results are consistent with the *in vitro* data showing that TNF, but not IFN-γ, markedly increases EC adhesiveness for lymphocytes and stimulates EC metabolism (Cavender et al., 1987b, 1989).

VI. The Effects of Cytokines on Endothelial Cell Expression of MHC Antigens and Their Possible Role in Endothelial Cell Antigen Presentation

A. DO ENDOTHELIAL CELLS FUNCTION AS ANTIGEN-PRESENTING CELLS *In Vivo*?

It is believed that activation of CD4+ helper T cells is the necessary first step for an effective immune response. Because CD4+ T cells recognize antigen only when it is presented in the context of class II antigens on an antigen-presenting cell, it is important to note that most ECs in the body do not normally express class II antigens. However, class II+ ECs have been noted at sites of immune-mediated disease in both man and experimental animals (Sobel et al., 1984; Traugott et al., 1985; Antoniou et al., 1987; Bottazzo et al., 1985). The factors involved in the induction of class II antigens on ECs will be discussed in a subsequent section.

There is general agreement that cultured ECs are fully capable of acting as accessory cells for mitogen-induced T cell proliferation (Wilcox et al., 1989; Hashimoto et al., 1989; Ashida et al., 1981; Roska et al., 1984). Similarly, they appear to be functional APCs for alloreactive T cells, especially when preincubated with IFN-γ in order to induce class II expression (Geppert and Lipsky,

1985; Wilcox et al., 1989; Hirschberg et al., 1975; Pober et al., 1983b). However, the ability of ECs to present soluble protein antigen to T cells remains controversial. Early studies indicated that cultured human umbilical vein ECs, thought to constitutively express class II antigens, could present native (unfragmented) soluble antigens to primed T cells *in vitro*, in a class II-restricted fashion (Hirschberg et al., 1980; Burger et al., 1981). Subsequent studies were unable to confirm that cultured ECs were class II+, although activated T cells, impure cytokine-containing supernatants, or treatment of the ECs with IFN-γ induced class II expression (Pober et al., 1983b). As noted above, several groups of investigators have observed that ECs at sites of inflammation often express Ia antigens prior to the formation of a large mononuclear cell infiltrate. This suggests that IFN-γ producing, presumably antigen-specific, T cells have been activated, and that IFN-γ and other cytokines secreted by those cells may be important in the subsequent non-antigen-specific recruitment of mononuclear cells. Based on the *in vitro* adhesion data discussed above, it would be predicted that the lymphocyte products TNF-β and IL-4 may be important cytokines at this initial stage of such a lesion.

A second requirement for effective APC function is the production of IL-1 and perhaps other soluble factors that are necessary for T cell activation. Many laboratories have reported that ECs can produce IL-1 in response to LPS, TNF, or thrombin (Stern et al., 1985; Nawroth et al., 1986a; Libby et al., 1986; Kurt-Jones et al., 1987; Locksley et al., 1987; Wagner et al., 1985; Miossec et al., 1986). Evidence for EC production of both IL-1α and IL-1β has been published (Libby et al., 1986; Kurt-Jones et al., 1987). In addition, ECs can apparently produce a cell surface form of IL-1 (Kurt-Jones et al., 1987).

Most of the *in vitro* experiments described above were performed with macrovascular ECs. Thus, the question of whether microvascular ECs function as APCs *in vivo* remains open, particularly as it relates to antigen-specific activation of unprimed T cells. Two groups have reported that cultured microvascular ECs (MVECs) derived from rat (Pryce et al., 1989) or guinea pig (Wilcox et al., 1989) brain are poor APCs for ovalbumin or PPD-reactive T cells, even when the ECs were pretreated with IFN-γ, exogenous IL-1 was provided, indomethacin was present to decrease production of inhibitory arachidonic acid metabolites by the ECs, and antigen-specific T cell lines were used (Pryce et al., 1989). However, brain-derived MVECs from strain 13 guinea pigs, which are susceptible to the induction of experimental autoimmune encephalomyelitis (EAE), can present myelin basic protein (MBP) to *in vivo*-primed MBP-specific T cells (Wilcox et al., 1989). Similar data have been obtained in a murine EAE model (McCarron et al., 1986). It was suggested that this apparently antigen-specific ability to present antigen could be related to possible differences in the degree of antigen processing required for the various antigens (Wilcox et al., 1989). It is of interest to note here that bidirectional transfer of cytoplasmic components can occur between ECs and bound lymphocytes (Guinan *et al.*, 1988). Whether this interaction is involved in the act of antigen presentation by ECs is not known.

Two groups have examined the possible APC function of brain vascular ECs *in vivo*. Doherty *et al.* (1988) studied the recruitment of mononuclear cells into the brain of mice infected with lymphocytic choriomeningitis (LCM) virus. The induction of disease in such animals is mediated by CD8+, class I-restricted T cells. Using lethally irradiated, bone marrow-reconstituted chimeric mice, they demonstrated that induction of disease in such mice required class I-restricted recognition of radiation-resistant cells at the blood–brain barrier; because the virus is known to be present in ECs, it is reasonable to assume that the vascular EC is the relevant cell. However, the secondary recruitment of donor T cells and monocytes, and the remaining (radioresistant) host monocytes, occurred regardless of the degree of MHC compatibility between donor and host. The simplest explanation of these findings is that there is a requirement for MHC-restricted recognition of radioresistant cells at the blood–brain interface but that, following migration of the CD8+ immune effector T cells into the parenchyma of the brain, cytokines secreted by the activated T cells and/or by resident host APCs act on nearby ECs to increase their adhesiveness for circulating mononuclear cells in a non-MHC-restricted fashion. Although the results of this study do not prove that microvascular ECs can function as APCs *in vivo*, they do suggest that MHC-restricted T cell recognition of EC-bound antigen may be important in the selective recruitment of antigen-specific T cells into inflammatory lesions. Consistent with this idea is the observation from other studies that MBP, following its injection into the cerebral spinal fluid of rats, can be found on the luminal surface of vascular ECs in the brain (Vass *et al.*, 1984).

However, adoptive transfer studies in the EAE model led to a different conclusion. Hinrichs *et al.* (1987) used F_1 to parent bone marrow chimeras as recipients of parental-derived MBP-sensitized spleen cells. It was observed that the presence of semisyngeneic F_1 bone marrow-derived accessory cells was sufficient for disease induction, even when the transferred lymphocytes were allogeneic to the central nervous system cells in the host. These results suggest that the requirement for MHC compatibility between donor and host for transfer of disease is confined to cells of bone marrow derivation and that there is no requirement for MHC compatibility between the transferred T cells and the vascular ECs of the host. Further studies are obviously necessary to determine whether vascular ECs are important APCs *in vivo*.

B. Endothelial Cell Expression of MHC Antigens: Regulation by Cytokines

Endothelial cells, like most other nucleated cells in the body, constitutively express class I major histocompatibility complex antigens. However, it has been demonstrated that several cytokines can up-regulate class I expression on macrovascular and/or microvascular ECs; these include IFN-α, IFN-β1, TNF-α, and TNF-β (LaPierre *et al.*, 1988; Leeuwenberg *et al.*, 1987, 1988; Collins *et al.*, 1986; Male and Pryce, 1988) (see Table III). However, IL-1 (LaPierre *et al.*, 1988) and IFN-β2 (Leeuwenberg *et al.*, 1987; LaPierre *et al.*, 1988) (also known as IL-6) had little or no effect. The effects on class I expression of IFN-α and IFN-β1, on the one hand, and TNF on the other hand, could be distinguished by comparing their influence on IFN-γ-increased class I expression. Both TNF-α and TNF-β synergized with IFN-γ to further increase expression of class I molecules. In contrast, either IFN-α or IFN-β1, when combined with IFN-γ, had a less than additive effect on class I levels (LaPierre *et al.*, 1988).

For both IFN-γ and TNF, it has been shown that the increased surface expression of class I antigens was associated with increased mRNA levels (Collins *et al.*, 1984, 1986). Interestingly, however, the protein synthesis inhibitor cycloheximide inhibited the increase in class I mRNA induced by TNF (Collins *et al.*, 1986), suggesting that TNF increased class I expression in an indirect fashion, by acting through an intermediate protein. Leeuwenberg *et al.* (1987) have provided evidence that this intermediate protein is IFN-β1.

TABLE III
Effects of Cytokines on EC Expression of MHC Antigens

Cytokine	Class I	Class II	Reference
IFN-α	Increase	No effect	LaPierre *et al.* (1988), Carlsen *et al.* (1988)
IFN-β	Increase	No effect	LaPierre *et al.* (1988), Carlsen *et al.* (1988)
IFN-γ	Increase	Increase	Collins *et al.* (1984), Leeuwenberg *et al.* (1988), Pober *et al.* (1983a)
TNF-α	Increase	No effect	Collins *et al.* (1986), Leeuwenberg *et al.* (1987)
LT (TNF-β)	Increase	No effect	LaPierre *et al.* (1988)
IFN-α + IFN-γ	Additive or less	Inhibit	LaPierre *et al.* (1988), Leeuwenberg *et al.* (1988)
IFN-β + IFN-γ	Additive or less	Inhibit	LaPierre *et al.* (1988), Leeuwenberg *et al.* (1988)
IFN-γ + TNF-α	Additive or more	Same as IFN-γ alone	LaPierre *et al.* (1988), Leeuwenberg *et al.* (1988)
		TNF-α inhibits when added before or at same time as IFN-γ; TNF stimulates further if added after IFN-γ.	Leeuwenberg *et al.* (1988)

Of all the cytokines tested, only IFN-γ has been shown to increase class II expression on ECs. The DP, DQ, DR, and invariant chain mRNA levels all increased in HUVECs to maximal levels within 24–48 hours in the presence of IFN-γ (Collins et al., 1984). Cell surface expression, however, did not peak until day 5 or 6 after the addition of IFN-γ (Collins et al., 1984). Of the three types of class II antigens, HLA-DR was most strongly induced (Geppert and Lipsky, 1985). DP was also induced, but at a lower density, and DQ expression was barely detectable. Similar effects of IFN-γ on rat brain microvascular ECs have been reported (Male and Pryce, 1988). Interestingly, IL-1 has recently been shown to inhibit the stimulatory effect of IFN-γ on MHC class II expression on rat heart EC, and to also inhibit the effect of TNF on class I expression (Leszczynski, 1990).

TNF has been reported to either have no effect (LaPierre et al., 1988) or an inhibitory effect (Leeuwenberg et al., 1988) on the IFN-γ-induced expression of class II molecules on HUVECs. The group that found an inhibitory effect reported that the inhibitory effect was blocked by MAb to IFN-β1, again suggesting that the effect of TNF on MHC antigen expression may be mediated through IFN-β1 (Leeuwenberg et al., 1988). Interestingly, they further reported that TNF inhibited the effect of IFN-γ only when it was added to the ECs prior to or at the same time as the IFN-γ. In contrast, when TNF was added 24 hours after the addition of IFN-γ, and class II expression was evaluated 24 hours later, a significant enhancement of class II expression was observed (Leeuwenberg et al., 1988). As noted by the authors (Leeuwenberg et al., 1988), the experiments using a combination of IFN-γ and TNF are complicated by the toxic effect of this particular combination of cytokines on ECs when used at sufficiently high concentrations (Saegusa et al., 1990; Stolpen et al., 1986). Both groups of investigators reported that IFN-β1 was a potent inhibitor of the induction of class II antigens by IFN-γ. LaPierre et al. (1988) further showed that this inhibitory effect of IFN-β1 on IFN-γ-induced HLA-DR expression occurred at the level of transcription; no DR mRNA was observed in the presence of both IFNs.

Injection of IFN-γ into rats (Leszczynski et al., 1986), or incubation of human skin organ cultures with IFN-γ (Messadi et al., 1988), has also been demonstrated to induce class II expression on microvascular ECs. The induction of class II on ECs in the rat study was a transient effect because class II expression returned to baseline levels by day 7. Because simultaneous injection of methylprednisolone completely inhibited the IFN-γ-induced increase in class II expression by ECs (Leszczynski et al., 1986), it was suggested that the immunosuppressive effect of glucocorticoids in organ transplantation may, in part, be mediated by inhibition of class II expression on passenger leukocytes in the graft. In the human study, some notable differences were observed regarding the responsiveness of ECs in the organ cultures compared to EC monolayers *in vitro*. First, HLA-DR expression was maximally induced within 24 hours (Messadi *et al.*, 1988), as opposed to several days for cultured ECs (LaPierre *et al.*, 1988). Second, HLA-DR expression slowly declined over time, even with the continual presence of IFN-γ, as was observed *in vivo* in the rat study. In contrast, DQ expression continued to increase up to 72 hours (Messadi *et al.*, 1988).

VII. Endothelial Cell Proliferation and Angiogenesis

Endothelial cell proliferation and angiogenesis occur infrequently under normal conditions (Hobson and Denekamp, 1984). However, vascular proliferation and angiogenesis have been repeatedly observed at sites of immune reactions (Dvorak *et al.*, 1976; Clark *et al.*, 1981; Polverini *et al.*, 1977b; Sidky and Auerbach, 1975). Subsequent studies suggested that activated mononuclear cells and/or impure cytokine-containing supernatants could stimulate EC proliferation *in vitro* (Martin *et al.*, 1981; Watt and Auerbach, 1986) or angiogenesis *in vivo* (Leibovich *et al.*, 1987; Polverini *et al.*, 1977a). With the recent development of recombinant cytokines, it is now possible to examine the effects of single, purified cytokines for their involvement in angiogenesis.

It should be kept in mind that the process of angiogenesis can be divided into at least five discrete steps: degradation of the preexisting subendothelial basement membrane, migration of the ECs (presumably toward an angiogenic stimulus), proliferation of the ECs, organization of the ECs into vessels, and reformation of a subendothelial basement membrane. Therefore, *in vitro* assays of EC proliferation measure only one aspect of the angiogenic process; to more completely study angiogenesis *in vitro*, assays of EC migration, chemotaxis, and tube formation are necessary. However, as noted by Folkman and Klagsbrun (1987) in their recent review of angiogenic factors, the interpretation of *in vivo* studies is also difficult because one cannot easily distinguish direct effects of the cytokine on the vascular endothelium from indirect effects mediated through other cell types and/or cytokines. An excellent example of this was given above when evidence was presented that certain effects of TNF on EC expression of MHC antigens may be mediated by IFN-β1.

In 1977, Polverini *et al.* (1977a) reported that neovascularization was induced in guinea pig corneas by the injection of murine macrophages that had been activated *in vivo* or *in vitro*. Furthermore, cell-free supernatants were also effective (Polverini *et al.*, 1977a). These results were subsequently duplicated with activated human peripheral blood monocytes (Koch *et al.*, 1986). Based on the observations that (1) injection of TNF also induced angiogenesis (Leibovich *et al.*, 1987; Frater-Schroder *et al.*, 1987) and (2) the angiogenic effect of supernatants from cultures of activated macrophages was completely blocked by an antiserum to TNF (Leibovich et al., 1987), it was concluded that TNF is responsible for the angiogenic effect of activated macrophages. There is general agreement, however, that both TNF and IL-1 inhibit EC proliferation *in vitro*, particularly in the presence of known EC mitogens (Frater-Schroder et al., 1987; Norioka et al., 1987; Saegusa et al., 1990; Sato et al., 1986; Stolpen et al., 1986). However, TNF has also been reported to be chemotactic for capillary ECs *in vitro* and to stimulate the formation of tube-like structures (Leibovich et al., 1987). These observations may explain why TNF is angiogenic *in vivo*, despite its antiproliferative effect *in vitro*. Similarly, it has been demonstrated that TGF-β inhibits EC proliferation *in vitro* but is angiogenic *in vivo* (Madri et al., 1988; Muller et al., 1987; Roberts et al., 1986). Like TNF, TGF-β has also been reported to induce tube formation *in vitro*, at least on certain substrates (Madri et al., 1988). Because TGF-β is chemotactic for monocytes (Wahl et al., 1987), it is possible that monocytes recruited by TGF-β are involved in *in vivo* effects of TGF-β. Interestingly, it has recently been reported that TGF-β alters the cell surface expression of all three classes of integrin adhesion molecules on various human cell lines (Heino et al., 1989; Ignotz et al., 1989). If a similar phenomenon occurs on ECs, one can easily imagine how TGF-β could have marked effects on angiogenesis. In view of the data that cytokines can alter both EC morphology (Montesano et al., 1985; Fitzgerald et al., 1987; Groenewegen et al., 1985; Stolpen et al., 1986) and EC production of extracellular matrix materials (Montesano et al., 1984; Stolpen et al., 1986) *in vitro*, and that EC proliferation is influenced by the matrix on which the ECs are plated (Form et al., 1986; Madri et al., 1988), it seems likely that cytokines may indirectly affect angiogenesis *in vivo* by altering the production by ECs of ECM molecules. Consistent with this hypothesis are the observations made by several groups that subendothelial basement membranes are often abnormal at sites of inflammation *in vivo* (Espinoza et al., 1982; Dvorak et al., 1976; Clark et al., 1981; Matsubara and Ziff, 1987; Roberts et al., 1986).

Finally, both inhibitory and stimulatory effects of IFN-γ on EC proliferation *in vitro* have been reported (Friesel et al., 1987; Saegusa et al., 1990). The reason for this discrepancy is unclear, although the stimulatory effect of IFN-γ was observed only at relatively low concentrations of IFN-γ (Saegusa et al., 1990); both groups reported inhibition at relatively high concentrations.

VIII. Effects of Endothelial Cell Products on the Function of Immune System Cells

Human ECs can be stimulated by cytokines to release a number of factors with chemotactic or activating properties on leukocytes. As noted above, several laboratories have reported EC secretion of IL-1, which, as recently reviewed by others (di Giovine and Duff, 1990), has multiple activating effects on B and T cells. In addition, both monocyte-derived IL-1 (Miossec et al., 1984) and EC-derived IL-1 (Miossec et al., 1988) have been reported to have chemotactic activity for T cells, and both stimulate EC adhesiveness for T cells (Cavender et al., 1986; Miossec et al., 1988). TNF and IL-1 also induce ECs to produce an ~ 8 kDa protein that both activates PMN and induces their chemotaxis (Matsushima et al., 1988; Strieter et al., 1989). As reviewed by others (Matsushima and Oppenheim, 1989), this molecule has been given various acronyms, including neutrophil-activating protein (NAP-1), neutrophil-activating factor (NAF), monocyte-derived neutrophil chemotactic factor (MDNCF), and IL-8. This cytokine is also chemotactic for T cells; in fact, it has been reported that T cells are about 10-fold more sensitive than PMNs (Larsen et al., 1989). As noted in a previous section, IL-8 also inhibits the adhesion of PMNs to cultured ECs (Gimbrone et al., 1989). In addition, TNF and IL-1 induce ECs to produce a heparin-binding chemotactic/activating factor for monocytes known as monocyte chemotactic and -activating factor (MCAF) (Furutani et al., 1989). MCAF and NAP-1/IL-8 are members of two separate families of cytokines that are nevertheless similar enough to be considered together as a superfamily (Matsushima and Oppenheim, 1989; Wolpe and Cerami, 1989). Similar proteins have been also described in mice (Brown et al., 1989). IL-1 also stimulates the production of granulocyte–macrophage colony-stimulating factor (GM-CSF) by EC (Babgy et al., 1986). GM-CSF has chemotactic activity for PMNs, monocytes (Wang et al., 1987), and ECs (Bussolino et al., 1989), and also stimulates EC proliferation *in vitro* (Bussolino et al., 1989). Thus, ECs produce at least four different factors—IL-1, IL-8, MCAF, and GM-CSF—that have chemotactic activity for PMNs, T cells, or monocytes. Finally, it has been reported that IL-1 and TNF stimulate IL-6 production by ECs (May et al., 1989; Sironi et al., 1989), which, as reviewed recently (Zielasek et al., 1990), also has stimulatory effects on lymphocyte proliferation and differentiation. Interestingly, EC-derived IL-6 was also shown to inhibit EC proliferation *in vitro* (May et al., 1989).

IX. Conclusions

As a result of rapid advances in the techniques of cell culture, cell biology, and molecular biology, our understanding of the functions of the vascular endothelium has greatly increased in recent years. It is now clear that vascular ECs and the cells of the immune system interact in many ways that markedly affect the function of both systems. A large number of those interactions appear to be mediated not by direct cell contact but by means of cytokines.

The challenge that remains is to delineate how the effects that have been described are regulated and controlled *in vivo*. Combinations of human and animal studies, both *in vitro* and *in vivo*, will be necessary.

Acknowledgments

The author would like to thank Dr. Morris Ziff for his encouragement to enter this line of research, and for his previous collaboration and support. This work was supported by NIH grants AI27809 and AI23285.

References

Albrightson, C. R., Baenziger, N. L., and Needleman, P. (1985). *J. Immunol.* **135,** 1872.
Anderson, N. D., Anderson, A. O., and Wyllie, R. G. (1976). *Immunology* **31,** 455.
Antoniou, A. V., El-Sady, H., Butter, C., and Turk, J. L. (1987). *J. Neuroimmunol.* **15,** 57.
Ashida, E. R., Johnson, A. R., and Lipsky, P. E. (1981). *J. Clin. Invest* **67,** 1490.
Bagby, G. C., Jr. Dinarello, C. A., Wallace, P., Wagner, C., Hefeneider, S., and McCall, E. (1986). *J. Clin. Invest.* **78,** 1316.
Bar-Shavit, R., Kahn, A., Fenton, J. W., II, and Wilner, G. D. (1983). *J. Cell Biol.* **96,** 282.
Bender, J. R., Pardi, R., Karasek, M. A., and Engleman, E. G. (1987). *J. Clin. Invest.* **79,** 1679.
Bevilacqua, M. P., Pober, J. S., Majeau, G. R., Cotran, R. S., and Gimbrone, M. A., Jr. (1984). *J. Exp. Med.* **160,** 618.
Bevilacqua, M. P., Pober, J. S., Wheeler, M. E., Cotran, R. S., and Gimbrone, M. A., Jr. (1985). *J. Clin. Invest.* **76,** 2003.
Bevilacqua, M. P., Pober, J. S., Majeau, G. R., Fiers, W., Cotran, R. S., and Gimbrone, M. A., Jr. (1986a). *Proc. Natl. Acad. Sci. U.S.A.* **83,** 4533.
Bevilacqua, M. P., Schleef, R. R., Gimbrone, M. A., Jr., and Loskutoff, D. J. (1986b). *J. Clin. Invest.* **78,** 587.
Bevilacqua, M. P., Stengelin, S., Gimbrone, M. A., Jr., and Seed, B. (1989). *Science* **243,** 1160.
Bochner, B. S., Peachell, P. T., Brown, K. E., and Schleimer, R. P. (1988). *J. Clin. Invest.* **81,** 1355.
Bottazzo, G. F., Dean, B. M., McNally, J. M., MacKay, E. H., Swift, P. G. F., and Gamble, D. R. (1985). *N. Engl. J. Med.* **313,** 353.
Bowen, B. R., Nguyen, T., and Lasky, L. A. (1989). *J. Cell Biol.* **109,** 421.
Brett, J., Gerlach, H., Nawroth, P., Steinberg, S., Godman, G., and Stern, D. (1989). *J. Exp. Med.* **169,** 1977.
Brown, K. D., Zurawski, S. M., Mosmann, T. R., and Zurawski, G. (1989). *J. Immunol.* **142,** 679.
Budd, R. C., Cerottini, J.-C., Horvath, C., Bron, C., Pedrazzini, T., Howe, R. C., and MacDonald, H. R. (1987). *J. Immunol.* **138,** 3120.
Burger, D. R., Ford, D., Vetto, R. M., Hamblin, A., Goldstein, A., Hubbard, M., and Dumonde, D. C. (1981). *Hum. Immunol.* **3,** 209.
Bussolino, F., Wang, J. M., Defilippi, P., Turrini, F., Sanavio, F., Edgell, C.-J. S., Aglietta, M., Arese, P., and Mantovani, A. (1989). *Nature* **337,** 471.
Camerini, D., James, S. P., Stamenkovic, I., and Seed, B. (1989). *Nature (London)* **342,** 78.
Carlsen, E., Flatmark, A., and Prydz, H. (1988). *Transplantation* **46,** 575.
Carter, W. G., and Wayner, E. A. (1988). *J. Biol. Chem.* **263,** 4193.
Cavender, D. E. (1989). *J. Invest. Dermatol.* **93,** 88S.
Cavender, D. E., and Edelbaum, D. (1988). *J. Immunol.* **141,** 3111.
Cavender, D. E., Haskard, D. O., Joseph, B., and Ziff, M. (1986). *J. Immunol.* **136,** 203.

Cavender, D., Haskard, D., Foster, N., and Ziff, M. (1987a). *J. Immunol.* **138,** 2149.
Cavender, D. E., Saegusa, Y., and Ziff, M. (1987b). *J. Immunol.* **139,** 1855.
Cavender, D. E., Haskard, D. O., Maliakkal, D., and Ziff, M. (1988). *Cell. Immunol.* **117,** 111.
Cavender, D. E., Edelbaum, D., and Ziff, M. (1989). *Am. J. Pathol.* **134,** 551.
Chin, Y.-H., Rasmussen, R. A., Woodruff, J. J., and Easton, T. G. (1986). *J. Immunol.* **136,** 2556.
Chin, Y.-H., Falanga, V., Taylor, J. R., Cai, J.-P., and Bax, J. (1990). *J. Invest. Dermatol.* **94,** 413.
Cines, D. B. (1989). *Rev. Infect. Dis.* **11** (Suppl. 4), S705.
Clark, R. A. F., Dvorak, H. F., and Colvin, R. B. (1981). *J. Immunol.* **126,** 787.
Collins, T., Korman, A. J., Wake, C. T., Boss, J. M., Kappes, D. J., Fiers, W., Ault, K. A., Gimbrone, M. A., Jr., Strominger, J. L., and Pober, J. S. (1984). *Proc. Natl. Acad. Sci. U.S.A.* **81,** 4917.
Collins, T., LaPierre, L. A., Fiers, W., Strominger, J. L., and Pober, J. S. (1986). *Proc. Natl. Acad. Sci. U.S.A.* **83,** 446.
Colvin, R. B., and Dvorak, H. F. (1975). *J. Immunol.* **114,** 377.
Colvin, R. B., Mosesson, M. W., and Dvorak, H. F. (1979). *J. Clin. Invest.* **63,** 1302.
Cotran, R. S., Gimbrone, M. A., Jr., Bevilacqua, M. P., Mendrick, D. L., and Pober, J. S. (1986). *J. Exp. Med.* **164,** 661.
Crutchley, D. J., Ryan, U. S., and Ryan, J. W. (1980). *J. Clin. Invest.* **66,** 29.
Damle, N. K., and Doyle, L. V. (1990). *J. Immunol.* **144,** 1233.
di Giovine, F. S., and Duff, G. W. (1990). *Immunol. Today* **11,** 13.
Doherty, P. E., Ceredig, R., and Allan, J. E. (1988). *Clin. Immunol. Immunopathol.* **47,** 19.
Downs, E. C., Cornwell, D. G., Proctor, V. K., and Whistler, R. L. (1987). *Lymphokine Res.* **6,** 351.
Doyle, C., and Strominger, J. L. (1987). *Nature (London)* **330,** 256.
Drake, T. A., Morrissey, J. H., and Edgington, T. S. (1989). *Am. J. Pathol.* **134,** 1087.
Drickamer, K. (1988). *J. Biol. Chem.* **263,** 9557.
Dumonde, D. C., Pulley, M. S., Paradinas, F. J., Southcott, B. M., O'Connell, D., Robinson, M. R. G., den Hollander, F., and Schuurs, A. H. (1982). *J. Pathol.* **138,** 289.
Dunn, C. J., and Fleming, W. E. (1984). *Eur. J. Rheumatol. Inflammation* **7,** 80.
Dustin, M. L., and Springer, T. A. (1988). *J. Cell Biol.* **107,** 321.
Dvorak, A. M., Mihm, M. C., Jr., and Dvorak, H. F. (1976). *Lab. Invest.* **34,** 179.
Dvorak, H. F., Senger, D. R., Dvorak, A. M., Harvey, V. S., and McDonagh, J. (1985). *Science* **227,** 1059.
Dvorak, H. F., Galli, S. J., and Dvorak, A. M. (1986). *Hum. Pathol.* **17,** 122.
Edwards, R. L., and Hicks, F. R. (1978). *Science* **200,** 541.
Elices, M. J., Osborn, L., Takada, Y., Crouse, C., Luhowskyj, S., Hemler, M. E., and Lobb, R. R. (1990). *Cell* **60,** 577.
Emeis, J. J., and Kooistra, T. (1986). *J. Exp. Med.* **163,** 1260.
Esmon, N. L. (1987). *Semin. Thromb. Hemostasis* **13,** 454.
Espinoza, L. R., Vasey, F. B., Espinoza, C. G., Bocanegra, T. S., and Germain, B. F. (1982). *Arthritis Rheum.* **25,** 677.
Fitzgerald, O. M., Hess, E. V., Chance, A., and Highsmith, R. F. (1987). *J. Leukocyte Biol.* **41,** 421.
Folkman, J., and Klagsbrun, M. (1987). *Science* **235,** 442.
Form, D. M., Pratt, B. M., and Madri, J. A. (1986). *Lab. Invest.* **55,** 521.
Frater-Schroder, M., Risau, W., Hallmann, R., Gautschi, P., and Bohlen, P. (1987). *Proc. Natl. Acad. Sci. U.S.A.* **84,** 5277.
Freemont, A. J., and Ford, W. L. (1985). *J. Pathol.* **147,** 1.
Freemont, A. J., and Jones, C. J. P. (1983a). *J. Anat.* **136,** 349.
Freemont, A. J., and Jones, C. J. P. (1983b). *J. Rheumatol.* **10,** 801.
Friesel, R., Komoriya, A., and Maciag, T. (1987). *J. Cell Biol.* **104,** 689.
Furutani, Y., Nomura, H., Notake, M., Oyamada, Y., Fukui, T., Yamada, M., Larsen, C. G., Oppenheim, J. J., and Matsushima, K. (1989). *Biochem. Biophys. Res. Commun.* **159,** 249.

Gallatin, W. M., Weissman, I. L., and Butcher, E. C. (1983). *Nature (London)* **304,** 30.
Gallatin, M., St.John, T. P., Siegelman, M., Reichert, R., Butcher, E. C., and Weissman, I. L. (1986). *Cell* **44,** 673.
Gallatin, W. M., Wayner, E. A., Hoffman, P. A., St.John, T., Butcher, E. C., and Carter, W. G. (1989). *Proc. Natl. Acad. Sci. U.S.A.* **86,** 4654.
Gamble, J. R., and Vadas, M. A. (1988). *Science* **242,** 97.
Geoffroy, J. S., and Rosen, S. D. (1989). *J. Cell Biol.* **109,** 2463.
Geppert, T. D., and Lipsky, P. E. (1985). *J. Immunol.* **135,** 3750.
Gerlach, H., Lieberman, H., Bach, R., Godman, G., Brett, J., and Stern, D. (1989). *J. Exp. Med.* **170,** 913.
Giddings, J. C., and Small, L. (1987). *Thromb. Res.* **47,** 259.
Gimbrone, M. A., Jr., Obin, M. S., Brock, A. F., Luis, E. A., Hass, P. E., Hebert, C. A., Yip, Y. K., Leung, D. W. Lowe, D. G., Kohr, W. J., Darbonne, W. C., Bechtol, K. B., and Baker, J. B. (1989). *Science* **246,** 1601.
Goldstein, L. A., Zhou, D. F. H., Picker, L. J., Minty, C. N., Bargatze, R. F., Ding, J. F., and Butcher, E. C. (1989). *Cell* **56,** 1063.
Gowans, J. L., and Knight, E. J. (1964). *Proc. R. Soc. London, Ser. B* **159,** 257.
Graham, R. C., Jr., and Shannon, S. L. (1972). *Am. J. Pathol.* **69,** 7.
Groenewegen, G., Buurman, W. A., and van der Linden, C. J. (1985). *Clin. Immunol. Immunopathol.* **36,** 378.
Guinan, E. C., Smith, B. R., Davies, P. F., and Pober, J. S. (1988). *Am. J. Pathol.* **132,** 406.
Hamann, A., Jablonski-Westrich, D., Duijvestijn, A., Butcher, E. C., Baisch, H., Harder, R., and Thiele, H.-G. (1988). *J. Immunol.* **140,** 693.
Hashimoto, Y., Nakano, K., Yoshinoya, S., Tanimoto, K., and Miyamoto, T. (1989). *Int. Arch. Allergy Appl. Immunol.* **89,** 11.
Haskard, D. O., Cavender, D., Beatty, P., Springer, T., and Ziff, M. (1986). *J. Immunol.* **137,** 2901.
Haskard, D. O., Cavender, D., Fleck, R. M., Sontheimer, R. D., and Ziff, M. (1987). *J. Invest. Dermatol.* **88,** 340.
Haskard, D. O., Strobel, S., Thornhill, M., Pitzalis, C., and Levinsky, R. J. (1989). *Immunology* **66,** 111.
Haynes, B. F., Harden, E. A., Telen, M. J., Hemler, M. E., Strominger, J. L., Palker, T. J., Scearce, R. M., and Eisenbarth, G. S. (1983). *J. Immunol.* **131,** 1195.
Haynes, B. F., Telen, M. J., Hale, L. P., and Denning, S. M. (1989). *Immunol. Today* **10,** 423.
Heino, J., Ignotz, R. A., Hemler, M. E., Crouse, C., and Massague, J. (1989). *J. Biol. Chem.* **264,** 380.
Hemler, M. E. (1990). *Annu. Rev. Immunol.* **8,** 365.
Hemler, M. E., Glass, D., Coblyn, J. S., and Jacobson, J. G. (1986). *J. Clin. Invest.* **78,** 696.
Hendriks, H. R., and Eestermans, I. L. (1983). *Eur. J. Immunol.* **13,** 663.
Hendriks, H. R., Duijvestijn, A. M., and Kraal, G. (1987). *Eur. J. Immunol.* **17,** 1691.
Heng, M. C. Y., Allen, S. G., and Chase, D. G. (1988). *Br. J. Dermatol.* **118,** 315.
Hinrichs, D. J., Wegmann, K. W., and Dietsch, G. N. (1987). *J. Exp. Med.* **166,** 1906.
Hirschberg, H., Evensen, S. A., Henriksen, T., and Thorsby, E. (1975). *Transplantation* **19,** 191.
Hirschberg, H., Bergh, O. J., and Thorsby, E. (1980). *J. Exp. Med.* **152,** 249s.
Hobson, B., and Denekamp, J. (1984). *Br. J. Cancer* **49,** 405.
Holzmann, B., and Weissman, I. L. (1989). *EMBO J.* **8,** 1735.
Holzmann, B., McIntyre, B. W., and Weissman, I. L. (1989). *Cell* **56,** 37.
Hughes, C. C. W., Male, D. K., and Lantos, P. L. (1988). *Immunology* **64,** 677.
Hughes, E. N., Mengod, G., and August, J. T. (1981). *J. Biol. Chem.* **256,** 7023.
Idzerda, R. L., Carter, W. G., Nottenburg, C., Wayner, E. A., Gallatin, W. M., and St.John, T. (1989). *Proc. Natl. Acad. Sci. U.S.A.* **86,** 4659.
Ignotz, R. A., Heino, J., and Massague, J. (1989). *J. Biol. Chem.* **264,** 389.

Iguchi, T., and Ziff, M. (1986). *J. Clin. Invest.* **77,** 355.
Issekutz, T. B. (1990). *J. Immunol.* **144,** 2140.
Issekutz, T. B., Stoltz, J. M., and van der Meide, P. (1988). *Clin. Exp. Immunol.* **73,** 70.
Jalkanen, S., Bargatze, R. F., de los Toyos, J., and Butcher, E. C. (1987). *J. Cell Biol.* **105,** 983.
Kabel, P. J., Voorbij, H. A. M., de Haan-Meulman, M., Pals, S. T., and Drexhage, H. A. (1989). *J. Clin. Endocrinol. Metab.* **68,** 744.
Kansas, G. S., Wood, G. S., and Dailey, M. O. (1989). *J. Immunol.* **142,** 3050.
Kaplan, G., Nusrat, A., Sarno, E. N., Job, C. K., McElrath, J., Porto, J. A., Nathan, C. F., and Cohn, Z. A. (1987). *Am. J. Pathol.* **128,** 345.
Keller, R., Pratt, B. M., Furthmayr, H., and Madri, J. A. (1987). *Am. J. Pathol.* **128,** 299.
Kishimoto, T. K., Larson, R. S., Corbi, A. L., Dustin, M. L., Staunton, D. E., and Springer, T. A. (1989). *Adv. Immunol.* **46,** 149.
Klein, L. M., Lavker, R. M., Matis, W. L., and Murphy, G. F. (1989). *Proc. Natl. Acad. Sci. U.S.A.* **86,** 8972.
Knapp, W., Rieber, P., Dorken, B., Schmidt, R. E., Stein, H., and von dem Borne, A. E. G. K. (1989). *Immunol. Today* **10,** 253.
Koch, A. E., Polverini, P. J., and Leibovich, S. J. (1986). *J. Leuk. Biol.* **39,** 233.
Koh, C.-S., and Paterson, P. Y. (1987). *Cell. Immunol.* **107,** 52.
Kurt-Jones, E. A., Fiers, W., and Pober, J. S. (1987). *J. Immunol.* **139,** 2317.
Lamas, A. M., Mulroney, C. M., and Schleimer, R. P. (1988). *J. Immunol.* **140,** 1500.
LaPierre, L. A., Fiers, W., and Pober, J. S. (1988). *J. Exp. Med.* **167,** 794.
Larsen, C. G., Anderson, A. O., Appella, E., Oppenheim, J. J., and Matsushima, K. (1989). *Science* **243,** 1464.
Lasky, L. A., Singer, M. S., Yednock, T. A., Dowbenko, D., Fennie, C., Rodriquez, H., Nguyen, T., Stachel, S., and Rosen, S. D. (1989). *Cell* **56,** 1045.
Leeuwenberg, J. F. M., Van Damme, J., Jeunhomme, G. M. A. A., and Buurman, W. A. (1987). *J. Exp. Med.* **166,** 1180.
Leeuwenberg, J. F. M., Van Damme, J., Jeunhomme, T. M. A. A., and Buurman, W. A. (1988). *Eur. J. Immunol.* **18,** 1469.
Leibovich, S. J., Polverini, P. J., Shepard, H. M., Wiseman, D. M., Shively, V., and Nuseir, N. (1987). *Nature (London)* **329,** 630.
Leszczynski, D. (1990). *Am. J. Pathol.* **136,** 229.
Leszczynski, D., Ferry, B., Schellekens, H., Meide, P. H. V. D., and Häyry, P. (1986). *J. Exp. Med.* **164,** 1470.
Leung, D. Y. M., Collins, T., LaPierre, L. A., Geha, R. S., and Pober, J. S. (1986a). *J. Clin. Invest.* **77,** 1428.
Leung, D. Y. M., Geha, R. S., Newburger, J. W., Burns, J. C., Fiers, W., LaPierre, L. A., and Pober, J. S. (1986b). *J. Exp. Med.* **164,** 1958.
Levine, J. D., Harlan, J. M., Harker, L. A., Joseph, M. L., and Counts, R. B. (1982). *Blood* **60,** 531.
Lewis, R. E., Buchsbaum, M., Whitaker, D., and Murphy, G. F. (1989). *J. Invest. Dermatol.* **93,** 672.
Libby, P., Ordovas, J. M., Auger, K. R., Robbins, A. H., Birinyi, L. K., and Dinarello, C. A. (1986). *Am. J. Pathol.* **124,** 179.
Locksley, R. M., Heinzel, F. P., Shepard, H. M., Agosti, J., Eessalu, T. E., Aggarwal, B. B., and Harlan, J. M. (1987). *J. Immunol.* **139,** 1891.
Lyberg, T., Galdal, K. S., Evensen, S. A., and Prydz, H. (1983). *Br. J. Haematol.* **53,** 85.
Madri, J. A., Pratt, B. M., and Tucker, A. M. (1988). *J. Cell Biol.* **106,** 1375.
Male, D., and Pryce, G. (1988). *Immunology* **63,** 37.
Marchesi, V. T., and Gowans, J. L. (1964). *Proc. R. Soc. London, Ser. B* **159,** 283.
Marcum, J. A., and Rosenberg, R. D. (1984). *Biochemistry* **23,** 1730.
Martin, B. M., Gimbrone, M. A., Jr., Unanue, E. R., and Cotran, R. S. (1981). *J. Immunol.* **126,** 1510.

Martin, S., Maruta, K., Burkart, V., Gillis, S., and Kolb, H. (1988). *Immunology* **64,** 301.
Maruyama, I., Bell, C. I., and Majerus, P. W. (1985). *J. Cell Biol.* **101,** 363.
Masuyama, J.-I., Minato, N., and Kano, S. (1986). *J. Clin. Invest.* **77,** 1596.
Matis, W. L., Lavker, R. M., and Murphy, G. F. (1990). *J. Invest. Dermatol.* **94,** 492.
Matsubara, T., and Ziff, M. (1987). *Arthritis Rheum.* **30,** 18.
Matsushima, K., and Oppenheim, J. J. (1989). *Cytokine* **1,** 2.
Matsushima, K., Morishita, K., Yoshimura, T., Lavu, S., Kobayashi, Y., Lew, W., Appella, E., Kung, H., Leonard, E. J., and Oppenheim, J. J. (1988). *J. Exp. Med.* **167,** 1883.
May, L. T., Torcia, G., Cozzolino, F., Ray, A., Tatter, S. B., Santhanam, U., Sehgal, P. B., and Stern, D. (1989). *Biochem. Biophys. Res. Commun.* **159,** 991.
McCarron, R. M., Spatz, M., Kempski, O., Hogan, R. N., Muehl, L., and McFarlin, D. E. (1986). *J. Immunol.* **137,** 3428.
Mentzer, S. J., Burakoff, S. J., and Faller, D. V. (1986). *J. Cell Physiol.* **126,** 285.
Mentzer, S. J., Crimmins, M. A. V., Burakoff, S. J., and Faller, D. V. (1987). *J. Cell Physiol.* **130,** 410.
Messadi, D. V., Pober, J. S., and Murphy, G. F. (1988). *Lab. Invest.* **58,** 61.
Miossec, P., Yu, C.-L., and Ziff, M. (1984). *J. Immunol.* **133,** 2007.
Miossec, P., Cavender, D., and Ziff, M. (1986). *J. Immunol.* **136,** 2486.
Miossec, P., Cavender, D., and Ziff, M. (1988). *Clin. Exp. Immunol.* **73,** 250.
Modlin, R. L., Melancon-Kaplan, J., Young, S. M. M., Pirmez, C., Kino, H., Convit, J., Rea, T. H., and Bloom, B. R. (1988). *Proc. Natl. Acad. Sci. U.S.A.* **85,** 1213.
Montesano, R., Mossaz, A., Ryser, J.-E., Orci, L., and Vassalli, P. (1984). *J. Cell Biol.* **99,** 1706.
Montesano, R., Orci, L., and Vassalli, P. (1985). *J. Cell Physiol.* **122,** 424.
Moore, K. L., Esmon, C. T., and Esmon, N. L. (1989). *Blood* **73,** 159.
Morimoto, C., Romain, P. L., Fox, D. A., Anderson, P., DiMaggio, M., Levine, H., and Schlossman, S. F. (1988). *Am. J. Med.* **84,** 817.
Mountz, J. D., Gause, W. C., Finkelman, F. D., and Steinburg, A. D. (1988). *J. Immunol.* **140,** 2943.
Muller, G., Behrens, J., Nussbaumer, U., Bohlen, P., and Birchmeier, W. (1987). *Proc. Natl. Acad. Sci. U.S.A.* **84,** 5600.
Munro, J. M., Pober, J. S., and Cotran, R. S. (1989). *Am. J. Pathol.* **135,** 121.
Nachman, R. L., Hajjar, K. A., Silverstein, R. L., and Dinarello, C. A. (1986). *J. Exp. Med.* **163,** 1595.
Nawroth, P. P. and Stern, D. M. (1986). *J. Exp. Med.* **163,** 740.
Nawroth, P. P., Bank, I. Handley, D., Cassimeris, J., Chess, L., and Stern, D. (1986a). *J. Exp. Med.* **163,** 1363.
Nawroth, P. P., Handley, D. A., Esmon, C. T., and Stern, D. M. (1989b). *Proc. Natl. Acad. Sci. U.S.A.* **83,** 3460.
Neale, T. J., Carson, S. D., Tipping, P. G., and Holdsworth, S. R. (1988). *Lancet* **2,** 421.
Nightingale, G., and Hurley, J. V. (1978). *Pathology* **10,** 27.
Norioka, K., Hara, M., Kitani, A., Hirose, T., Hirose, W., Harigai, M., Suzuki, K., Kawakami, M., Tabata, H., Kawagoa, M., and Nakamura, H. (1987). *Biochem. Biophys. Res. Commun.* **145,** 969.
Oppenheimer-Marks, N., and Ziff, M. (1988). *Cell. Immunol.* **114,** 307.
Osborn, L., Hession, C., Tizard, R., Vassallo, C., Luhowskyj, S., Chi-Rosso, G., and Lobb, R. (1989). *Cell* **59,** 1203.
Pals, S. T., den Otter, A., Miedema, F., Kabel, P., Keizer, G. D., Scheper, R. J., and Meijer, C. J. L. M. (1988). *J. Immunol.* **140,** 1851.
Pals, S. T., Hogervorst, F., Keizer, G. D., Thepen, T., Horst, E., and Figdor, C. C. (1989). *J. Immunol.* **143,** 851.
Parrott, D. M. V., de Sousa, M. A. B., and East, J. (1966). *J. Exp. Med.* **123,** 191.
Picker, L. J., de los Toyos, J., Telen, M. J., Haynes, B. F., and Butcher, E. C. (1989). *J. Immunol.* **142,** 2046.

Pitzalis, C., Kingsley, G., Haskard, D., and Panayi, G. (1988). *Eur. J. Immunol.* **18,** 1397.
Pober, J. S., Collin, T., Gimbrone, M. A., Jr., Cotran, R. S., Gitlin, J. D., Fiers, W., Clayberger, C., Krensky, A. M., Burakoff, S. J., and Reiss, C. S. (1983a). *Nature (London)* **305,** 726.
Pober, J. S., Gimbrone, M. A., Jr., Cotran, R. S., Reiss, C. S., Burakoff, S. J., Fiers, W., and Ault, K. A. (1983b). *J. Exp. Med.* **157,** 1339.
Polverini, P. J., Cotran, R. S., Gimbrone, M. A., Jr., and Unanue, E. R. (1977a). *Nature (London)* **269,** 804.
Polverini, P. J., Cotran, R. S., and Sholley, M. M. (1977b). *J. Immunol.* **118,** 529.
Prieto, J., Beatty, P. G., Clark, E. A., and Patarroyo, M. (1988). *Immunology* **63,** 631.
Pryce, G., Male, D., and Sedgwick, J. (1989). *Immunology* **66,** 207.
Rasmussen, R. A., Chin, Y.-H., Woodruff, J. J., and Easton, T. G. (1985). *J. Immunol.* **135,** 19.
Rice, G. E., and Bevilacqua, M. P. (1989). *Science* **246,** 1303.
Rice, G. E., Munro, J. M., and Bevilacqua, M. P. (1990). *J. Exp. Med.* **171,** 1369.
Roberts, A. B., Sporn, M. B., Assoian, R. K., Smith, J. M., Roche, N. S., Wakefield, L. M., Heine, U. I., Liotta, L. A., Falanga, V., Kehrl, J. H., and Fauci, A. S. (1986). *Proc. Natl. Acad. Sci. U.S.A.* **83,** 4167.
Rosen, S. D., and Yednock, T. A. (1986). *Mol. Cell Biochem.* **72,** 153.
Rosen, S. D., Singer, M. S., Yednock, T. A., and Stoolman, L. M. (1985). *Science* **228,** 1005.
Rosenbaum, J. T., Howes, E. L., Jr., Rubin, R. M., and Samples, J. R. (1988). *Am. J. Pathol.* **133,** 47.
Roska, A. K., Johnson, A. R., and Lipsky, P. E. (1984). *J. Immunol.* **132,** 136.
Rossi, V., Breviario, F., Ghezzi, P., Dejana, E., and Mantovani, A. (1985). *Science* **229,** 174.
Rothlein, R., Dustin, M. L. Marlin, S. D., and Springer, T. A. (1986). *J. Immunol.* **137,** 1270.
Ruoslahti, E., and Pierschbacher, M. D. (1987). *Science* **238,** 491.
Ryan, U. S. (1986). *Fed. Proc., Fed. Am. Soc. Exp. Biol.* **45,** 101.
Ryan, J., and Geczy, C. (1987). *Immunol. Cell Biol.* **65,** 127.
Sackstein, R., Falanga, V., Streilein, J. W., and Chin, Y.-H. (1988). *J. Invest. Dermatol.* **91,** 423.
Saegusa, Y., Cavender, D., and Ziff, M. (1988). *J. Immunol.* **141,** 4140.
Saegusa, Y., Ziff, M., Welkovich, L., and Cavender, D. (1990). *J. Cell Physiol.* **142,** 488.
Sanders, M. E., Makgoba, M. W., Sharrow, S. O. Stephany, D., Springer, T. A., Young, H. A., and Shaw, S. (1988a). *J. Immunol.* **140,** 1401.
Sanders, M. E., Makgoba, M. W., and Shaw, S. (1988b). *Immunol. Today* **9,** 195.
Sato, N., Goto, T., Haranaka, K., Satomi, N., Nariuchi, H., Mano-Hirano, Y., and Sawasaki, Y. (1986). *JNCI, J. Natl. Cancer Inst.* **76,** 1113.
Schleef, R. R., Bevilacqua, M. P., Sawdey, M., Gimbrone, M. A., Jr., and Loskutoff, D. J. (1988). *J. Biol. Chem.* **263,** 5797.
Schleimer, R. P., and Rutledge, B. K. (1986). *J. Immunol.* **136,** 649.
Schorer, A. E., Moldow, C. F., and Rick, M. E. (1987). *Br. J. Haematol.* **67,** 193.
Sidky, Y. A., and Auerbach, R. (1975). *J. Exp. Med.* **141,** 1084.
Siegelman, M. H., Van de Rijn, M., and Weissman, I. L. (1989). *Science* **243,** 1165.
Siegelman, M. H., and Weissman, I. L. (1989). *Proc. Natl. Acad. Sci. U.S.A.* **86,** 5562.
Sironi, M., Breviario, F., Proserpio, P., Biondi, A., Vecchi, A., Van Damme, J., Dejana, E., and Mantovani, A. (1989). *J. Immunol.* **142,** 549.
Sobel, R. A., Blanchette, B. W., Bhan, A. K., and Colvin, R. B. (1984). *J. Immunol.* **132,** 2402.
Stamenkovic, I., Amiot, M., Pesando, J. M., and Seed, B. (1989). *Cell* **56,** 1057.
Stamper, H. B., Jr., and Woodruff, J. J. (1976). *J. Exp. Med.* **144,** 828.
Staunton, D.E., Dustin, M. L., and Springer, T. A. (1989). *Nature (London)* **339,** 61.
Stern, D. M., Bank, I., Nawroth, P. P., Cassimeris, J., Kisiel, W., Fenton, J. W., II, Dinarello, C., Chess, L., and Jaffe, E. (1985). *J. Exp. Med.* **162,** 1223.
Stern, D. M., Kaiser, E., and Nawroth, P. P. (1988). *Haemostasis* **18,** 202.
Stolpen, A. H., Guinan, E. C., Fiers, W., and Pober, J. S. (1986). *Am. J. Pathol.* **123,** 16.

Stoolman, L. M. (1989). *Cell* **56,** 907.
Stoolman, L. M., Tenforde, T. S., and Rosen, S. D. (1984). *J. Cell Biol.* **99,** 1535.
Streeter, P. R., Berg, E. L., Rouse, B. T. N., Bargatze, R. F., and Butcher, E. C. (1988). *Nature (London)* **331,** 41.
Streiter, R. M., Kunkel, S. L., Showell, H. J., Remick, D. G., Phan, S. H., Ward, P. A., and Marks, R. M. (1989). *Science* **243,** 1467.
Tannebaum, S. H., Finko, R., and Cines, D. B. (1986). *J. Immunol.* **137,** 1532.
Tedder, T. F., Isaacs, C. M., Ernst, T. J., Demetri, G. D., and Adler, D. A. (1989). *J. Exp. Med.* **170,** 123.
TeVelde, A. A., Keizer, G. D., and Figdor, C. G. (1987). *Immunology* **61,** 261.
Thornhill, M. H., Williams, D. M., and Speight, P. M. (1989). *Br. J. Exp. Pathology* **70,** 59.
Thornhill, M. H., Kyan-Aung, U., and Haskard, D. O. (1990a). *J. Immunol.* **144,** 3060.
Thornhill, M. H., Kyan-Aung, U., Lee, T. H., and Haskard, D. O. (1990b). *Immunology* **69,** 287.
Traugott, U., Scheinberg, L. C., and Raine, C. S. (1985). *J. Neuroimmunol.* **8,** 1.
van Hinsbergh, V. W. M., Sprengers, E. D., and Kooistra, T. (1987). *Thromb. Haemostasis* **57,** 148.
van Hinsbergh, V. W. M., Kooistra, T., van den Berg, E. A., Princen, H. M. G., Fiers, W., and Emeis, J. J. (1988). *Blood* **72,** 1467.
Vass, K., Lassmann, H., Wisniewski, H. M., and Iqbal, K. (1984). *J. Neurol. Sci.* **63,** 423.
Wagner, C. R., Vetto, R. M., and Burger, D. R. (1985). *Cell Immunol.* **93,** 91.
Wahl, S. M., Hunt, D. A., Wakefield, L. M., McCartney-Francis, N., Wahl, L. M., Roberts, A. B., and Sporn, M. B. (1987). *Proc. Natl. Acad. Sci. U.S.A.* **84,** 5788.
Wallis, W. J., Beatty, P. G., Ochs, H. D., and Harlan, J. M. (1985). *J. Immunol.* **135,** 2323.
Wang, J. M., Colella, S., Allavena, P., and Mantovani, A. (1987). *Immunology* **60,** 439.
Watt, S. L., and Auerbach, R. (1986). *J. Immunol.* **136,** 197.
Wayner, E. A., Garcia-Pardo, A., Humphries, M. J., McDonald, J. A., and Carter, W. G. (1989). *J. Cell Biol.* **109,** 1321.
Wenk, E. J., Orlic, D., Reith, E. J., and Rhodin, J. A. G. (1974). *J. Ultrastruct. Res.* **47,** 214.
Wheeler, M. E., Luscinskas, F. W., Bevilacqua, M. P., and Gimbrone, M. A., Jr. (1988). *J. Clin. Invest.* **82,** 1211.
Wilcox, C. E., Healey, D. G., Baker, D., Willoughby, D. A., and Turk, J. L. (1989). *Immunology* **67,** 435.
Wolpe, S. D., and Cerami, A. (1989). *FASEB J.* **3,** 2565.
Woodruff, J. J., Clarke, L. M., and Chin, Y.-H. (1987). *Annu. Rev. Immunol.* **5,** 201.
Wright, S. D., Craigmyle, L. S., and Silverstein, S. C. (1983). *J. Exp. Med.* **158,** 1338.
Yednock, T. A., Butcher, E. C., Stoolman, L. M., and Rosen, S. D. (1987). *J. Cell Biol.* **104,** 725.
Yu, C.-L., Haskard, D. O., Cavender, D., Johnson, A. R., and Ziff, M. (1985). *Clin. Exp. Immunol.* **62,** 554.
Yu, C.-L., Haskard, D., Cavender, D., and Ziff, M. (1986). *J. Immunol.* **136,** 569.
Zielasek, J., Burkart, V., Naylor, P., Goldstein, A., Kiesel, U., and Kolb, H. (1990). *Immunology* **69,** 209.

Molecular Biology of Cytokine Effects on Vascular Endothelial Cells

HIROSHI SUZUKI and HEIHACHIRO KASHIWAGI

Department of Rheumatology, Institute of Clinical Medicine, University of Tsukuba, Ibaraki-ken 305, Japan

I. Introduction

II. Molecular Basis of Cytokine Responsiveness of Vascular Endothelial Cells
   A. Interleukin 1
   B. Tumor Necrosis Factor
   C. Interferon-γ
   D. Transforming Growth Factor β

III. Regulation and Induction of Endothelial Gene Expression by Cytokines
   A. Genes Related to Blood Coagulation and Fibrinolysis
   B. Genes of Leukocyte Adhesion Molecules
   C. Major Histocompatibility Antigen Complex
   D. Production of Cytokines
   E. Protooncogene Expression
   F. Endothelin

IV. Endothelial Gene Expression in *in Vivo* and *in Situ* Hybridization

V. Future Directions of Research
   References

I. Introduction

Vascular endothelial cells constitute the luminal surface of the vascular system and play an active role in normal hemostasis and in various pathophysiological responses, such as inflammation, wound healing, selective transfer of substances to and from the circulation, and regulation of vascular tonus. Positioned at the interface between circulating blood and the subendothelial vascular structures, endothelial cells (ECs) mediate the effects of products and signals released from ECs to the vascular wall. For these reasons, functional and structural abnormalities of ECs may contribute significantly to vascular pathology such as thrombosis, atherosclerosis, and vasculitis.

The demonstration that hemostasis, inflammation, and immunity involve close interactions between immunocompetent cells and vascular ECs has marked an important advance in understanding the role of ECs. Cytokines, produced by and acting on ECs, are mediators of the complex bidirectional interactions between immunocompetent cells and ECs. Cytokines affect EC function in inflammation, thrombosis, angiogenesis, and immune responses.

Cytokines are the biologically potent polypeptides with molecular weights of up to 30,000; they are produced by a variety of cells and act on many different cell types. Interleukins IL-1α, IL-1β, and IL-2 through IL-8 are important members of the cytokine family. No less important than ILs in the study of EC functions are tumor necrosis factors TNF-α and TNF-β (lymphotoxin), interferons (IFNs), transforming growth factors TGF-α and TGF-β, and platelet-derived growth factor (PDGF).

Common features of these cytokines are that minute quantities are enough to bring about biological effects that include the regulation of cell proliferation and differentiation, the stimulation of new protein synthesis, and the induction of the production of inflammatory metabolites. In addition, various inhibitors of cytokines in body fluids have been reported. Because of these features, cytokines are considered to be primarily active only within short ranges of distances, such as in cell–cell interactions. From this point of view, vascular ECs at the sites of, or in close proximity to, inflammatory or immune responses may be regarded as the direct targets of cytokines. In addition, several cytokines (IL-1, IL-6, IFN-α, and IFN-γ) have been demonstrated to be increased in the circulating blood of hosts with inflammatory diseases. These cytokines may affect EC functions at sites distant from inflammatory lesions. In contrast to the wealth of knowledge gained by a number of studies revealing the effects of various cytokines on vascular ECs *in vitro*, the roles of cytokines in the functions of vascular endothelium *in vivo* have been incompletely understood.

Methodological improvements for culturing ECs *in vitro* have enabled us to study the effects of cytokines on vascular ECs *in vitro* at the molecular level. Compared with bovine and porcine aortic ECs, which can be propagated in a long-term culture with relative ease, human ECs demand more fastidious growth conditions. With the use of heparin and endothelial cell growth factor (ECGF) as growth supplements, a long-term serial cultivation of human umbilical vein ECs has become possible for investigative purposes (Thornton *et al.*, 1983). Techniques of isolation and cultivation of capillary ECs have been also established (Folkman *et al.*, 1979). With these techniques, the functions of ECs induced by cytokines *in vitro* have been studied by a number of investigators and our understanding of endothelial functions has rapidly progressed.

To date, a number of cytokines have been cloned molecularly and their primary amino acids sequences have been determined. Using purified or recombinant materials, some cytokines have been demonstrated to share certain biological activities on ECs in spite of their binding to different receptors. IL-1 and TNF stimulate the synthesis of the same molecules (e.g., tissue factor, IL-1, and IL-6) and induce similar functions, such as the adherence of ECs to neutrophils. Among several cytokines, synergistic or antagonistic effects on ECs have also been found with purified and recombinant materials. Several, but not all, cytokines have been demonstrated to affect EC functions. In this article we review recent findings relative to the multiplex effects of various cytokines on the vascular endothelium in terms of molecular biology.

II. Molecular Basis of Cytokine Responsiveness of Vascular Endothelial Cells

Several cytokines have been demonstrated to affect EC functions. Each cytokine binds to its specific receptor and appears to use distinct intracellular signaling pathways. Several cytokine receptors have been purified and cloned, but details of signal transduction pathways evoked by binding of the cytokine to its receptor have been incompletely understood. In spite of clear differences of the receptor and the postreceptor events evoked by each cytokine, some of these cytokines induce similar or overlapping effects on vascular ECs. Though most of the past studies on cytokine receptors and signal transduction pathways have dealt with lymphocytes or fibroblasts or cell lines, ECs are increasingly used today for the same purposes because common receptor systems are thought to be operative in these cells.

A. INTERLEUKIN 1

A variety of effects of IL-1 on vascular ECs indicate the presence of IL-1 receptors on their surface. Thieme *et al.* (1987), in their study of the binding of radiolabeled human recombinant IL-1 and murine recombinant IL-1α to human umbilical vein ECs, demonstrated a binding constant of $7 \times 10^{10}\ M^{-1}$ and approximately 630 sites per cell for human IL-1α by Scatchard analysis. Almost the same affinity and receptor molecules on ECs were observed for murine IL-1. In spite of equal affinity of human and murine IL-1α for receptors on human ECs, the human IL-1α was 1000-fold more active than the murine IL-1α in increasing endothelial adherence to lymphocytes. There was no difference in IL-1 activity in human and murine IL-1α assayed by murine thymocyte proliferation, thus Thieme *et al.* (1987) questioned whether IL-1 receptors on ECs were identical with those on other cell types because of their ability to respond differently to human and murine IL-1. More recently, however, the same group (Thieme and Wagner, 1988) has isolated IL-1 receptor molecules from human umbilical vein ECs by immunoprecipitation and chemical cross-linking to the ligand, and found that the molecular weight of the human endothelial IL-1 receptor was 78,000, a value not different from that of the IL-1 receptor on human lung fibroblasts and a human T cell line. Several groups have already reported almost identical molecular weights of IL-1 receptors on human fibroblasts (Chin *et al.*, 1987) and murine T cells and fibroblasts (Dower *et al.*, 1986).

In contrast, the molecular weights of IL-1 receptors on human B cell lines (Matsushima *et al.*, 1986; Horuk *et al.*, 1987) and a murine B lymphoid cell line, 70Z/3 (Bomsztyk *et al.*, 1989), have been reported to be significantly smaller (i.e., 60,000–68,000). Bomsztyk *et al.* (1989) have investigated the IL-1 receptors on the 70Z/3 B lymphoid cell line and those on a T lymphoid cell line, EL-4 6.1 C10, to explore possible differences at the molecular level. They found that a monoclonal antibody against the IL-1 receptor on EL-4 cells does not bind to the IL-1 receptor on 70Z/3 cells. Affinity cross-linking studies showed that the molecular mass of the IL-1 receptors on EL-4 cells in significantly higher than that of the receptors on 70Z/3 cells. Furthermore, different effects of a phorbol ester, phorbol myristate acetate (PMA), on the expression and phosphorylation of the two kinds of IL-1 receptor molecules suggested that the cytoplasmic domains of the IL-1 receptor molecules of 70Z/3 and EL-4 cell lines might be also different. Finally, a probe containing the entire coding region of the murine T cell IL-1 receptor gene was shown to hybridize with mRNA from EL-4 cells, but not with mRNA from 70Z/3 cells under highly stringent conditions. These results led the authors to conclude that major structural differences exist among the IL-1 receptors on B and T lymphocytes.

Chizzonite *et al.* (1989) have also examined the difference in the two classes of IL-1 receptors at the molecular level. Equilibrium binding studies have demonstrated a class of IL-1 receptors on T cells, fibroblasts, and epithelial cells that have two- to five-fold higher affinity than do the receptors on bone marrow cells, pre-B cells, and macrophage cell lines. A difference in molecular weights of the two IL-1 receptors has also been observed. Hybridization studies of mRNA to a full-length cDNA probe of mouse EL-4 IL-1 receptor gene demonstrated that mouse T cells, fibroblasts, and epithelial cells expressed an identical IL-1 receptor, whereas the IL-1 receptor on pre-B cells, macrophages, and bone marrow cells was found to be a different gene product. It seems now generally accepted that IL-1 receptors on human ECs are the same at those on T cells and fibroblasts, as suggested by the results of the studies on molecular weight and affinity (Thieme et al., 1987; Thieme and Wagner, 1988).

Mouse and human IL-1 receptor genes of the T cell type have been cloned (Sims et al., 1988, 1989). The human and murine receptors are very similar molecules, both containing an extracellular segment of three immunoglobulin light-chain domains, a transmembrane region, and a cytoplasmic portion of approximately 215 amino acids. The IL-1 receptor is glycosylated on asparagine residues, and the removal of the carbohydrate with N-glycanase decreases the size of the receptor on murine T cells from 80 to 62 kDa (Urdal et al., 1988), close to the 64,598 Da predicted from the cDNA sequence of murine T cell IL-1 receptors.

The recombinant murine IL-1 receptor expressed in COS cells after transfection possesses IL-1 binding characteristics and signal transduction properties similar to those of native receptors (Sims et al., 1988). In addition, a secreted, soluble form of the IL-1 receptor, containing only the extracellular part of the molecule, binds IL-1 with an affinity identical to the native receptor on EL-4 cells, indicating that this is the only molecule involed in IL-1 binding in these cells (Dower et al., 1989). Therefore, this IL-1 receptor molecule appears to be functionally complete without association of other molecules in IL-1 binding and in signal transduction. However, several groups have shown data supporting the possibility that the IL-1 receptor has a second chain (Bird et al., 1987; Kroggel et al., 1988), similar to the situation with the IL-2 receptor, which has two components, the so-called TAC 55-kDa antigen and a higher affinity polypeptide chain of 75 kDa. The function and structure of the second receptor chain of the IL-1 receptor remain to be determined.

Biochemical and molecular events following the binding of IL-1 to the receptor have been studied only recently. A few groups of investigators have used vascular ECs to study signal transduction pathways of IL-1. Magnuson et al. (1989) assessed the effects of two protein kinase inhibitors, H-7 and HA-1004, on EC adherence to neutrophils induced by 3 hours of stimulation with IL-1, TNF, and lipopolysaccharide (LPS). Both H-7 and HA-1004 inhibited a similar spectrum of protein kinases, and H-7 was an effective inhibitor of protein kinase C but HA-1004 was not. H-7 markedly inhibited the adherence of neutrophils to IL-1-, TNF-, and LPS-stimulated human umbilical vein ECs. In contrast, HA-1004 did not inhibit EC adherence. Based on these results, these investigators suggested that protein kinase C could be an essential component common to EC activation by IL-1, TNF, and LPS.

Likewise, Goldgaber et al. (1989), in their study of the regulation of amyloid β-protein precursor mRNA expression in human ECs, reported inhibition of an IL-1-mediated increase of amyloid β-protein precursor mRNA levels by H-7. They also showed data indicating that the induction of this gene in ECs by IL-1 utilizes the upstream AP-1-binding site of the gene promoter.

Because IL-1 induces c-*jun* gene transcript in human ECs (Dixit *et al.*, 1989) and c-*jun* gene products may function as an AP-1 transcription factor, it may be a crucial question whether H-7 blocks the induction of c-*jun* expression in ECs by IL-1. Summarizing these results, these investigators have postulated that IL-1 up-regulates amyloid β-protein precursor gene expression through a pathway mediated by protein kinase C. These studies also suggest the participation of protein kinase C in some endothelial functions induced by IL-1 or TNF. Because H-7 is relatively nonspecific as a protein kinase C inhibitor, more direct evidence may be necessary to establish the participation of protein kinase C in endothelial activation by IL-1 or TNF. However, proof of participation of protein kinase C in some IL-1-induced EC functions does not necessarily mean that IL-1 directly activates protein kinase C. Activation of protein kinase C by IL-1 is questionable at least in other cell systems.

It is well known that mitogens and growth factors stimulate the production of diacylglycerol and increase intracytoplasmic calcium in resting cells. These two second messengers are considered to arise from enhanced phosphatidylinositol turnover. Whereas the release of diacylglycerol during phosphatidylinositol, 4,5-biphosphate hydrolysis has been shown to mediate the activation of protein kinase C (Berridge, 1987), IL-1 does not cause translocation or activation of protein kinase C, nor does it cause an increase in levels of intracellular calcium or generation of inositol triphosphate in IL-1-induced activation of T cells and other cells (Abraham *et al.*, 1987; Rosoff *et al.*, 1988; Kester *et al.*, 1989; Matsushima *et al.*, 1987). Rosoff *et al.* (1988) have shown that IL-1 stimulates rapid diacylglycerol and phosphorylcholine production from phosphatidylcholine in the absence of phosphatidylinositol turnover in a human T cell leukemia cell line and other T cell sources. The hydrolysis of phosphatidylcholine occurs at very low concentrations of IL-1, reaching maximal levels at 10^{-13} M. A similar IL-1-induced phosphatidylcholine turnover was found in the D10.G4.1 T helper cell line, the EL-4 cell line, and human peripheral T cells.

Protein kinase C exists as a family of isozymes, at least seven of which are now well characterized (Nishizuka, 1988). Dinarello (1989) has proposed the hypothesis that a mitogen that stimulates diacylglycerols through phosphatidylinositol turnover results in activation of one type of protein kinase C, whereas IL-1, which stimulates the production of phosphatidylcholine-specific diacylglycerols through phosphatidylcholine turnover, activates another isoenzyme. Several other signal transduction pathways for IL-1 have been reported. IL-1 stimulates the production of cAMP in a variety of cell types, including lymphocytes and fibroblasts (Shirakawa *et al.*, 1988). Chedid *et al.* (1989) have observed that IL-1 activates adenyl cyclase through the involvement of a pertussis toxin-sensitive GTP-binding protein, resulting in increased intracellular levels of cAMP. IL-1, in addition, induces the phosphorylation of a cytosolic 65-kDa protein in human peripheral blood mononuclear cells (Matsushima et al., 1987) and the phosphorylation of the IL-1 receptor molecules on murine T cells (Gallis et al., 1989). The relation of each signaling pathway to individual cellular functions is still obscure, but it is possible that different functions may be mediated by different signal transduction pathways. Whether similar phenomena may be observed in human vascular ECs remains to be determined.

B. Tumor Necrosis Factor

Vascular ECs express high-affinity receptors for TNF-α on their surface. Nawroth et al. (1986) first reported the presence of saturable and high-affinity binding sites for TNF-α on human umbilical vein ECs. They observed that the affinity of ^{125}I-labeled TNF for the EC surface (105 pM) was similar to the affinity of the ligand previously reported by Baglioni et al. (1985) and by Tsujimoto et al. (1985) for other cell surfaces with specific binding sites (100–300 pM). The expression of the receptors for TNF appears to be up-regulated by IFN-γ. An increase in the number of TNF receptors, with no demonstrable change in binding affinity, has been reported in several cell lines (Tsujimoto et al., 1986). The up-regulation of TNF receptors by IFN-γ may explain synergistic effects observed among these cytokines on vascular ECs. Another cytokine, epidermal growth factor (EGF), also increases the expression of TNF receptors. Mawatari et al. (1989) have observed that morphologic changes of human microvascular ECs induced by simultaneous addition of TNF-α and EGF into cell cultures are more dramatic than those induced by TNF-α alone. They reported that the number of TNF receptors increased about threefold and the affinity also increased twofold when microvascular ECs were treated with EGF for 24 hours. Enhanced expression of TNF receptors may reflect a synergistic effect of EGF and TNF on the morphologic changes of these microvascular ECs.

The affinity of receptors for TNF on vascular ECs appears to change according to culture conditions. Gerlach et al. (1989) have observed that bovine aortic ECs cultured in a growing state display an extended, motile form and express high-affinity receptors for TNF, with a K_d of approximately 0.1 nM, whereas only lower affinity sites (K_d of approximately 1.8 nM) are detected on postconfluent cultures. To elucidate the mechanisms underlying the change in the affinity of ECs for TNF, these investigators carried out crosslinking experiments with ^{125}I-labeled TNF. Though they could demonstrate new polypeptide chains of approximately 66 and 84 kDa with subconfluent cultures, they were unable to detect the two polypeptides with postconfluent cultures. The absence of these polypeptides with postconfluent cultures suggests that subconfluent cells express new polypeptides on the cell surface, with which TNF becomes associated. Results of *in vitro* wounding study, in which a late postconfluent monolayer was wounded by physically removing a section of the culture, then was allowed to recover for 36 hours, with subsequent exposure to TNF, demonstrated that enhanced binding and responsiveness to TNF were associated with the proliferating and/or motile cells. These results support the concept that local stimulation of endothelial growth and/or motility *in vivo* should result in expression of high-affinity TNF receptors and targeting of the effects of this cytokine to a particular locus in the vasculature.

Several components of TNF receptors on the surface of various cell types have also been detected by cross-linking experiments. Tsujimoto *et al.* (1985) described 95- and 75-kDa polypeptides in a fibroblast (L-M) cell line. Likewise, Kull *et al.* (1985) and Israel *et al.* (1986) confirmed two polypeptides of similar sizes in mouse L929 fibroblasts and in human cells. Creasey *et al.* (1987) have reported that TNF binds mainly to four cellular polypeptides (138, 90, 75, and 54 kDa, respectively), three of which are found in every cell type. In addition, recent studies suggest that there are two different types of TNF receptors that are differentiated by their compositions and structures of polypeptide chains and that these are differentially expressed by cells of different types (Engelmann *et al.*, 1990). Two groups (Loetscher *et al.*, 1990; Schall *et al.*, 1990) recently succeeded in molecular cloning of a human TNF receptor. The predicted sequence of the receptor molecule showed N-terminal homology to one of the two polypeptides reported by Engelmann *et al.* (1990). Molecular structures and the type of the receptor for TNF on ECs have not yet been determined.

C. INTERFERON-γ

Responsiveness to IFN-γ is common to many cells and tissues, indicating that IFN-γ receptors are probably ubiquitous. At the receptor level it is known that IFN-α and IFN-β cross-react with common receptors, whereas IFN-γ mediates its biological effects through its own receptor system. Most binding studies with ^{125}I-labeled INF-γ have suggested only one class of IFN-γ binding site with a K_d of about 10^{-11} to 10^{-10} M (Sarkar and Gupta, 1984; Littman *et al.*, 1985).

A human IFN-γ receptor gene has been cloned (Auget *et al.*, 1988). The cDNA encodes a protein of 489 amino acids with the N-terminal signal peptide (14 amino acids). The deduced amino acid sequence indicates seven potential N-linked glycosylation sites, explaining the discrepancy between the apparent molecular weight of approximately 90,000 for the purified natural receptor protein and the approximately 54 kDa predicted from the cDNA-deduced protein.

Protein kinase C appears to be involved in IFN-γ-induced class II antigen expression in vascular ECs (Mattila *et al.,* 1989). Selective inhibitors of protein kinase C, H-7 as well as sphingosine, inhibited the induction of class II antigen expression by IFN-γ. Involvement of protein kinase C in IFN-γ-induced functions has been demonstrated in other cell systems. Fan *et al.* (1988) have concluded that IFN-γ-induced transcriptional activation of a human macrophage-specific gene, $\gamma.1$, is mediated by protein kinase C based on the following grounds: (1) PMA, a direct activator of protein kinase C, effectively induces $\gamma.1$ expression; (2) intracellular translocation of protein kinase C from cytosol to membrane induced by IFN-γ treatment is an essential step of the enzyme activation; (3) induction of $\gamma.1$ mRNA by IFN-γ is blocked by the inhibitors of protein kinase C. These investigators also observed that the expression of several other genes, including the major histocompatibility complex (MHC) class II genes in human macrophages, was mediated by protein kinase C. Several other reports suggest that IFN-γ enhances the potential activity of protein kinase C (Hamilton *et al.,* 1985; Becton *et al.,* 1985). Activation of protein kinase C may be one of the several signal transduction pathways evoked by IFN-γ in various cells, including ECs (Adams and Hamilton, 1987).

D. Transforming Growth Factor β

TGF-β, originally described by its ability to confer anchorage-independent growth on nonmalignant fibroblasts, is now known to have many different biologic effects on a wide spectrum of target cells, including stimulation and inhibition of cell proliferation and modulation of cellular functions (Massaguè, 1985). TGF-β is a homodimeric polypeptide (25 kDa) that is principally found in platelets and bone; it is synthesized and secreted by a variety of cells. Recent reports describe several functionally and structurally related forms of TGF-β, of which TGF-β1 and TGF-β2 are the most abundant forms (Cheifetz *et al.,* 1987).

Receptors for TGF-β are ubiquitous (Tucker *et al.,* 1984), and three types of receptors have been reported: type I (65 kDa), type II (85–110 kDa), and type III (280–330 kDa) (Massaguè, 1985; Cheifetz *et al.,* 1987; Boyd and Massaguè, 1989). Affinity cross-linking studies with ^{125}I-labeled TGF-β demonstrated high-affinity receptors for TGF-β, consisting of the 280-, 85-, and 72-kDa components, on bovine capillary and fetal heart ECs (Müller *et al.,* 1987). The large receptors (280 kDa) are only observed in subconfluent cultures, whereas the two smaller receptors (85 and 72 kDa) are seen in confluent cultures. Therefore, three types of receptors can be detected on cultured EC surfaces. In addition, the appearance of these receptors seems to be dependent on the confluency of the cells.

Cheifetz et al. (1987) have reported that a 280-kDa receptor displays high affinity for both TGF-β1 and TGF-β2, whereas 65- and 85-kDa receptors have high affinity for TGf-β1 but lower affinity for TGF-β2. Although the 85- and 65-kDa TGF-β receptors are similar to their affinity for both types of TGF-β, these two receptors have distinct structural and kinetic properties (Cheifetz et al., 1986; Massaguè et al., 1986). It has been suggested that these different types of TGF-β receptors may convey different signals to the cells (Cheifetz et al., 1986). However, Boyd and Massaguè (1989) recently proposed the hypothesis that the type I receptor (65 kDa) may be essential for signal transduction on the grounds that the cells that lost this receptor could not respond to TGF-β.

TGF-β exhibits diverse effects on vascular ECs. A prominent effect of TGF-β on ECs is inhibition of *in vitro* angiogenesis at several steps. TGF-β antagonizes the proliferation of both aortic and capillary ECs induced by fibroblast growth factor (Fràter-Schröder et al., 1986; Baird and Durkin, 1986). TGF-β also blocks the locomotion of ECs and prevents tube formation after treatment with PMA (Müller et al., 1987). Molecular events evoked after the binding of TGF-β to the receptors on ECs are poorly understood, however.

III. Regulation and Induction of Endothelial Gene Expression by Cytokines

A. Genes Related to Blood Coagulation and Fibrinolysis

Increasing experimental evidence supports an active role of the vascular ECs in a "hemostatic balance" between procoagulant and anticoagulant activities (Rosenberg and Rosenberg, 1984; Stern et al., 1985a). Perturbation of endothelium may induce procoagulant activity and suppress antifibrinolytic systems, allowing ECs to promote the so-called coagulation cascade leading to the formation of fibrin. Procoagulant properties of ECs are mediated mainly by the surface expression of tissue factor (Colucci et al., 1983) and the synthesis and secretion of tissue plasminogen activator inhibitor 1 (Loskutoff et al., 1983) and von Willebrand factor (Jaffe et al., 1974).

Anticoagulant activities of ECs, on the other hand, are dependent on the synthesis and the secretion of prostacyclin (Moncada et al., 1976) and tissue-type plasminogen activator (Levin and Loskutoff, 1982). ECs also express on their surface heparin-like molecules (Marcum et al., 1984) and thrombomodulin (Esmon and Owen, 1981), the latter being a potent activator of circulating protein C. Under physiological conditions, the anticoagulant properties are dominant on the surface of the endothelium. In some pathological states, however, the balance between the anticoagulant and procoagulant properties of endothelium is disturbed.

For example, the delayed-type hypersensitivity response, in which various inflammatory cytokines have been demonstrated, includes the induction of procoagulant activity (PCA) of vascular endothelium (Edwards and Rickles, 1978). Gram-negative sepsis is frequently associated with disseminated intravascular coagulation (DIC), which is thought to be triggered by endotoxemia. Although originally attributed directly to endotoxin, it is now accepted that most, if not all, of the metabolic derangements, including DIC, evoked by endotoxic shock are mediated by endogenous cytokines, mainly TNF (Sherry and Cerami, 1988). Therefore, inflammatory cytokines may play a central role in the regulation of these endothelial activities.

An increase of tissue-factor-like PCA by IL-1 was first demonstrated by Bevilacqua *et al.* (1984). IL-1-induced PCA was relatively short-lived, being maximal at 4–8 hours after treatment with the cytokine, followed by a gradual decline to pretreatment levels within 24 hours. It was observed that the increase of PCA was inhibited by cycloheximide and actinomycin D, suggesting a requirement for transcription and protein synthesis. It has been also demonstrated that TNF produces similar effects on vascular ECs (Nawroth and Stern, 1986; Bevilacqua *et al.*, 1986a).

Tissue factor cDNA has been recently cloned by two groups (Morrissey *et al.*, 1987; Fisher *et al.*, 1987). Messenger RNA expression of the tissue factor gene was examined in several cell types, including human umbilical vein ECs. A major hybridizing band (2.4 kb) and two more weakly hybridizing bands (3.5 and 3.1 kb) were observed, though the nature of the latter of these two larger bands was not known (Fisher *et al.*, 1987). Boeri *et al.* (1989) have demonstrated that PCA induced by IL-1-stimulated umbilical vein ECs is accompanied by induction of the accumulation of tissue factor mRNA.

Vascular ECs also play an important role in fibrinolysis through synthesis and secretion of tissue plasminogen activator (tPA) and tissue plasminogen activator inhibitor 1 (tPAI-1), a fast-acting inhibitor of tPA (Loskutoff *et al.*, 1983; Levin, 1983; Philips *et al.*, 1984). A number of reports have demonstrated that IL-1 suppresses the fibrinolytic activity of vascular ECs by increasing tPAI activity (Bevilacqua *et al.*, 1986a; Emeis and Kooistra, 1986; Nachman *et al.*, 1986). Likewise, TNF has been also demonstrated to increase endothelial tPAI activity (Schleef *et al.*, 1988).

Both IL-1 and TNF decrease tPA activity in umbilical vein ECs in a dose- and time-dependent manner (Bevilacqua *et al.*, 1986a; Schleef *et al.*, 1988). Bevilacqua *et al.* (1986b) have shown that, in contrast to the rapid and transient effect of the cytokines on PCA, the changes in tPA and tPAI activity were not detected until 6 hours and were maximal at 24 hours. After a 24-hour treatment with IL-1β, the ECs secreted only one-quarter of the control value of tPA, but released PAI at a rate that was fivefold higher than control. Two other groups, however, observed a slight or no decrease of tPA antigen in IL-1-stimulated umbilical vein ECs in spite of a remarkable increase of the secretion of tPAI by these cells (Nachman et al., 1986; Emeis and Kooistra, 1986). Therefore, increased tPAI expression in IL-1-stimulated ECs *in vitro* may be regarded as a constant phenomenon, whereas the levels of tPA expression by these cells appear to be variable according to the condition of cultures and experiments.

Several other factors influence tPA and tPAI activities of vascular ECs. Thrombin increases both tPA antigens and tPAI activity (Dickek and Quertermous, 1989). Endotoxin markedly increases PAI-1 activity but does not affect tPA levels (Hanss and Collen, 1987). The addition of heparin and endothelial cell growth factor (ECGF) to EC cultures results in a decrease in the tPAI-1 activity without changes in tPA antigen and mRNA levels (Konkle and Ginsburg, 1988).

Transcriptional regulation of tPA and tPAI-1 genes in vascular ECs has not been fully evaluated. Schleef *et al.* (1988) have found that treatment of umbilical vein ECs with IL-1 or TNF for 16 hours increased the steady-state levels of the 3.2- and 2.3-kb tPAI-1 mRNA species by three- to ninefold with a preferential increase in the larger mRNA form. A number of studies have demonstrated that human cells produce the two distinct mRNA species for tPAI-1; these two species are encoded by a single gene and arise by alternative polyadenylation (Ny et al., 1986; Lund et al., 1987; Van de Berg et al., 1987). These authors have not determined whether the preferential increase of the larger form of tPAI-1 mRNA reflects a control mechanism at the posttranscription level or at the level of transcription, resulting in more frequent polyadenylation at the downstream site to generate the larger transcript. The 3'-untranslated regions of the larger tPAI-1 mRNA species contain AU-rich sequences that are 75 bp long (Ginsburg et al., 1986). Similar sequences have been noted in the 3'-untranslated regions of the mRNAs for a number of cytokine-inducible genes, including IL-1α, IL-β, and TNF genes (Caput et al., 1986). These findings suggest that a common regulatory pathway may control the accumulation of tPAI-1 and other inflammatory mediator-gene mRNAs in response to cytokines. The changes in the mRNA levels of tPA in cytokine-stimulated vascular ECs remain to be clarified.

B. GENES OF LEUKOCYTE ADHESION MOLECULES

1. *Cytokine Effect on Leukocyte Adherence to Human Vascular Endothelial Cells*

Leukocyte adhesion to the vascular endothelium is an essential event in inflammatory response related to the pathogenesis of certain vascular diseases. Recent *in vitro* studies with cultured vascular ECs have provided new insights into the effects of inflammatory cytokines on endothelial–leukocyte interactions. Bevilacqua *et al.* (1985) have found enhanced adherence of IL-1-stimulated human umbilical vein ECs to neutrophils, monocytes, and related leukocyte cell lines. The induction of endothelial adhesivity by IL-1 was concentration (maximum 10 U/ml) and time dependent (peak 4–6 hours). In addition, the increase of endothelial adherence was blocked by cycloheximide or actinomycin D, indicating a requirement for transcription and protein synthesis.

Pober *et al.* (1986a) have developed monoclonal antibodies (H4/18 and H18/7) against cytokine-stimulated umbilical vein ECs. The molecules recognized by one of the monoclonal antibodies (H4/18) are not detected on unstimulated ECs. The majority of ECs stimulated with IL-1 can be induced to express the H4/18-binding proteins, but the expression is transient (peak 4–6 hours) and decreases to near basal levels over the subsequent 24 hours. These investigators have also observed that one of the two monoclonal antibodies (H18/7) blocks the adhesion of human neutrophils and HL-60 to IL-1- or TNF-stimulated ECs by almost 60% (Bevilacqua *et al.*, 1987). The same molecule on cytokine-activated ECs was detected by both antibodies with immunoprecipitation and was designated as ELAM-1 (endothelial leukocyte adhesion molecule 1).

In contrast to the EC-dependent effect of IL-1 in leukocyte–endothelial adherence, certain stimuli such as complement components enhance leukocyte adherence to the endothelium by acting principally on leukocytes (Tonnesen *et al.*, 1984). Gamble *et al.* (1985) have demonstrated that the enhancement of leukocyte adherence to ECs by TNF is mediated by the effect of the cytokine on both neutrophils and ECs. Whereas the effect on neutrophils is maximally induced within 5 minutes and does not require protein and RNA synthesis, the maximal effect on ECs takes 4 hours to develop and requires *de novo* protein and RNA synthesis.

In studies of the leukocyte surface molecules involved in leukocyte-dependent adhesion to ECs, Harlan *et al.* (1985) demonstrated that a CD11/CD18 complex was involved. The same investigators also reported that coincubation of neutrophils with a monoclonal antibody against the CD11/CD18 complex, 60.3, produced a 70% inhibition of neutrophil adherence to LPS-pretreated ECs, a 59% inhibition of adherence to IL-1-pretreated ECs, and a 65% inhibition of adherence to TNF-α-pretreated ECs (Pohlman *et al.*, 1986). They concluded that LPS, IL-1, and TNF-α induced synthesis of EC surface factors that mediate neutrophil adherence primarily by a mechanism involving a CD11/CD18 complex.

Monoclonal antibodies against a CD11/CD18 complex have been demonstrated to block the adhesion of neutrophils to ECs *in vivo* (Arfors *et al.*, 1987;

Price et al., 1987). The CD11/CD18 complex consists of three molecules with distinct α subunits, LFA-1α, Mo-1 (OKM1/Mac-1)α, and p150 complexed with a common β-chain subunit (Sanchez-Madrid et al., 1983). The individual α subunits have been designated as CD11a, CD11b, and CD11c, respectively, and the common β subunit, as CD18, by the Third International Workshop on Leukocyte Differentiation Antigens (Shaw, 1987). LFA-1 (CD11a/18) is expressed on all murine and human leukocytes, and CD11b/18 and CD11c/18 are present on the surface of neutrophils, monocytes, macrophages, and large granular lymphocytes (Stoolman, 1989). The respective contributions of these cell surface structures to the enhanced adherence of neutrophils to cytokine-activated ECs have been studied by a number of investigators.

A novel intercellular adhesion molecule 1 (ICAM-1) has been described by Rothlein et al. (1986). ICAM-1 is a cell surface glycoprotein that is involved in LFA-1 (CD11a/CD18 complex)-dependent cell aggregation of phorbol ester-stimulated peripheral bood lymphocytes and several lymphoid cell lines. Marlin and Springer (1987) as well as Simmons et al. (1988) provided direct evidence that ICAM-1 was an adhesion ligand for LFA-1.

The expression of ICAM-1 on umbilical vein ECs has been shown to be increased by IFN-γ, IL-1, and TNF-α (Pober et al., 1986b). Hence, the involvement of ICAM-1 in the adherence of neutrophils to ECs may be postulated. Smith et al. (1989) have demonstrated that attachment of unstimulated neutrophils to IL-1-stimulated ECs involves ICAM-1–LFA-1 interactions. They showed that the anti-ICAM-1 monoclonal antibody, R6.5.D6, profoundly inhibited the adherence of unstimulated neutrophils to ECs stimulated with IL-1 for 18 hours. In addition, the anti-CD11a monoclonal antibody, R3.1, inhibited the same adherence by 83.4%. These findings suggest that unstimulated neutrophil adherence to IL-1-activated ECs is dependent on ICAM-1–LFA-1 interactions to a significant degree.

Luscinskas et al. (1989) have examined the contributions of the endothelial surface molecule, ELAM-1, and leukocyte surface structures, CD11/CD18 complexes, in the adhesion of neutrophils to IL-1-stimulated ECs. They have demonstrated that neutrophil adherence to IL-1-activated ECs involves, in addition to a CD11/CD18-dependent mechanism, an ELAM-1-dependent mechanism. Moreover, the relative contributions of ELAM-1-dependent versus CD11/CD18-dependent mechanisms vary at different times during IL-1-induced EC activation. After 4 hours of IL-1 treatment of EC, both ELAM-1-dependent and CD11/CD18-dependent mechanisms are involved, whereas at 24 hours, the leukocyte CD11/CD18-dependent mechanism predominates. Because CD11/CD18 surface adhesive complexes on neutrophils are not functioning as obligatory ligands for ELAM-1, still undefined neutrophil surface structures may be a prerequisite for ELAM-1-dependent neutrophil adherence to vascular ECs.

The relative contributions of the leukocyte molecules LFA-1, Mac-1 (Mo-1), and p150,95 in the adhesion of neutrophils to human umbilical vein ECs have been studied with subunit-specific monoclonal antibodies by Arnaout et al. (1988). Phorbol myristate acetate-induced neutrophil adhesion to unstimulated ECs was significantly inhibited by anti-Mo-1α and anti-common β, but not by anti-LFAα or anti-p150, suggesting that the adhesion was mainly dependent on Mo-1 molecules. When ECs were prestimulated with IL-1, every monoclonal antibody against each of the three α subunits as well as the common β subunit inhibited neutrophil adherence to ECs at least partially. Furthermore, the inhibitory effect of the three anti-α subunit monoclonal antibodies on neutrophil–EC adherence was additive. These findings led the authors to conclude that all three neutrophil surface structures, LFA-1, Mo-1, and p150,95, contributed to the adherence of neutrophils to IL-1-stimulated ECs.

Luscinskas et al. (1989) have also provided evidence that all three CD11 heterodimers are involved in neutrophil adherence to IL-1-activated human umbilical vein ECs. Smith et al. (1989), however, observed that the adherence of neutrophils to IL-1-stimulated ECs was mainly dependent on LFA-1. It is conceivable that the relative importance of each CD11/18 heterodimer in the adherence of neutrophils to IL-1-stimulated ECs may be variable to some extent, according to the difference in experimental conditions, such as time of IL-1 stimulation. At present, the requisite receptor or structure on the neutrophil surface for the binding to ELAM-1 on ECs has not been determined. MO-1 (MAC-1, CD11b/18) is known to function as a receptor for surface-bound C2bi (Wright et al., 1983). However, the ligands on human umbilical vein ECs recognized by Mo-1 are not known. Neither is it known whether CD11b/CD18 or CD11c/CD18 can recognize ICAM-1. Figure 1 lists the leukocyte adhesion molecules and ligands that have been demonstrated to be necessary for leukocyte–EC adhesion.

2. Cytokine Regulation of Gene Expression of Endothelial Adhesion Molecules

ICAM-1 is a glycoprotein with molecular weights ranging between 76,000–114,000. The difference in molecular weights is due to the variable extent of glycosylation in different cell types (Dustin et al., 1986; Clark et al., 1986). Staunton et al. (1988) have isolated ICAM-1 cDNA clones from LPS-stimulated human umbilical vein ECs and the myelomonocytic cell line, HL-60. The molecular weight of the mature polypeptide predicted from the cDNA clones is 55,219, which is in excellent agreement with the observed molecular weight of 55,000 for the deglycosylated form (Dustin et al., 1986). Eight N-linked glycosylation sites have been predicted.

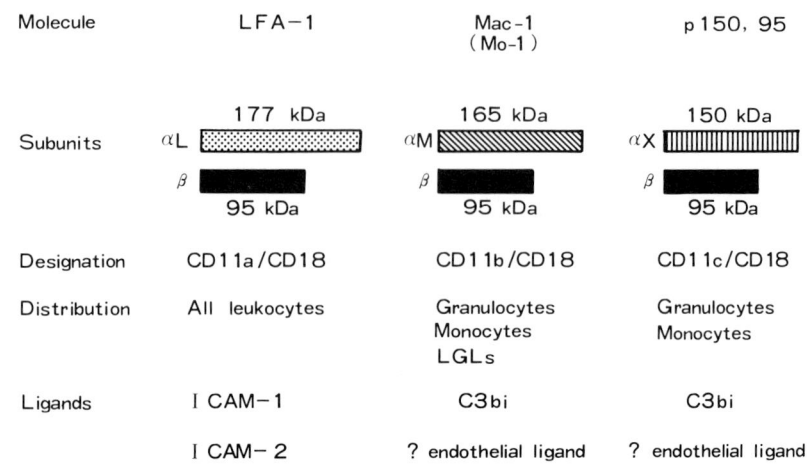

Molecule	LFA−1	Mac−1 (Mo−1)	p150, 95
Subunits	αL 177 kDa / β 95 kDa	αM 165 kDa / β 95 kDa	αX 150 kDa / β 95 kDa
Designation	CD11a/CD18	CD11b/CD18	CD11c/CD18
Distribution	All leukocytes	Granulocytes Monocytes LGLs	Granulocytes Monocytes
Ligands	ICAM−1, ICAM−2	C3bi, ? endothelial ligand	C3bi, ? endothelial ligand

FIG. 1. Structure of leukocyte adhesion molecules and their ligands.

Staunton et al. (1988) have found that the predicted amino acid sequence of ICAM-1 fulfills all criteria proposed for membership in the immunoglobulin (Ig) supergene family (Williams and Barclay, 1988). The entire extracellular domain is constructed of five homologous Ig-like domains. ICAM-1 has been found to be strikingly homologous with two adhesion molecules of the nervous system, the NCAM and MAG glycoproteins, which also belong to the Ig supergene family. NCAM is involved in neuron–neuron and neuron–muscular interactions (Cunningham et al., 1987), and MAG is reported to be involved in neuron–oligodendrocyte and oligodendrocyte–oligodendrocyte interactions during myelination (Poltorak et al., 1987). The expression of ICAM-1 mRNA in various cells, including human vascular ECs, has also been examined. Hybridization with poly(A) mRNA has revealed a 3.3-kb mRNA in LPS-stimulated ECs. A second mRNA of 2.4 kb appears to be present in smaller quantities.

Staunton et al. (1989) have isolated the cDNA clone of a second LFA-1 ligand, designated ICAM-2, from a cDNA library prepared from LPS-stimulated human umbilical vein ECs. The predicted mature sequence consists of a putative extracellular domain (amino acids 1–202), followed by a 26-residue hydrophobic putative transmembrane domain and a 26-residue cytoplasmic domain. The predicted molecular weight of the mature ICAM-2 is 28,393. Six N-linked glycosylation sites are predicted. The 202-amino acid extracellular domain of ICAM-2 consists of two Ig-like domains. The Ig-like domains of ICAM-2 have 34% identity in their amino acid sequence with the first and second N-terminal Ig-like domains of ICAM-1, and 27% identity with the third and fourth Ig-like domains of ICAM-1. The mRNA levels of ICAM-1 and ICAM-2 have been examined in various cells, including vascular ECs. ICAM-2 cDNA hybridizes to a 1.4-kb mRNA and weakly to a 3.0-kb mRNA, both of which are distinct from the 3.3- and 2.4-kb ICAM-1 mRNA. ICAM-1 mRNA is strongly induced in ECs by LPS. In contrast, the basal expression of ICAM-2 mRNA is high in ECs and is not induced further by LPS. ICAM-2 mRNA has been reported to be present in a variety of cell types, including B cell, macrophage, and T cell lines in addition to vascular ECs. High basal expression of ICAM-2 mRNA in vascular ECs is consistent with the findings of an LFA-1-dependent, ICAM-1-independent pathway of adhesion to unstimulated ECs (Dustin and Springer, 1988).

A cDNA clone for ELAM-1 has been isolated by Bevilacqua *et al.* (1989). The translated amino acid sequence predicts a mature polypeptide of 589 amino acids and a signal peptide of 21 amino acids. The extracellular domain of the mature polypeptide contains 11 potential sites of N-linked glycosylation. The putative transmembrane region (residue 536–557) is followed by a cytoplasmic portion of 32 amino acids. The extracellular portion of ELAM-1 can be divided into three segments (Fig. 2). Approximately 120 amino acids at the N-terminus are related to the carbohydrate-binding domain of a variety of lectins (Drickamer, 1988). A second segment (residue 121–150) is related to proteins containing the epidermal growth factor (EGF) motif (Cooke *et al.*, 1987). The EGF-like domain is followed by six tandem repetitive motifs of approximately 60 amino acids that are homologous to a variety of complement-binding proteins (Lasky *et al.*, 1989; Siegelman *et al.*, 1989). The structure of the ELAM-1 molecule resembles that of two other cell surface proteins, the Mel-14 antigen and granule membrane protein 140 (GMP-140) (Fig. 2).

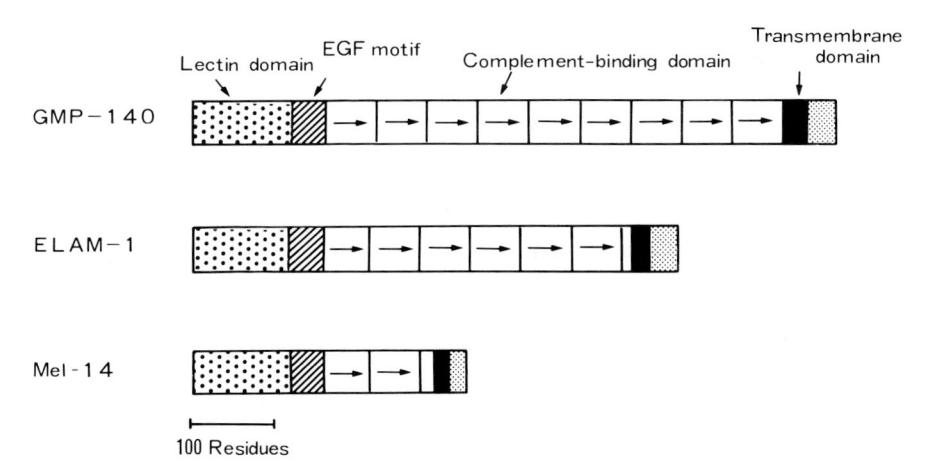

FIG. 2. Structure of ELAM-1 molecule and other related adhesion molecules (GMP-140 and Mel-14).

The murine Mel-14 antigen, which is expressed on lymphocytes, monocytes, and neutrophils, was originally proposed to be the homing receptor mediating the interaction of lymphocytes with peripheral node high endothelial venules (Gallatin et al., 1983; Lewinsohn et al., 1987). The primary sequence of Mel-14 consists of an N-terminal lectinlike domain (approximately 120 amino acids) contiguous with an EGF-like domain of 33 amino acids and two identical repeats homologous to the complement-binding proteins (Lasky et al., 1989; Siegelman et al., 1989).

GMP-140, a 140-kDa glycoprotein, is present in the membranes of secretory granules of platelets and ECs and can be rapidly mobilized to the cell surface by stimulants such as thrombin (McEver and Martin, 1984; Stenberg et al., 1985). The recently completed sequence of GMP-140 similarly predicts a structure that contains an N-terminal lectinlike domain, an EGF-like domain, and nine repetitive motifs of complement-binding proteins (Johnston et al., 1989). The identification of similar domain structures of the three cell surface molecules appears to constitute a new gene family (Stoolman, 1989).

Bevilacqua et al. (1989) have examined the regulation of ELAM-1 gene expression in human umbilical vein ECs by cytokines. Treatment of ECs for 2 hours with IL-1 or TNF induces a single 3.9-kb mRNA that hybridizes with ELAM-1 cDNA. ELAM-1 mRNA is not detected in unstimulated ECs or IFN-γ-stimulated ECs. Expression of ELAM-1 mRNA in IL-1-stimulated ECs is maximum at 2–4 hours after stimulation and declines close to basal levels 24 hours after stimulation. Expression of ELAM-1 protein on the surface of ECs is well correlated with the expression of ELAM-1 mRNA. Also, ELAM-1 mRNA contains multiple AT-rich sequences, including the consensus sequence TTATTTAT described in cDNAs encoding various inflammatory mediators, including cytokines (Caput et al., 1986).

C. Major Histocompatibility Antigen Complex

The major histocompatibility antigen complex, or HLA system, encodes cell surface molecules involved in the regulation of immune responses. The class I loci (HLA-A, HLA-B, and HLA-C loci) encode 44-kDa glycoproteins that are associated with a 12-kDa polypeptide, β_2-microglobulin, and are present on nearly all somatic cells (Hood et al., 1983).

Functionally, class I antigens are intimately involved in the recognition of target cells by cytotoxic T lymphocytes (Zinkernagel and Doherty, 1979). The class II antigens are also glycoproteins consisting of α and β chains that are encoded by a family of homogeneous genes clustered in the HLA-D region (HLA-DP, -DQ, and -DR) of the MHC (Trowsdale et al., 1985; Mach et al., 1986). The expression of class II genes is largely limited to certain cells of the immune system, primarily B lymphocytes, activated T cells, macrophages, and dendritic cells (Flavell *et al.*, 1986), though their expression can be induced in a number of class II-negative cells, including ECs, by stimulation with IFN-γ (Basham and Merigan, 1983; Collins *et al.*, 1984). The expression of class II antigens on antigen-presenting cells mediates the activation of T lymphocytes. Accordingly, the regulation of MHC class II gene expression plays a key role in the control of immune responses (Benacerraf, 1981).

Under unstimulated conditions, human umbilical vein ECs express class I MHC antigens but not class II MHC antigens (Pober and Gimbrone, 1982). Pober *et al.* (1983) first described the induction of HLA-DR antigens on the surface of cultured human umbilical vein ECs and of foreskin microvascular ECs by the stimulation of IFN-γ. The same group has examined the regulation of class II gene expression by IFN-γ in ECs at the molecular level (Collins *et al.*, 1984). Treatment of ECs with IFN-γ induces not only HLA-DR but also two other class II antigens, SB (DP) and DC. Time course studies have shown that maximal surface expression of all three antigens is reached 4–6 days after IFN-γ stimulation, and HLA-DR and -DP are induced to a higher level of expression than is HLA-DC. Expression of mRNA for class II genes has been also examined. Messenger RNA levels of the HLA-DRα chain increase from undetectable levels to a plateau 24–48 hours after stimulation with IFN-γ. HLA-DQα mRNA is also induced by treatment with IFN-γ. Class I mRNA levels and antigen expression are increased likewise by IFN-γ at a rate similar to that for class II mRNA and antigens.

The roles of class I and class II antigens on vascular ECs have been studied by many investigators. *In vitro* studies with canine and umbilical vein ECs have shown that lymphocytes are capable of recognizing antigenic determinants on ECs (Hirschberg *et al.*, 1975; Groenewegen *et al.*, 1984). Moreover, ECs can function as antigen-presenting cells to lymphocytes (Hirschberg *et al.*, 1980). Geppert and Lipsky (1985) have observed that IFN-γ-treated human umbilical vein ECs can stimulate allogeneic T4 cells to induce DNA synthesis.

MHC antigen expression on vascular ECs appears to have an active role in the development of pathological lesions in certain immunological disorders. Studies involving immunostaining of transplant tissues have shown that increased expression of class I and class II HLA antigens on vascular ECs is associated with allograft rejection (Häyry *et al.*, 1986; Rose *et al.*, 1986). The immunogenic activity of an allograft seems to be directly dependent on the expression of these class II HLA antigens on the EC surface (Ferry *et al.*, 1987). Another example implicating the immunopathogenetic role of the class II HLA antigens is the expression of HLA-DR on the vascular endothelium of rheumatoid synovium (Palmer *et al.*, 1985; Klareskog *et al.*, 1984).

Collins *et al.* (1986a) reported that TNF-α increased mRNA levels and surface expression of HLA-A and -B antigens in umbilical vein ECs. The increase of class I antigens by TNF-α was maximal 4 days after stimulation with TNF-α and the expression remained at elevated levels in the continuous presence of TNF-α. The increase of surface class I antigen expression was accompanied by the increase of steady-state mRNA levels for the class I antigens. Surface expression of or induction of mRNA for class II antigens was not induced in TNF-α-treated ECs. These effects of TNF-α on ECs were similar to those evoked by IFN-α and IFN-β (Lapierre et al., 1988), both of which increased surface antigens and mRNA expression for class I antigens, but not for class II antigens.

Lymphotoxin (TNF-β) has been also reported to increase steady-state mRNA levels and surface antigen expression for class I antigens without inducing class II transcripts or surface expression (Pober et al., 1987). Though TNF-α/β and IFN-α/β increase the expression of class I antigens on ECs, the responsible mechanism appears to be different. Cycloheximide led to enhancement of the IFN-α/β-mediated increase of class I mRNA and superinduction of class II mRNA in ECs, whereas this protein synthesis inhibitor blocked the action of TNF (Collins et al., 1986a). Furthermore, whereas both TNF-α and TNF-β at optimal concentrations do not affect IFN-γ-induced class II antigen expression on the surface of ECs, IFN-α and IFN-β markedly inhibit the induction of class II antigens by IFN-γ (Lapierre et al., 1988). In addition, TNF-α and TNF-β can further increase the expression of surface class I antigens on ECs that have been already stimulated maximally by IFN-α or IFN-β. These observations have led Lapierre et al. (1988) to conclude that there are at least three classes of regulatory cytokines, TNF-α/β, IFN-α/β, and IFN-γ, each of which has distinct effects on endothelial expression of MHC antigens.

The treatment of umbilical vein ECs with IFN-γ has been reported to induce the surface expression of HLA-DR and -DP, whereas the addition of IFN-α to IFN-γ-treated ECs remarkably inhibits the expression of class II MHC antigens (Manyak et al., 1988). Similar regulatory functions of MHC gene expression by cytokines have been demonstrated in ECs of other sources, such as human arterial ECs obtained from transplant donors (Markus et al., 1988). Using human capillary ECs obtained from omentum, Leeuwenberg et al. (1989) have reported induction of class II antigens by IFN-γ. They have also found that both IFN-β and TNF-α decrease IFN-γ-induced class II antigen expression when the cytokines are added before IFN-γ. In contrast, when added 24 hours after IFN-γ, TNF-α displays a remarkably enhancing activity on the IFN-γ-induced class II expression on ECs. In the opinion of these investigators, these findings are compatible with the previous reports showing similar phenomena in a murine macrophage cell line, some human tumor cell lines, and activated T cells (Chang and He Lee, 1986; Pfizenmaier et al., 1987; Scheurich et al., 1987).

Molecular mechanisms regulating the expression of HLA class II antigens have been studied by a number of groups. Several conserved DNA sequence motifs are found in the promoter region of HLA-DRA (previously called HLA-DRα) (Fig. 3). An octamer motif (ATTTGCAT) is found at position −45 to −52 upstream of the cap site. This sequence is detected in the promoter regions of several other genes, including Ig light and heavy chains (Parslow et al., 1984), human histone 2B, and human U2 small nuclear RNA genes (Sive and Roeder, 1986). Upstream of the octamer motif, there are two conserved sequences called the X (−95 to −108) and the Y (−63 to −74) boxes, which are highly conserved among all murine and human class II genes (Mathis et al., 1983; Saito et al., 1983; Kelly and Trowsdale, 1985).

The functional importance of these consensus sequences in constitutive and inducible expression has been demonstrated by transfection experiments (Boss and Strominger, 1986; Sherman et al., 1987). More recently, Reith et al. (1988) have identified three different DNA-binding proteins, an X-box-binding protein, a Y-box-binding protein, and an octamer-binding protein, in nuclear extracts of normal human B cells.

A specific sequence in the promoter region of HLA class II genes necessary for the IFN-γ-induced expression was studied by Basta et al. (1987). They constructed recombinant plasmids containing various segments of the promoter region of the HLA-DRA chain gene linked to the reporter gene, chloramphenicol acetyltransferase gene, and transfected them into human glioblastoma cells that could be induced to express class II antigens by IFN-γ. The DRA sequences present in the plasmid inducing the reporter gene included 267 bp of DNA immediately 5′ to the cap site, the cap site, and 27 bp 3′ of the cap site. In addition, they found a possible consensus sequence shared among different IFN-γ-inducible sequences in promoter regions of several other genes. In the HLA-DRA chain gene, this consensus sequence (AGAAGTCAG) was present at positions −264 to −256 upstream of the cap

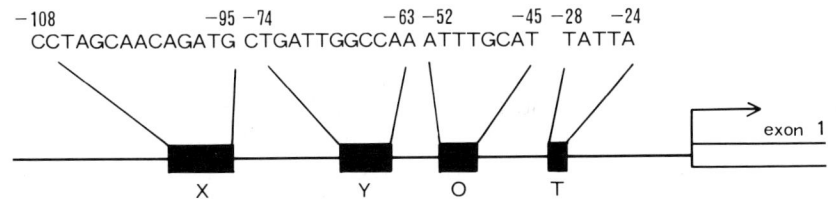

FIG. 3. Map of the HLA-DRA promoter region. The transcriptional start site is indicated by an arrow. The solid black boxes represent potential regulatory elements; the conserved class II boxes (X and Y), the octamer motif (O), and the TATA box (T). The sequence of these elements and their position in nucleotides relative to the cap site are indicated. (Adapted from Reith et al., 1988.)

site. Precise roles of this sequence in the cellular response to IFN-γ, however, have not been demonstrated.

In addition to transcriptional regulation, several studies have proposed putative posttranscriptional regulation through the specific stabilization of class II gene mRNA by IFN-γ. Rosa and Fellous (1988), in assessing the effect of IFN-γ treatment on HLA-DR gene expression of a melanoma cell line, VAL, demonstrated that the steady-state levels of HLA-DRA mRNA were increased 100-fold, whereas the transcription rate was increased only 5-fold, indicating the relative importance of posttranscriptional regulations. For further elucidation of the molecular mechanisms of HLA class II gene expression in ECs, it will be necessary to isolate and clone the trans-acting factors and to reconstitute *in vitro* the tissue-specific transcription system.

C. Production of Cytokines

Vascular ECs are important producers of various cytokines that regulate the differentiation and proliferation of T and B cells, the proliferation of smooth muscle cells, the recruitment of leukocytes at sites of inflammation, and hematopoiesis (Table I). Countless studies have demonstrated that the synthesis and release of cytokines from vascular ECs are also regulated by several cytokines that mediate inflammatory responses, such as IL-1 and TNF-α.

1. *IL-1*

IL-1, first described as a monocyte product that induces thymocyte proliferation and activates T and B cells, has been demonstrated to be released from a number of cell types, including vascular ECs (Wagner *et al.*, 1985; Stern *et al.*, 1985a). Various cytokines regulate the release of IL-1 from ECs. TNF-α as well as IL-1 itself stimulate the release of IL-1 from vascular ECs (Libby *et al.*, 1986;

TABLE I
Cytokines Produced by Cultured Endothelial Cells

Cytokine[a]	Stimulus
IL-1 (IL-1α, IL-1β)	LPS, IL-1, TNF-α, TNF-β
Il-6	Spontaneous, LPS, IL-1, TNF-α
CSFs (GM-CSF, M-CSF, and G-CSF)	LPS, IL-1, TNF-α
PDGF (PDGF-A chain and PDGF-B chain)	Spontaneous, TGF-β, IL-1, TNF-α
MDNCF (IL-8) and MGSA/gro	LPS, IL-1, TNF-α

[a] MDNCF, Monocyte-derived neutrophil chemotactic factor; MGSA, melanoma growth stimulatory activity.

Nawroth *et al.*, 1986; Warner *et al.*, 1987). Though IFN-γ alone has no effect on intracellular IL-1 content or on the amount of IL-1 released from ECs, it enhances the release of IL-1 from ECs in association with a second signal from LPS (Miossec and Ziff, 1986).

Recently, TNF-α and IL-1 have been shown to induce the release of IL-1 from ECs synergistically (Howells *et al.*, 1988). TNF-β is also capable of inducing the release of IL-1 from ECs, but is a relatively poor stimulus in comparison with TNF-α (Locksley *et al.*, 1987). With approximately 30% homology in its amino acid sequence with TNF-α, TNF-β demonstrates similar biological effects on various cells and has been shown to bind to the same receptor as TNF-α (Aggarwal *et al.*, 1985). Locksley *et al.* (1987) pointed out that the lower activity of TNF-β in the release of IL-1 from ECs might be due to the lower affinity of TNF-β for binding to endothelial monolayers.

Sequence analysis of cDNA and of purified IL-1 proteins has revealed that human IL-1 consists of at least two separate gene products, IL-1α and IL-1β (Auron *et al.*, 1984; March *et al.*, 1985). The two types of IL-1 have only 26% identity in amino acid sequence, but share biological activities and use the same receptors (Kilian *et al.*, 1986; Dower *et al.*, 1986; Matsushima *et al.*, 1986). Libby *et al.* (1986) assessed the expression of IL-1 mRNA in cytokine-treated human saphenous vein ECs. The treatment of ECs with TNF-α and endotoxin resulted in the accumulation of IL-1β mRNA. The accumulation of IL-1β mRNA in ECs was induced soon after stimulation (4 hours). IL-1α mRNA was detected only when the ECs were exposed to endotoxin in the presence of cycloheximide. The same group has also reported the induction of IL-1 mRNA in IL-1-treated human saphenous vein ECs (Warner *et al.*, 1987). Time course studies showed that IL-1β mRNA was detected within 1 hour of exposure to recombinant IL-1, reaching a peak after 24 hours, and declining thereafter. IL-1α mRNA was only induced when ECs were stimulated with IL-1 in the presence of cycloheximide.

Suzuki *et al.* (1989a) have demonstrated an increase in IL-1β mRNA accumulation in LPS-stimulated human umbilical vein ECs in contrast to profound suppression of c-*sis* mRNA by IFN-γ (Fig. 4). These findings support the contention that stimulation with both LPS and IFN-γ enhances greater release of IL-1 from ECs than stimulation with LPS alone (Miossec and Ziff, 1986). The indication is that induction of IL-1β mRNA is greater than induction of IL-1α in cytokine-stimulated ECs. Kurt-Jones *et al.* (1987), however, reported that stimulation of human umbilical vein ECs with TNF-α or TNF-β for 72 hours induced more IL-1α mRNA expression than IL-1β mRNA expression. Stimulation of these cells with IL-1α or IL-1β for 72 hours also increased the levels of IL-1α and IL-1β mRNA. It is conceivable that the longer exposure (72 hours) of ECs to these cytokines may preferentially induce IL-1α mRNA, in contrast to predominant induction of IL-1β mRNA soon (several hours) after stimulation.

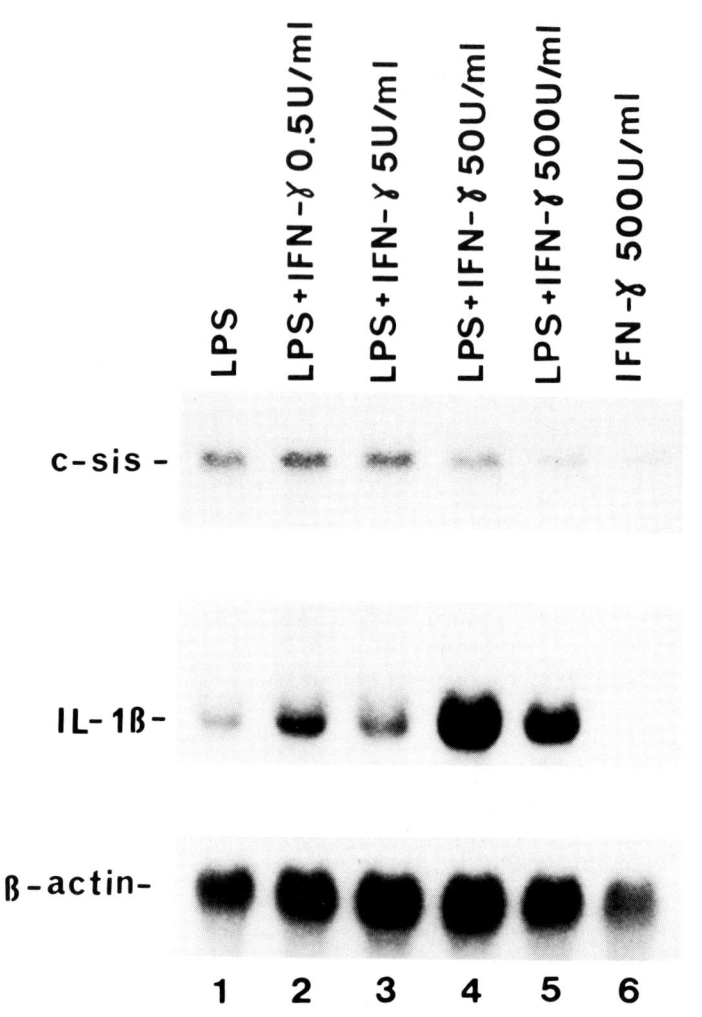

FIG. 4. Changes of IL-1β and c-sis mRNA levels in human umbilical vein ECs after a 24-hour treatment with lipopolysaccharide (LPS) in the presence of various concentrations of IFN-γ. (Reproduced from Suzuki et al., 1989a.)

The dominant type of IL-1 mRNA induced in cells seems to differ depending on the cell type and the condition of stimulation. In monocytes and macrophages, cells best equipped to secrete IL-1, most of the IL-1 mRNA and secreted IL-1 are of the β type (Demczuk et al., 1987). In keratinocytes, however, mainly α-type IL-1 mRNA is induced (Kuper et al., 1986). On the other hand, Epstein–Barr virus (EBV)-transformed B cell lines have been reported to produce either IL-1α or IL-1β, but not both (Acres *et al.*, 1987). The two forms of IL-1 are initially synthesized as 31-kDa precursor peptides, but neither contains a signal peptide sequence that would indicate a cleavage site for the N-terminus. This observation has raised the possibility that IL-1 may follow a metabolic pathway that is not typical of most secreted proteins.

Several studies have shown that IL-1β is rapidly secreted from activated cells whereas IL-1α remains cell associated. In human vascular ECs, several groups have examined which form of IL-1, i.e., IL-1α or IL-1β, can be produced by treatment with cytokines. Miossec *et al.* (1986) observed two peaks of IL-1 activity at pI 5 (IL-1α) and 7 (IL-1β) in chromatofocused LPS-stimulated EC supernatants. IL-1 activities of the two peaks were comparable, suggesting that similar amounts of IL-1α and IL-1β were produced by cytokine-stimulated ECs. Similar findings have also been obtained by Howells *et al.* (1988), who reported that IL-1 activity in the supernatants of IL-1α- or IL-1β-stimulated ECs was only partially blocked by anti-IL-1α or anti-IL-1β antibody alone, whereas simultaneous treatment with both types of antibodies blocked the IL-1 activity almost completely. These reports suggest that IL-1α and IL-1β may be secreted in similar amounts by cytokine-activated ECs.

There has been some controversy about the distinction between secreted and membrane-associated forms of IL-1. Several studies have suggested that IL-1 is expressed in both secreted and membrane-associated forms by macrophages, monocytes, and B cells (Kurt-Jones *et al.*, 1985; Matsushima *et al.*, 1986; Gerrard and Volkman, 1985). Membrane-associated IL-1 has been reported to be biologically active and may be the form that participates in activating lymphocytes (Kurt-Jones *et al.*, 1985). The same investigators (Kurt-Jones *et al.*, 1987) have reported that membrane-associated IL-1, which is structurally related to IL-1α but not IL-1β, is induced on TNF-α-stimulated human vascular ECs.

However, the concept of a membrane-associated form of IL-1 is not generally accepted. Several groups were unable to demonstrate the presence of IL-1 on the surface of cells (Singer *et al.*, 1988; Sisson and Dinarello, 1988). The evidence against a membrane-associated form of IL-1 has been provided by Suttles *et al.* (1990), who recently suggested that IL-1 activity attributed to "membrane IL-1" may be caused by leakage from an inadequately fixed intracytoplasmic site, rather than being due to a membrane-bound source. The authors have shown that, though IL-1β released from paraformaldehyde-treated cells remains predominantly as an inactive, precursor molecule, IL-1α is functionally mature. These results are consistent with the previous reports that membrane-associated IL-1 is mainly α type (Fuhlbrigge *et al.*, 1988; Eugui and Almquist, 1989). Therefore, it is still uncertain whether cell-associated IL-1, including EC-associated IL-1, is capable of participating in the activation of lymphocytes.

2. Platelet-Derived Growth Factor

Platelet-derived growth factor (PDGF) is a major mitogen for connective tissue cells *in vitro* (Ross *et al.*, 1986). Originally purified from human platelets (Deuel *et al.*, 1981; Heldin *et al.*, 1981), the functionally active PDGF molecule consists of two polypeptide dimers termed A chain and B chain; their mature parts share 60% amino acid sequence similarity, with conservation of eight cysteine residues (Betsholtz *et al.*, 1986). More recently, PDGF homodimers composed of two A chains (PDGF-AA) or two B chains (PDGF-BB) have been isolated from osteosarcoma cells and porcine platelets, respectively (Stroobant and Waterfield, 1984; Heldin *et al.*, 1986). The B chain is the normal cellular homolog to the oncogene v-*sis* of simian sarcoma virus (SSV) (Waterfield *et al.*, 1983; Doolittle *et al.*, 1983). A cDNA for the A chain of PDGF has been also cloned from a human glioma cell line cDNA library (Betsholtz *et al.*, 1986).

Although the exact physiologic role of PDGF remains to be elucidated, it has been suggested that PDGF is involved in some physiological and pathological processes, including wound healing, atherosclerosis, neoangiogenesis, and carcinogenesis (Ross *et al.*, 1986). DiCorleto and co-workers were the first to demonstrate that cultured ECs could produce a PDGF-like protein in addition to other growth factors (DiCorleto and Bowen-Pope, 1983). Approximately 25% of the mitogenic activity in the supernatant of the EC culture has been specifically attributed to a PDGF-like protein, as determined by radiolabeled PDGF receptor competitive assay as well as by the inhibition of the PDGF-like activity by anti-PDGF antiserum (Bowen-Pope *et al.*, 1984). Release of PDGF—like protein from cultured ECs was further confirmed by the demonstration of c-*sis* (PDGF-B chain gene) mRNA expression (Barrett *et al.*, 1984). Cultured human umbilical vein ECs gave a single band at 3.7 kb of PDGF-B (c-*sis*) mRNA that was 10 times more intense in cultured cells than it was in *in vivo* umbilical vein endothelium obtained by trypsinization.

Jaye *et al.* (1985) examined the expression of c-*sis* mRNA levels in ECs during their differentiation *in vitro*. ECs organize into tubular structures in environments that limit cell proliferation. Jaye *et al.* (1985) found that the amount of c-*sis* mRNA decreased approximately 77% after 5 weeks of continuous culture in the absence of ECGF, when 80% of the cells were organized into a tubular network. THe organized cells, however, could be induced again to increase c-*sis* mRNA levels when these cells were subcultured in the presence of ECGF. They considered that an increase in c-*sis* expression during cell proliferation, in contrast to organized ECs, suggests the importance of a PDGF-like protein released from ECs during neovascularization. ECs are the first vascular cells to appear during neovascularization. PDGF is a potent chemotactic polypeptide for monocytes and neutrophils as well as fibroblasts and smooth muscle cells, in addition to being mitogenic for fibroblasts and smooth muscle cells. It therefore appears likely that during the development of neovascularization the c-*sis* product may act as a paracrine biological mediator of mesenchymal cell migration and proliferation.

PDGF-A chain gene expression has been observed in human umbilical vein ECs by Collins *et al.* (1986b). Hybridization analysis of total RNA from cultured human umbilical vein ECs has revealed that ECs contain three PDGF-A chain transcripts (2.8, 2.2, and 1.4 kb). A 2.2-kb mRNA is about twice as prevalent as either the larger (2.8 kb) or smaller (1.4 kb) species. The amounts of A chain and B chain mRNA in human umbilical vein ECs appear to be almost at the same level. Transcripts of both PDGF genes, i.e., A chain and B chain genes, have been confirmed in cultured microvascular ECs (Starksen *et al.*, 1987) and in human iliac artery ECs (Sitaras *et al.*, 1987).

The expression of PDGF genes in vascular ECs is modulated by several cytokines. Hajjar *et al.* (1987) assessed the effect of TNF-α on the EC-derived mitogenic activity for smooth muscle cells. The mitogenic activity in the supernatants of TNF-α-stimulated ECs increased by 90% compared with controls. The mitogenic activity was completely inhibited by anti-PDGF antiserum. This effect of TNF was accompanied with a 2.5-fold increase in the amount of PDGF-B chain (c-*sis*) mRNA. It was also observed that stimulation of ECs with IL-1 resulted in the increase of the mitogenic activity for smooth muscle cells. It must be remembered that TNF-α is an important inducer of IL-1 release from ECs. However, the mitogenic activity for smooth muscle cells by TNF-α-treated ECs was only partially reduced in the presence of anti-IL-1 antibodies. These results suggested that the induction of proliferative activity of smooth muscle cells by the TNF-α-stimulated ECs was partly mediated by TNF-α-induced secretion of autocrine IL-1 by ECs.

Daniel *et al.* (1987) examined the agents that can modulate c-*sis* expression in human renal microvascular ECs. TFG-β as well as thrombin increased c-*sis* mRNA levels. The c-*sis* mRNA levels peaked at 10-fold basal level 30 hours after stimulation with TGF-β, though some increase was apparent after 2 hours. They also observed that agents that increased cAMP accumulation, such as isoproterenol and epinephrine, blocked the expression of c-*sis* mRNA under the influence of both TFG-β and thrombin. The release of PDGF activity correlated well with the changes of c-*sis* mRNA levels (Daniel *et al.*, 1987).

In contrast to these enhancing effects of TNF-α and TFG-β on c-*sis* expression, we have recently observed that IFN-γ blocks the induction of c-*sis* in cultured human umbilical vein ECs (Suzuki *et al.*, 1989a). Treatment of ECs with IFN-γ profoundly suppressed the accumulation of c-*sis* mRNA not only in unstimulated cells, but also in cells stimulated with IL-1, TNF-α, or LPS (Fig. 5).

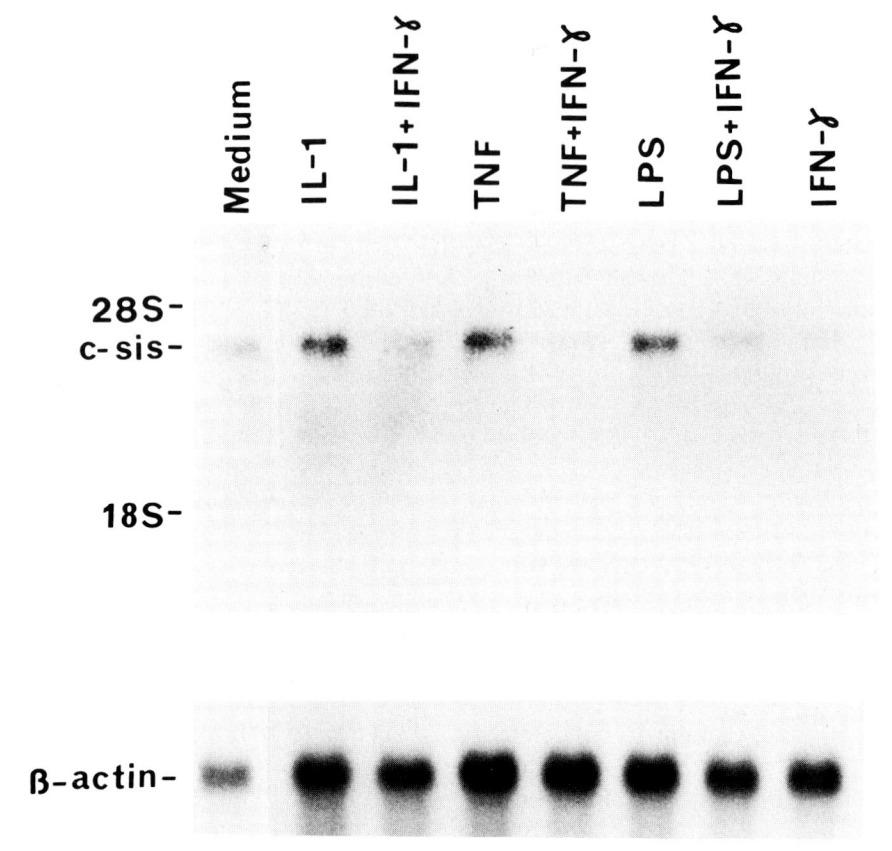

FIG. 5. Inhibition of c-*sis* expression in ECs by treatment with IFN-γ. Umbilical vein ECs were treated for 24 hours with IL-1α (10 U/ml), IL-1α + IFN-γ (500 U/ml), TNF (200 U/ml), TNF + IFN-γ, LPS (10 μg/ml), LPS + IFN-γ, or IFN-γ alone. (Reproduced from Suzuki *et al.*, 1989a.)

Kourembanas and Faller (1989) have reported that basic fibroblast growth factor (bFGF), a growth factor for ECs in culture, significantly decreases the amount of PDGF-like protein secreted by these cells. The levels of c-*sis* mRNA also decreased in ECs exposed to bFGF. The c-*sis* mRNA levels increased 12 hours after the removal of bFGF as the cells began to accumulate in G_0 stage of the cell cycle. These investigators suggest that bFGF may regulate c-*sis* mRNA levels and PDGF production by ECs either directly, or indirectly via cell cycle arrest at G_0. It remains unclear whether the suppression of the accumulation of c-*sis* mRNA in IFN-γ-treated ECs is mediated through the same intracellular signaling pathway as that in bFGF-treated cells.

Regulation of PDGF-A chain gene expression in microvascular ECs by cytokines has also been examined. PDGF-A chain mRNA levels were increased 5- to 25-fold by a phorbol ester (PMA), thrombin, and TGF-β (Starksen et al., 1987). The amount of PDGF-A chain mRNA in TGF-β-stimulated ECs reached maximal levels 4 hours after stimulation and remained significantly high 50 hours after stimulation. Agents that elevated cAMP, known to block induction of PDGF-B chain mRNA, blocked A chain mRNA induction by TGF-β. PDGF-A chain mRNA levels appear to be regulated by the same agents that regulate B chain mRNA levels (Starksen et al., 1987). The mechanisms by which different cytokines induce similar changes of PDGF gene mRNA levels are obscure. For example, biological effects on ECs evoked by IL-1, TNF-α, and TGF-β and intracellular signaling pathways of these cytokines are different from each other. A possible common effect on ECs of these cytokines and other agents that increase PDGF gene expression, such as thrombin (Harlan et al., 1986) and factor Xa (Gajdusek et al., 1986), may be found in the stimulation of IL-1 production by ECs (Hajjar et al., 1987).

3. Colony-Stimulating Factors

Hematopoiesis is dependent on the production of hematopoietic growth factors, including colony-stimulating factors (CSFs). These factors have been demonstrated to be produced by a variety of cell types, including T lymphocytes, fibroblasts, and ECs, all of which are components of the hematopoietic microenvironment. It is generally accepted that ECs in the microenvironment of bone marrow have important roles in the production of growth factors.

Quesenberry and Gimbrone (1980) first reported the production of CSF activity by cultured human ECs. The CSF activity was assayed by the capacity to promote the growth of hematopoietic progenitor cells, thus giving rise to colonies made of differentiated cells. The CSF activity released by ECs induced the appearance of colonies consisting of granulocytes and macrophages (Quesenberry and Gimbrone, 1980). Recently, three CSFs acting on granulocytes and/or macrophages have been purified and their cDNAs have been cloned: granulocyte–macrophage CSF (GM-CSF) (Cantrell et al., 1985), which promotes the development of colonies made of both granulocytes and macrophages, and G-CSF (Nagata et al., 1986) and M-CSF (or CSF-1) (Kawasaki et al., 1985), which promote the appearance of colonies consisting of either granulocytes or macrophages, respectively.

Bagby et al. (1983) have found that the supernatants of cultured peripheral blood monocytes stimulate human vascular ECs to release multilineage CSF activity. These investigators tried to characterize a mononuclear phagocyte-derived factor that stimulates ECs to release CSF activity. Exposure of monocytes to endotoxin markedly enhanced the release of the CSF activity, which peaked at 24 hours after stimulation (McCall and Bagby, 1985). They purified the monocyte-derived factor and found it to be identical with IL-1 (Bagby et al., 1986). In fact, both purified native IL-1 and recombinant IL-1 stimulated ECs to release CSF activities. These activities were initially detected by bioassay for colony-stimulating activity, but were subsequently demonstrated to be specifically the products of the G-CSF and GM-CSF genes by several investigators (Zsebo et al., 1988; Sieff et al., 1987; Broudy et al., 1986).

It has been shown that TNF-α also stimulates ECs to release GM-CSF (Broudy et al., 1986; Munker et al., 1986). It is now generally accepted that the two cytokines, IL-1 and TNF-α, induce CSF production by various cells, including ECs.

Seelentag et al. (1987) examined the regulation of CSF gene expression in human umbilical vein ECs by IL-1 and TNF-α. Whereas GM-CSF mRNA and G-CSF mRNA were not detectable in unstimulated ECs, a small amount of M-CSF mRNA could be detected. After addition of IL-1, GM-CSF mRNA became detectable after 8 hours, reaching a maximal level at 24 hours and decreasing somewhat at 48 hours. The TNF-α-induced expression of GM-CSF mRNA in ECs was slower, with the highest expression 48 hours after stimulation. Simultaneous treatment of ECs with maximally stimulating concentrations of both IL-1 and TNF-α resulted in an additive effect on the accumulation of GM-CSF mRNA. G-CSF mRNA was similarly induced in ECs by IL-1 and TNF-α. M-CSF (CSF-1) mRNA was more quickly induced in ECs by IL-1 and TNF-α, and was of comparable intensity at 4 and 28 hours. An additive effect of the two cytokines was observed on the accumulation of G-CSF, M-CSF, and GM-CSF. The authors believe that the two cytokines act via different pathways in the induction of GM-CSF mRNA accumulation by ECs. The same authors also found, in their assessment of the rate of transcription of the GM-CSF gene by nuclear run-on experiments, that both IL-1 and TNF-α increased the rate of GM-CSF, G-CSF, and M-CSF gene transcription to a varying degree.

In contrast to GM-CSF and G-CSF mRNA and M-CSF protein have been shown to be constitutively produced in cultured mesenchymal cells, including human umbilical vein ECs (Sieff et al., 1988). IL-3, another hematopoietic growth factor, was not detected in any of these mesenchymal cells.

Interestingly, the induction of GM-CSF transcription by IL-1 in human umbilical vein ECs seems to be different from that in fibroblasts. Bagby et al. (1989) have assessed the activity of transcription by GM-CSF gene in cultured fibroblasts by DNase I hypersensitivity analysis. Their results suggested that GM-CSF transcription was not induced by IL-1, supporting the notion that GM-CSF gene transcription in bone marrow cells is constitutive. They found that the accumulation of GM-CSF mRNA in IL-1-stimulated cells mainly resulted from prolonged survival of mRNA of the gene, namely, posttranscriptional control being a major factor for the change in mRNA levels. In their opinion it seemed likely that IL-1 stabilized RNA by inducing inhibitors of ribonuclease. Relevant to this notion is the study by Malone et al. (1988), who found that rat microvascular ECs cultured in serum-free medium produced a substantial amount of GM-CSF and expressed GM-CSF mRNA at a high level. These findings present a contrast to the results of previous studies in which large-vessel ECs were used. Though it has not been examined whether IL-1 or TNF increases the accumulation of GM-CSF mRNA in microvascular ECs, the results suggest that a mechanism of GM-CSF gene expression similar to that seen in fibroblasts is operative in microvascular ECs, in contrast to hematopoietic progenitor cells in the bone marrow.

4. IL-6

IL-6 is a pleiotropic lymphokine originally known by various names, such as IFN-β2 (Weissenbach et al., 1980; Sehgal and Sagar, 1980), B-cell-stimulating factor 2 (Hirano et al., 1986), hepatocyte-stimulating factor (Gauldie et al., 1987), and hybridoma/plasmacytoma growth factor (Aarden et al., 1985). Three groups have independently succeeded in cloning the IL-6 gene (Zilberstein et al., 1986; Haegeman et al., 1986; Hirano et al., 1986). We now know that various cell types, including vascular ECs, can produce IL-6.

Astaldi et al. (1980) first reported that a growth factor for hybridomas was present in the conditioned medium used in culturing ECs. Sironi et al. (1989) examined a hybridoma growth factor activity in the supernatants of human umbilical vein ECs. They found that ECs produce hybridoma growth factor in the absence of stimulation and that IL-1 increases the release of the growth factor by these cells. The identification of the hybridoma growth factor as IL-6 was confirmed with anti-IL-6 antibodies. Enhanced IL-6 activity released from IL-1-stimulated ECs was associated with increased IL-6 mRNA expression.

Podor et al. (1988) have assessed the effect of several cytokines on the secretion of IL-6 from cultured human umbilical vein ECs. ECs were stimulated with cytokines, and IL-6 activity in 48-hour supernatants was tested by the hybridoma growth factor assay. IL-1β and TNF-α significantly increased the production of IL-6 from ECs up to levels greater than 200 pg/ml. TNF-β was a much weaker IL-6 inducer than TNF-α. They also observed that IFN-γ was a potent stimulus for IL-6 secretion by human ECs. Enhanced secretion of IL-6 from IL-1- or TNF-α-stimulated human vascular ECs has been confirmed by several other groups (Shalaby et al., 1989; May et al., 1989; Mawatari et al., 1989).

In contrast to the results of Podor et al. (1988), two groups (Shalaby et al., 1989; Loppnow and Libby, 1989) did not find an increase of IL-6 production by human ECs treated with IFN-γ alone, though they observed that significantly greater quantities of IL-6 were produced by ECs treated with IFN-γ together with TNF-α. Addition of TGF-β to EC cultures resulted in a dose-related inhibition of IL-1β- and TNF-α-induced IL-6 production by ECs (Shalaby et al., 1989).

Ray et al. (1988a) examined the molecular mechanism by which IL-6 gene expression is regulated. The activation by cytokines, viruses, and second messenger agonists, such as PMA and forskolin, of the IL-6 promoter linked to the bacterial chloramphenicol acetyltransferase (CAT) gene was studied after transfection of the plasmids into HeLa cells. Ray et al. (1988a) found that 5′-flanking sequences of IL-6 DNA between −225 and +13 from the transcription start site mediate the responsiveness of the promoter to exogenous signals such as cytokines and viruses. Deletion of IL-6 DNA from −225 to −112 led to a marked decrease in the ability of all of the inducers to activate the chimeric gene. Therefore, the 113-nucleotide portion in the 5′-flanking region of IL-6 DNA appears to be involved in regulating the expression of the cytokine.

The same investigators have examined the similarity of the nucleotide sequence in the 5′-flanking region of the human IL-6 gene to the nucleotide sequence of the growth-factor-responsive enhancer element in the human c-fos gene (Ray et al., 1988b). There was a striking similarity in the human c-fos enhancer element and the IL-6 gene in the region between residues −169 to −124. A 70% nucleotide sequence identity across a 50-nucleotide long stretch of the c-fos enhancer was observed. In another report, Ray et al. stated that there are similarities in the regulation of expression of the human IL-6 and the c-fos genes: both are induced by a number of identical agents, including TNF, IL-1, PMA, serum, EGF, and Sendai virus (Ray et al., 1988b). They raise the possibility that the agents that turn on the c-fos gene automatically also turn off IL-6 gene transcription through the similar DNA regulatory elements, suggesting thereby that some transcription factors regulating the expression of both genes are identical.

5. IL-8 and Melanoma Growth Stimulatory Activity

A novel polypeptide chemotactic factor produced by LPS-activated monocytes has been described by several investigators (Yoshimura et al., 1987; Schröder et al., 1987; Walz et al., 1987). Matsushima et al. (1988) recently purified the polypeptide chemotactic factor and succeeded in molecular cloning. The molecular weight determined by SDS–PAGE of purified material is approximately 8000, which is consistent with a calculated molecular weight of 8000 (72 amino acids) as deduced from cDNA of the monocyte-derived neutrophil chemotactic factor. This factor seems to belong to the category of inflammatory cytokines and was named IL-8 at the International Symposium on Novel Neutrophil Stimulating Peptides (December, 9, 1988, London).

Small amounts of IL-8 mRNA are detectable in unstimulated human peripheral blood mononuclear cells, but mRNA levels of IL-8 increase within 1 hour and reach maximal levels at 3 hours, persisting as long as 16 hours after stimulation with LPS. Both IL-1 and TNF induce similarly high levels of IL-8 mRNA (Matsushima *et al.*, 1988). Strieter *et al.* (1989) have reported that human umbilical vein ECs are also able to produce monocyte-derived neutrophil chemotactic factor (IL-8) in response to TNF-α, IL-1β, and LPS stimulation. They demonstrated that the chemotactic factor produced by LPS-stimulated ECs was IL-8 based on the following results: concomitant induction of IL-8 mRNA, similar molecular weights of the chemotactic factor and of IL-8, and chemotactic activity characteristic of IL-8 for neutrophils, but not for monocytes. IL-8 mRNA was induced within 1 hour after stimulation and peaked between 4 and 8 hours of stimulation.

A recently isolated factor that stimulates the proliferation of melanoma cells, named melanoma growth stimulatory activity (MGSA), has recently been cloned and found to be identical to a growth-regulated gene product (gro) in transformed cells (Anisowicz *et al.*, 1988). The gro mRNA was initially detected as mRNA that was elevated in several tumor cell lines and could be transiently induced in certain normal cells by serum (Anisowicz *et al.*, 1987). At present, no other functions except stimulatory activity for melanoma cells have been assigned to the products of the "gro" gene. However, elucidation of its sequence has demonstrated that the MGSA/gro protein is structurally related to various factors, including IL-8 (Matsushima *et al.*, 1988). Other factors related to MGSA/gro are platelet factor 4 and platelet basic protein, which is proteolytically processed into β-thromboglobulin and connective-tissue-activating peptide 3 (CTP-III).

Recently, Wen *et al.* (1989) have reported that human umbilical vein ECs are capable of producing MGSA/gro. The mRNA expression and release of MGSA/gro are strongly induced by IL-1, TNF, LPS, and thrombin. Furthermore, addition of MGSA to EC cultures induces MGSA/gro expression, which is evidence for the expression of the receptor on ECs and the presence of the autocrine mechanism for the factor. Wen *et al.* (1989) suggested the possibility that the protein encoded by the MGSA/gro gene plays a role in inflammatory responses and exerts its effect on ECs in an autocrine fashion. The findings that MGSA/gro and IL-8 are structurally related and that their expression is induced in ECs by similar stimuli put this suggestion within the bounds of probability.

6. *Common Nucleotide Sequences in 3'-Untranslated Regions of mRNA for Cytokine-Induced Genes in Endothelial Cells*

Caput *et al.* (1986) have identified a consensus sequence (UUAUUUAU) in the 3'-untranslated region of both human and mouse TNF mRNA, as well as in mRNAs for human lymphotoxin (TNF-β), human CSF, human and mouse IL-1α and IL-1β, human and rat fibronectin, and most of the sequenced human and mouse IFNs. Because this consensus sequence in the 3'-untranslated region of mammalian mRNA is uncommon, they consider that it may serve a specific regulatory function in the mRNA in which it is found. They also indicate that the genes containing the consensus sequence in their mRNA are related to the inflammatory responses.

Shaw and Kamen (1986) have examined the function of the AU-rich sequences in 3'-untranslated regions of a human cytokine gene mRNA, GM-CSF mRNA. They constructed chimeric plasmids containing a 51-nucleotide AT-rich sequence of the 3'-untranslated region of cytokine cDNA ligated to the rabbit β-globin gene and transfected the plasmids into NIH3T3 cells. Their results revealed that insertion of the AT-rich sequence, identical to that found in the human GM-CSF cDNA, into the 3'-untranslated region of the β-globin gene reduced the accumulation of mRNA to approximately 3% of wild-type levels. Analysis of the transcription rates of the β-globin gene containing the insertion of the AT-rich sequence and of the control β-globin gene by a nuclear run-on assay indicated that both genes were transcribed at equivalent rates. In addition, studies of decay rates of both mRNAs, in the cells after treatment with actinomycin D revealed that the β-globin mRNA containing AU-rich sequences decayed much more quickly. Shaw and Kamen (1986) proposed from these results that the AU sequences are the recognition signal for an mRNA processing pathway in which the mRNA for certain cytokines and protooncogenes is specifically degraded.

The principal cause of instability of the mRNAs containing AU-rich sequences appears to be related to their content of the UpA dinucleotide (Beutler et al., 1989). Moreover, Kruys et al. (1989) recently reported that the AU-rich sequence decreases the translational efficiency. The levels of translation inhibition increased with the copy number of the AU-rich consensus sequence (AUUUA). IL-1- and TNF-inducible cytokine genes containing the consensus AU-rich sequences in their 3'-untranslated regions of mRNA by vascular ECs are listed in Fig. 6.

E. Protooncogene Expression

The cellular protooncogenes, c-*fos* and c-*myc*, are rapidly induced by growth factors or mitogens in various normal cells, suggesting that these genes play an important role in the control of cell proliferation and differentiation (Kelly et al., 1983; Greenberg and Ziff, 1984; Müller et al., 1984). The inhibitory effect of TGF-β on the growth of vascular ECs has been described by several investigators (Fràter-Schröder et al., 1986; Heimark et al., 1986; Baird and Durkin, 1986). Using a rat heart EC culture system, Takehara et al. (1987) further examined the effect of EGF and TGF-β on the expression of

Human IL-1α	UUUAAUUAUU<u>AUUUA</u>UAU<u>AUGUA</u><u>UUUA</u>UAAAU<u>AUUUA</u>AAGA
Human IL-1β	UUCCCU<u>AUUU</u><u>AUUU</u><u>AUUU</u><u>AUUU</u>AUUUGUU
Human GM-CSF	UAAU<u>AUUU</u>AUA<u>UAUUU</u>A<u>UAUUUU</u>UAAAAU<u>AUUU</u><u>AUUU</u><u>AUUU</u><u>AUUU</u>AA
Human G-GSF	U<u>AUUU</u>AUCUCU<u>AUUU</u>AAU<u>AUUU</u>AUGUCU<u>AUUU</u>AA
C-SIS (PDGF-B)	CCUUUU<u>AUUUUU</u>AAAUGUAAA<u>AUUU</u><u>AUUU</u>AUAUUUCGU<u>AUUU</u>AAA
Human IL-6	GGUUUUAAUAUUUUU<u>AAUUU</u>AUUAA<u>UAUUU</u>AAAUAUGUGAAGCUGAGUU<u>AAUUU</u>AUGUAAGUC<u>AUAUUU</u>AUAUUU
MDNCF (IL-8)	UAAAGU<u>AUUA</u><u>UUUA</u>UUUGAAUCUACAAAAAACAA
MGSA/gro	CU<u>AUUU</u><u>AUUU</u>AUGU<u>AUUU</u><u>AUUU</u>AUUUCA

FIG. 6. The AU-rich sequences found in the 3′-untranslated region of cytokine genes inducible in human umbilical vein ECs. The motif (AUUUA) common to all mRNAs is underlined. References: IL-1α (March et al., 1985); IL-1β (Auron et al., 1984); GM-CSF (Wong et al., 1985); G-CSF (Nagata et al., 1986); c-sis (Ratner et al., 1985); IL-6 (Hirano et al., 1986); MDNCF (Matsushima et al., 1988); MGSA/gro (Anisowicz et al., 1988).

c-fos and c-myc genes in ECs. Addition of optimal concentrations of EGF to confluent growth-arrested monolayers of rat heart ECs stimulated both DNA synthesis and cell division, whereas TGF-β-treated ECs did not respond to EGF as assayed by either DNA synthesis or cell division. Furthermore, the treatment of confluent rat heart ECs with EGF was found to induce the expression of both c-fos and c-myc. Very low levels of c-fos and easily detectable levels of c-myc mRNA are present in the growth-arrested ECs. The levels of expression of both genes after exposure of confluent ECs to EGF were similar to those described in 3T3 fibroblasts treated with PDGF or serum (Kelly et al., 1983; Greenberg and Ziff, 1984). After stimulation with EGF, the levels of c-fos mRNA increased within 30 minutes and then decreased to control levels within 2 hours, whereas the c-myc mRNA levels rose more slowly and remained at a maximal level from 2 to 6 hours after exposure to EGF. They have found that the maximal level of induction of c-fos is 20-fold and that of c-myc is 5-fold over baseline. Furthermore, these investigators have assessed the effect of TGF-β treatment on the EGF induction of c-fos and c-myc. In the confluent cultures of rat heart ECs pretreated with TGF-β for 24 hours, the absolute level of c-myc expression in both EGF-induced and noninduced ECs was approximately one-sixth of the cells without pretreatment with TGF-β. In contrast, TGF-β pretreatment of ECs had little effect on the EGF induction of c-fos. From these results, Takehara et al. (1987) proposed that TGF-β blocks the proliferation of ECs in the early phase of G_1; some of the earliest changes in gene expression (e.g., c-fos) occur in a normal fashion, whereas others, such as c-myc induction, are suppressed.

Colotta et al. (1988) have reported that IL-1 and TNF-α induce c-fos mRNA in cultured human umbilical vein ECs. The c-fos mRNA was not detectable in confluent human umbilical vein ECs and even in the cells treated with cycloheximide, an agent known to superinduce expression of this protooncogene primarily via stabilization of mRNA (Mitchell et al., 1985). However, exposure of ECs to both IL-1 and TNF-α in the presence of cycloheximide induced a substantial accumulation of c-fos mRNA. In contrast, c-fos transcripts were not easily detectable in the absence of cycloheximide in the cultures to which the cytokines had been added. IFN-γ did not induce a detectable accumulation of c-fos mRNA in the presence or absence of cycloheximide.

Dixit et al. (1989) have recently reported that c-jun mRNA is induced in human umbilical vein ECs by stimulation with TNF-α. Untreated ECs contain barely detectable levels of c-jun mRNA but the addition of TNF-α causes a 5- to 10-fold increase in the mRNA levels within 30 minutes. This high level of expression persists for up to 4 hours following addition of TNF-α. The degree and kinetics of induction of c-jun expression are equivalent to those seen during the G_0/G_1 transition of growth-factor-treated fibroblasts (Angel et al., 1988; Ryseck et al., 1988). The two different sizes of transcripts, estimated at 2.6 and 3.2 kb, respectively, are similar to those in stimulated fibroblasts (Angel et al., 1988) and appear to be coordinately regulated. IL-1 has been also shown to induce c-jun mRNA in ECs. In contrast, they could not detect c-myc and c-fos mRNA induction in TNF-α-treated ECs without cycloheximide, a finding compatible with the results of Colotta et al. (1988). Many of the TNF-induced responses of ECs, according to the view of Colotta et al., may be at least indirect results of AP-1/c-jun-mediated de novo transcriptional activation.

AP-1 was first identified as a transcription factor required for optimal activity of the human metallothionein gene promoter in vitro and in vivo (Lee et al., 1987; Karin et al., 1987). Then, it has been shown that AP-1 also mediates the induction of various cellular genes in response to serum, growth factors, and 12-O-tetradecanoylphorbol-13-acetate (TPA), a potent activator of protein kinase C (Angel et al., 1987; Lee et al., 1987; Imler et al., 1988). AP-1 accomplishes this activity by modulating the transcription of genes having the consensus octanucleotide sequence, namely, TGAGTCAG, in their promoter/enhancer region (Angel et al., 1987; Bohmann et al., 1987).

A number of recent experiments indicate that AP-1 is not a single protein, but a complex composed of the jun and fos genes. Landschulz et al. (1988) have found that various nuclear oncogene products and transcription factors such as those of myc, fos, and jun genes have a sequence motif that contains four to five leucines at every seventh position. These investigators suggest that leucine side chains that extend from one side of the α-helix of a polypeptide may interdigitate with other leucine side chains extending from the helix of another polypeptide. In fact, the "leucine zipper" region in jun and fos proteins allows dimerization among jun gene family proteins (homodimers and heterodimers) as well as among *jun* gene family proteins and *fos* gene family proteins via parallel interactions of the zipper regions (Gentz *et al.*, 1989). It has been demonstrated that jun homodimers are able to bind to the AP-1/*jun* DNA recognition sequence (TPA-responsive element, or TRE) and stimulate transcription, properties that have been found to be significantly enhanced by the cooperative formation of heterodimers between jun and the fos protein family, e.g., of c-fos and Fra-1 (Chiu *et al.*, 1988; Cohen *et al.*, 1989).

It has been demonstrated that AP-1 plays a role in gene activation by TNF-α (Brenner *et al.*, 1989) and by IL-1 (Muegge *et al.*, 1989). It is well known that addition of TNF-α to confluent human fibroblasts causes specific induction of collagenase mRNA. Brenner *et al.* (1989) have investigated the mechanism by which TNF-α activates the collagenase gene. Chimeric plasmids containing segments of the collagenase 5'-flanking region ligated to the chloramphenicol transferase gene were used to identify the TNF-α-responsive cis-acting element and were transfected in Hep G_2 cells. Brenner *et al.* (1989) found that the TPA-responsive element of the collagenase gene, through its function as a binding site for transcription factor AP-1, is necessary for the expression of the constructed gene by TNF-α. In addition, treatment of fibroblasts with TNF-α results in prolonged induction of c-*jun* mRNA lasting at least 6 hours. The induction of c-*jun* mRNA by TNF-α does not seem to require *de novo* protein synthesis, as it is not blocked by cycloheximide. TNF-α or TPA, moreover, elicits a rapid and transient induction of c-*fos* mRNA. Therefore, TNF-α stimulates the expression of both *fos* and *jun* genes, whose products interact and stimulate transcription of AP-1-responsive genes. Because the protein kinase C inhibitor, H7, inhibits the induction of collagenase mRNA by TPA and TNF-α, Brenner and co-workers have concluded that TNF-α, like TPA, activates protein kinase C, which in turn may result in increased AP-1 activity and induction of AP-1-responsive genes.

Muegge *et al.* (1989) have studied an IL-1-responsive element in the promoter region of the human IL-2 gene by transfection of chimeric genes containing the 5'-flanking region of the human IL-2 gene linked to the CAT gene into a mouse T lymphoma cell line, LBRM. They have found that the deletion of sequences −218 to −176 upstream of the transcription start site abrogates the IL-1 effect, indicating the presence of an IL-1-responsive element in this region. Position −185 has the sequence TCAGTCAG, which is similar to the motif TGAGTCAG of the AP-1-binding region. In fact, Muegge *et al.* have found that the nuclear factors induced by IL-1 and phytohemagglutinin (PHA) in the transfectants bind specifically to the AP-1-binding region-like sequence. The c-fos and c-jun mRNA are also induced without *de novo* protein synthesis in the LBRM cells by IL-1 and PHA. These findings suggest that many cellular functions induced by IL-1 and TNF-α may be mediated through AP-1.

Recently, Goldgaber *et al.* (1989) demonstrated that IL-1 upregulates the amyloid β-protein precursor (APP) gene expression through the pathway mediated by protein kinase C, utilizing the upstream AP-1-binding site of the APP gene promoter in human umbilical vein ECs. They have found that IL-1 and TPA induce a three- to fourfold increase in the level of APP mRNA transcripts in confluent monolayers of ECs. The increase in the level of APP mRNA with treatment of IL-1 is blocked by the protein kinase C inhibitor, H7, indicating that the effect of IL-1 on the level of APP mRNA is mediated by protein kinase C. To map the APP promoter-active region responsive to the induction of IL-1, a variety of the APP promoter fragments were linked to human growth hormone (hGH) cDNA, and each of the constructs was transfected into a mouse neuroblastoma cell line. The results suggested that IL-1 could induce hGH gene expression driven by the APP promoter and that the removal of the 180-bp fragment containing the upstream AP-1-binding site eliminated the induction of the reporter hGH gene by IL-1.

IL-1 and TNF-α induce c-jun in ECs (Dixit *et al.*, 1989). Therefore, it is highly probable that the transcription factor AP-1 that is induced by IL-1 in turn activates the promoter of the APP gene by binding to the AP-1-binding site (TPA-responsive element) in human ECs. A variety of activities of IL-1 and TNF-α on ECs may utilize the AP-1 factor in the activation of genes.

F. ENDOTHELIN

A novel vasoconstrictive peptide, endothelin, isolated and cloned by Yanagisawa *et al.* (1988), has recently attracted considerable interest. The number of articles devoted to the biology and pharmacology of endothelin has increased dramatically in the past year. Recent studies have shown that there may be three distinct members of an endothelin family, endothelin 1, endothelin 2, and endothelin 3, which may exert different profiles of biological functions possibly through action on distinct subtypes of endothelin receptors with different relative affinities (Yanagisawa and Masaki, 1989).

Endothelin 1 provokes a strong and sustained constrictive response in isolated vascular smooth muscle preparations. Vascular effects of endothelin 1 also include the stimulation of release of prostaglandins and endothelium-derived relaxing factor (EDRF) from perfused vascular beds (de Nucci *et al.*, 1988). Various extravascular activities of endothelin 1 include constriction of nonvascular smooth muscle cells such as airway, intestine, and uterus (Wright and Fozard, 1988; Lagente *et al.*, 1989; Kozuka *et al.*, 1989); a positive inotropic and chronotropic action (Ishikawa *et al.*, 1988; Fukuda *et al.*, 1988); and mitogenic actions on cultured vascular smooth muscle cells, mesangial cells, and Swiss 3T3 fibroblasts (Komuro *et al.*, 1989; Takuwa *et al.*, 1989).

The structure of the human endothelial 1 gene has been studied by Inoue et al. (1989). The 5'-flanking region of the gene contains octanucleotide sequences very similar to the AP-1/jun-binding element. When confluent monolayers of human ECs are stimulated with phorbol esters, endothelin 1 mRNA is quickly induced, suggesting the possibility that the human endothelin 1 gene is directly regulated by intracellular signaling mediated by protein kinase C via the trans-acting transcription factor AP-1. The 5'-flanking region of the gene also contains the consensus motifs for the binding site of nuclear factor 1, which mediates the responsiveness to TGF-β and hexanucleotide sequence for the acute-phase reactant regulator element that may be involved in the induction of endothelin 1 in response to acute physical stress *in vivo*. The 3'-untranslated region of endothelin 1 mRNA contains three AUUUA motifs that are found in various cytokines-inducible genes. These structural studies of the endothelin gene suggest that synthesis and release of endothelin from vascular EC may be regulated by various inflammatory mediators.

Regulation of endothelin gene expression by various agents has been studied by several groups. Yanagisawa *et al.* (1988) first reported the induction of endothelin mRNA in porcine aortic EC by thrombin, Ca ionophore, and epinephrine. Kurihara *et al.* (1989) have found that TGF-β1 stimulates the expression of endothelin mRNA in porcine aortic ECs. The mRNA levels of an endothelin gene increased within 1 hour following the addition of TGF-β1 and reached maximal levels at 2 hours. It remains to be determined whether the induction of nuclear factor 1 by TGF-β1 is involved in this response. The TGF-β1-induced expression of endothelin mRNA was associated with an increased synthesis and secretion of endothelin peptide from ECs. Expression of c-*sis* and production of PDGF-like proteins in ECs were also stimulated by thrombin and TGF-β. The investigators suggest that the production of PDGF and endothelin may be enhanced by the same stimulants in the process of thrombus formation and that these mediators may cooperatively cause smooth muscle proliferation in the vascular walls contributing to the development of atherosclerosis.

Recently, endotoxin has been shown to stimulate the release of endothelin *in vivo* and *in vitro* (Sugiura *et al.*, 1989). The level of immunoreactive endothelin in serum obtained from rats infused with endotoxin is increased more than 50 times compared with control rats. They have also observed a significant stimulation of endothelin release by endotoxin from cultured bovine transformed aortic ECs. In relation to this finding, Yoshizumi *et al.* (1990) reported enhanced expression of endothelin gene by IL-1-stimulated cultured procine ECs. Induction of endothelin mRNA started within 1 hour after exposure to IL-1α, peaked at 4 hours and again at 24 hours, and was followed by a decline thereafter. A similar profile of mRNA induction was observed by IL-1β-treated ECs, though IL-1α was a more potent inducer of endothelin mRNA. Immunoreactive endothelin in the culture medium also increased to nearly twice the levels in untreated culture medium 24 hours after stimulation. IL-1-induced activation of the endothelin gene was not unexpected, because the endothelin gene contains AP-1-binding sites in its promoter region, and the 3'-untranslated region of the mRNA has AUUUA motifs that are found in many cytokine-induced genes. It has not been determined yet whether IL-1-induced activation of this gene is mediated by the induction of the transcription factor AP-1, similar to IL-1-induced expression of the amyloid β-protein precursor mRNA in ECs (Goldgaber *et al.*, 1989). These observations, however, raise the important possibility that release of endothelin may be regulated by various inflammatory mediators and that this vasoconstrictive peptide may participate in the pathogenesis of inflammatory vascular disorders.

IV. Endothelial Gene Expression in *in Vivo* and *in Situ* Hybridization

Whereas most of the studies examining effects of cytokines on vascular ECs have used cultured ECs, studies of the expression of cytokines or cytokine-related genes in pathological sites may help elucidate the roles of cytokines and ECs in the pathogenesis of certain vascular diseases, such as atherosclerosis and vasculitis. The roles of PDGF genes in the pathogenesis of atherosclerosis have been studied mainly by the latter methodologic approach.

Barrett *et al.* (1984) first reported the expression of PDGF-B chain mRNA in freshly isolated human umbilical vein ECs and bovine aortic ECs and found that the levels of mRNA expression in ECs of these vessels were much less than those in cultured vascular ECs. Barrett *et al.* considered that low-level expression of the PDGF-B chain gene by bovine aortic endothelium *in vivo* may be necessary for maintenance of the integrity of vessel walls. A variety of cells, including macrophages, ECs, and arterial smooth muscle cells, can produce PDGF at least *in vitro*. Because cells of the same types are found in human atherosclerotic plaques, the so-called PDGF hypothesis for atherogenesis initially propounded by Ross has been modified to include the possible production of PDGF within the developing sites (Ross *et al.*, 1986).

Barrett and Benditt (1987) have demonstrated by Northern blots that c-*sis* (PDGF-B chain) transcript levels are higher in human carotid plaques removed at surgery than in normal artery walls. The same investigators (Barrett and Benditt, 1988) have further explored the expression of PDGF-A and -B chain genes in atherosclerotic plaques and tried to identify the transcriptionally active cell type. They quantitated PDGF-A and PDGF-B mRNA levels in dissected fractions derived from carotid atherosclerotic plaques and normal artery, and subsequently rehybridized these blots with three cDNA probes that could recognize cell type-specific markers: the *fms* gene for macrophages, the von Willebrand factor gene for ECs, and the smooth muscle actin gene for smooth muscle cells. In plaques, PDGF-A mRNA expression correlated well with smooth muscle actin mRNA, suggesting a major contribution of smooth muscle cells to the expression of the PDGF-A chain gene. Likewise, PDGF-B mRNA strongly correlated with *fms* mRNA, suggesting a major contribution of macrophages to the expression of PDGF-B mRNA. Furthermore, a minor fraction of PDGF-B mRNA appeared to be correlated with von Willebrand factor mRNA, supporting a possible contribution of ECs to the expression of PDGF-B mRNA.

Though the studies just discussed suggest relative contributions of respective cell types to the expression of PDGF genes in atherosclerotic plaques, *in situ* hybridization techniques may be a more direct method to identify the cell types expressing these genes in normal and pathologic tissues.

Wilcox et al. (1988) have examined mRNA of PDGF and PDGF receptor genes in human atherosclerotic plaques by *in situ* hybridization. By autoradiographic intensity, PDGF-B chain hybridization was most intense among the endothelial-appearing cells of plaques capillaries, and the largest number of cells positively hybridized to B and A chain gene probes were noncapillary, mesenchymal-appearing intimal cells. Some of the latter cells had the light microscopic appearance of smooth muscle cells. In contrast, macrophages, identified as either foam cells or hemosiderin-containing cells, did not appear to be a major site of PDGF mRNA biosynthesis in the plaques. Furthermore, many cells with morphologic features of mesenchymal cells that were positive for PDGF-A and -B mRNA in the intima of the plaques expressed PDGF receptor mRNA. No lymphocyte-like cells, no endothelial-like cells, and almost no foam cells or hemosiderin-containing cells were positive for PDGF receptor mRNA. In a separate study, they also detected PDGF-B chain mRNA in ECs of normal internal mammary arteries, whereas there was little hybridization to the PDGF-A chain probe and the PDGF receptor gene probe. These *in situ* hybridization studies demonstrate that human artery endothelium normally expresses the PDGF-B chain gene, which may be induced to increase its expression in certain vascular diseases, e.g., in atherosclerosis. It is not clear whether cytokines actually participate in *in vivo* induction of PDGF genes in ECs, but this possibility clearly deserves further study because transcripts of IL-1 and TNF can be detected in atherosclerotic lesions (Barrett and Benditt, 1987).

At least, most macrovessel ECs are devoid of receptors for PDGF, whereas some microvessel ECs appear to express PDGF receptors. Hermansson et al. (1988) have examined the expression of PDGF genes and the PDGF receptor gene in biopsy specimens from human glioma by *in situ* hybridization and

Northern blots. Hyperplasia of the vascular endothelium is a prominent characteristic of human glioblastoma multiforme. The *in situ* hybridization technique has revealed that the proliferating vascular ECs contain large quantities of mRNA for the PDGF-B chain and its receptor (B-type receptor), and small quantities of mRNA for the PDGF-A chain. The glioblastoma cells, in contrast, express more PDGF-A chain mRNA than PDGF-B chain mRNA and its receptor gene. This finding suggests the possibility that ECs, especially those of capillary origin, may be able to express PDGF receptors in certain conditions and may become targets of PDGF-like growth factors through autocrine and paracrine routes. The meaning of the expression of the PDGF receptor on some kinds of ECs will be evaluated by establishment of cultured ECs expressing the receptor. A recent study (Bar *et al.*, 1989) has described that two types of cultured microvessel ECs can bind PDGF and respond to the growth factor. *In situ* hybridization studies of the expression of other cytokine genes in blood vessels will be critically important for elucidating the roles of interactions between endothelium and cytokines at molecular levels in the pathogenesis of various vascular disorders, including atherosclerosis and vasculitis.

V. Future Directions of Research

Most of the studies examining EC functions have utilized cultured ECs monolayered on gelatin-coated plastic plates. ECs cultured under such conditions are, however, considered to have features similar to those of injured ECs in pathological vascular lesions, such as in atherosclerosis. In line with this view are the findings of enhanced expression in cultured ECs of several genes, including c-*sis* and endothelin genes, which are much less expressed, if at all, in normal vascular endothelium.

Microvascular ECs as well as large-vessel ECs have the ability to differentiate spontaneously and form capillary-like structures (Folkman and Haudenschild, 1980). When ECs are cultured on several extracellular components, including laminin and collagen IV, they rapidly align and form a hollow tubelike structure. Cells differentiating on such an extracellular matrix may be regarded as more physiological than cells cultured on plastic plates, hence the use of these materials is probably more desirable.

Studies of gene expression in ECs that have differentiated *in vitro* may be important, but further technological improvements should be stressed. For these studies, it will be necessary to pursue the development of techniques to isolate intact cells from a gel matrix and the method to detect the mRNA of specific genes in trace amounts of RNA extracted from limited numbers of ECs.

Recently, Rappolee et al. (1988) reported the expression of TGF-α, TGF-β, and PDGF-A genes in a small number of macrophages (about 100 cells) isolated from a wound with the aid of the polymerase chain reaction (PCR) combined with reverse transcription of macrophage RNA. With this method we are able to compare the relative levels of mRNA expression of several genes in one assay, an advantage over the Northern blot. It has been difficult to assess the changes of mRNA levels of various genes in ECs induced by a cytokine, but such a study may be feasible with the use of the PCR combined with reverse transcription of endothelial RNA.

In spite of countless studies investigating functions induced by cytokines, regulatory mechanisms of cytokine effects on vascular endothelium *in vivo* are still obscure. A number of regulatory proteins that modulate the effects of cytokines have been reported to be present in blood and to be produced by a variety of cells, including ECs (Larrick, 1989). Some of the factors may inhibit effects of cytokines on the vascular endothelium and some may potentiate cytokine functions.

An important group of cytokine regulatory substances consists of IL-1 inhibitors in blood and other body fluids. We have recently reported the presence of neutralizing anti-IL-1α autoantibodies in some sera from patients with rheumatoid arthritis (Suzuki et al., 1989b). IL-1 is regarded as one of the important factors in the pathogenesis of rheumatoid synovitis. The anti-IL-1α antibodies not only blocked IL-1α-induced IL-1β mRNA induction by human umbilical vein ECs, but also decreased LPS-induced IL-β mRNA accumulation (Fig. 7).

Several other inhibitory factors of IL-1 activity have been reported (Rosenstreich et al., 1988; Eisenberg et al., 1990). Recently, soluble forms of cytokine receptors, including IL-2 and TNF receptors that may inhibit the action of the cytokines, have been demonstrated (Rubin et al., 1985; Engelmann et al., 1990). Soluble forms of IL-2 receptors are increased in blood of patients with certain inflammatory diseases and adult T cell leukemia. The fact that ECs produce several cytokines in a paracrine and autocrine fashion raises the possibility that these regulatory molecules present in blood and various inflammatory sites may function as modulators of cytokine activities on vascular ECs *in vivo*. Studies of these regulatory factors are highly relevant to investigations of pathophysiological aspects of the interaction between cytokines and vascular ECs *in vivo*.

Though *in vivo* models such as rabbit corneal pocket assays for studying the process of neovascularization have been developed and widely used for the assay of angiogenic activity, further improvement of *in vivo* experimental systems for assessing EC functions will be of inestimable value. One approach may be by short-term organ cultures. Recently, Tozzi et al. (1989) reported

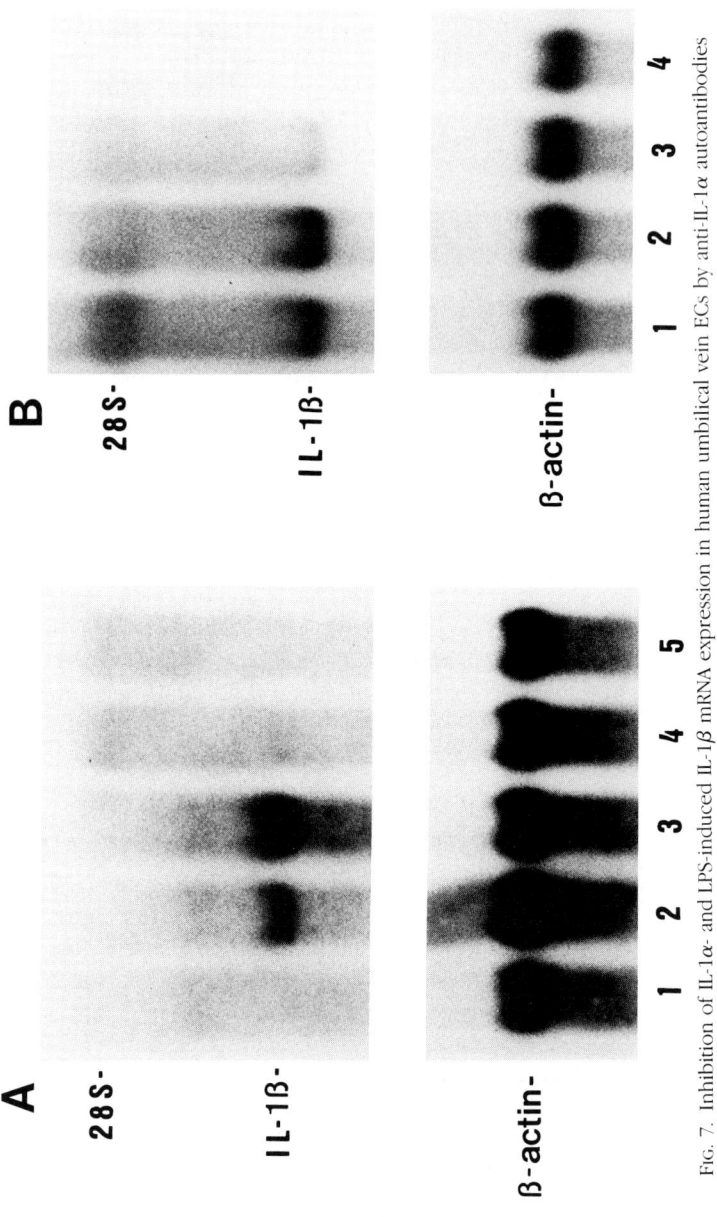

FIG. 7. Inhibition of IL-1α- and LPS-induced IL-1β mRNA expression in human umbilical vein ECs by anti-IL-1α autoantibodies from two patients with rheumatoid arthritis (RA). (A) IL-1β mRNA expression in ECs after 6 hours of treatment with IL-1α (5 U/ml) in the presence (10%) of normal serum #1 (lane 2), normal serum #2 (lane 3), patient serum #1 (lane 4), or patient serum #2 (lane 5). Both sera from patients with RA contain high titers of anti-IL-1α autoantibodies. (B) IL-1β mRNA expression in ECs after 6 hours of treatment with IL-1α (5 U/ml) (lanes 2 and 4) or LPS (10 μg/ml) (lanes 1 and 3) in the presence (10%) of normal serum #1 (lanes 1 and 2) or patient serum #1 (lanes 3 and 4).

pressure-induced, endothelium-dependent expression of pro α1(I) collagen and c-sis (PDGF-B chain) genes in intact vessel walls. They isolated fresh segments of large vessels (pulmonary artery, aorta, and jugular vein) from rats and incubated them in culture medium under static tension for 4 hours. They have observed that static tension induces synthesis of collagen and elastin and also induces the accumulation of pro α1(I) collagen mRNA in intact vessels. When endothelium had been removed from the isolated vessels, induction of collagen synthesis was no longer detected. Messenger RNA levels for c-sis were increased by static tension in intact but not in denuded vessels. Similar systems may be applicable to the studies of cytokine effects on vascular endothelium and may help elucidate the regulation of gene expression in the endothelium of intact blood vessels in the future.

References

Aarden, L., Lansdorp, P., and De Groot, E. (1985). *Lymphokines* **10,** 175.
Abraham, R. T., Ho, S. N., Barna, T. J., and McKean, D. J. (1987). *J. Biol. Chem.* **262,** 2719.
Acres, R. B., Larsen, A., Gillis, S., and Conlon, P. J. (1987). *Mol. Immunol.* **24,** 479.
Adams, D. O., and Hamilton, T. A. (1987). *Immunol. Rev.* **97,** 5.
Aggarwal, B. B., Eessalu, T. E., and Hass, P. E. (1985). *Nature (London)* **318,** 665.
Angel, P., Imagawa, M., Chiu, R., Stein, B., Imbra, R. J., Rahmsdorf, H. J., Jonat, C., Herrlich, P., and Karin, M. (1987). *Cell* **49,** 729.
Angel, P., Allegretto, E. A., Okino, S. T., Hattori, K., Boyle, W. J., Hunter, T., and Karin, M. (1988). *Nature (London)* **332,** 166.
Anisowicz, A., Bardwell, L., and Sager, R. (1987). *Proc. Natl. Acad. Sci, U.S.A.* **84,** 7188.
Anisowicz, A., Zajchowski, D., Stenman, G., and Sager, R. (1988). *Proc. Natl. Acad. Sci. U.S.A.* **85,** 9645.
Arfors, K. E., Lindberg, C., Lindbom, L., Lindberg, P., Beatty, P. G., and Harlan, J. M. (1987). *Blood* **69,** 338.
Arnaout, M. A., Lanier, L. L., and Faller, D. V. (1988). *J. Cell. Physiol.* **137,** 305.
Astaldi, G. C., Janssen, M. C., Lansdorp, P., Willems, W. P., Zeijlemaker, W. P., and Oosterhof, F. (1980). *J. Immunol.* **125,** 1411.
Auget, M., Dembic, Z., and Merlin, G. (1988). *Cell* **55,** 273.
Auron, P. E., Webb, A. C., Rosenwasser, L. J., Mucci, S. F., Rich, A., Wolff, S. M., and Dinarello, C. A. (1984). *Proc. Natl. Acad. Sci. U.S.A.* **81,** 7907.
Bagby, G. C., McCall, K. A., Bergstrom, K. A., and Burger, D. (1983). *Blood* **62,** 663.
Bagby, G. C., Dinarello, C. A., Wallace, P., Wagner, C., Hefeneider, S., and McCall, E. (1986). *J. Clin. Invest.* **78,** 1316.
Bagby, G. C., Shaw, G., Brown, M., and Segal, G. M. (1989). *J. Invest. Dermatol.* **93,** 48S.
Baglioni, C., McCandless, S., Tavernier, J., and Fiers, W. (1985). *J. Biol. Chem.* **260,** 13395.
Baird, A., and Durkin, T. (1986). *Biochem. Biophys. Res. Commun.* **138,** 476.
Bar, R. S., Boes, M., Booth, B. A., Dake, B. L., Henley, S., and Hart, M. N. (1989). *Endocrinology (Baltimore)* **124,** 1841.
Barrett, T. B., and Benditt, E. P. (1987). *Proc. Natl. Acad. Sci. U.S.A.* **84,** 1099.
Barrett, T. B., and Benditt, E. P. (1988). *Proc. Natl. Acad. Sci. U.S.A.* **85,** 2810.
Barrett, T. B., Gajdusek, C. M., Schwartz, S. M., McDougall, J. K., and Benditt, E. P. (1984). *Proc. Natl. Acad. Sci. U.S.A.* **81,** 6772.

Lewinsohn, D. M., Bargatze, R. F., and Butcher, E. C. (1987). *J. Immunol.* **138,** 4313.
Libby, P., Ordovas, J. M., Auger, K. R., Robbins, A. H., Birinyi, L. K., and Dinarello, C. A. (1986). *Am. J. Pathol.* **124,** 179.
Littman, S. J., Faltynek, C. R., and Baglioni, C. (1985). *J. Biol. Chem.* **260,** 1191.
Locksley, R. M., Heinzel, F. P., Shepard, H. M., Agosti, J., Eessalu, T. E., Aggarwal, B. B., and Harlan, J. M. (1987). *J. Immunol.* **139,** 1891.
Loetscher, H. L., Pan, Y-C. E., Lahm, H-W., Gentz, R., Brockhaus, M., Tabuchi, H., and Lesslauer, W. (1990). *Cell* **61,** 351.
Loppnow, H., and Libby, P. (1989). *Cell. Immunol.* **122,** 493.
Loskutoff, D. J., van Mourik, J. A., Erickson, L. A., and Lawrence, D. (1983). *Proc. Natl. Acad. Sci. U.S.A.* **80,** 2956.
Lund, L. R., Riccio, A., Andreason, P. A., Nielson, L. S., Kristensen, P., Laiho, M., Saksela, O., Blasi, F., and Dano, K. (1987). *EMBO J.* **6,** 1281.
Luscinskas, F. W., Brock, A. F., Arnaout, M. A., and Gimbrone, M. A., Jr. (1989). *J. Immunol.* **142,** 2257.
Mach, B., Gorski, J., Rollini, P., Berte, C., Amaldi, I., Berdoz, J., and Ucla, C. (1986). *Cold Spring Harbor Symp. Quant. Biol.* **51,** 67.
Magnuson, D. K., Maier, R. V., and Pohlman, T. H. (1989). *Surgery* **106,** 216.
Malone, D. G., Pierce, J. H., Falko, J. P., and Metcalfe, D. D. (1988). *Blood* **71,** 684.
Manyak, C. L., Tse, H., Fischer, P., Coker, L., Sigal, N. H., and Koo, G. C. (1988). *J. Immunol.* **140,** 3817.
March, C. J., Mosley, B., Larsen, A., Cerreti, D. P., Braedt, G., Price, V., Gillis, S., Henney, C. S., Kronheim, S. R., Grabstein, K., Conlon, P. J., Hopp, T. P., and Cosman, D. (1985). *Nature (London)* **315,** 641.
Marcum, J. A., McKenney, J. B., and Rosenberg, R. D. (1984). *J. Clin. Invest.* **74,** 341.
Markus, B. H., Colson, Y. L., Fung, J. J., Zeevi, A., and Duquesnoy, R. J. (1988). *Tissue Antigens* **32,** 241.
Marlin, S. D., and Springer, T. A. (1987). *Cell* **51,** 813.
Massaguè, J. (1985). *Trends Biochem. Sci. (Pers. Ed.)* **10,** 237.
Massaguè, J., Cheifetz, S., Endo, T., and Nadal-Ginard, B. (1986). *Proc. Natl. Acad. Sci. U.S.A.* **83,** 8206.
Mathis, D. J., Benoist, C. O., Williams, V. E., II, Kanter, M. R., and McDevitt, H. O. (1983). *Cell* **32,** 745.
Matsushima, K., Akahoshi, T., Yamada, M., Furutani, Y., and Oppenheim, J. J. (1986). *J. Immunol.* **136,** 4496.
Matsushima, K., Kobayashi, Y., Copeland, T. D., Akahoshi, T., and Oppenheim, J. J. (1987). *J. Immunol.* **139,** 3367.
Matsushima, K., Morishita, K., Yoshimura, T., Lavu, S., Kobayashi, Y., Lew, W., Appella, E., Kung, H., Leonard, E. J., and Oppenheim, J. J. (1988). *J. Exp. Med.* **167,** 1883.
Mattila, P., Häyry, P., and Renkonen, R. (1989). *FEBS Lett.* **250,** 362.
Mawatari, M., Kohno, K., Mizoguchi, H., Matsuda, T., Asoh, K., Damme, J., Welgus, H. G., and Kuwano, M. (1989). *J. Immunol.* **143,** 1619.
May, L. T., Torcia, G., Cozzolino, F., Ray, A., Tatter, S. B., Santhanam, U., Sehgal, P. B., and Stern, D. (1989). *Biochem. Biophys. Res. Commun.* **159,** 991.
McCall, E., and Bagby, G. C. (1985). *Blood* **65,** 689.
McEver, R. P., and Martin, M. N. (1984). *J. Biol. Chem.* **259,** 9799.
Miossec, F., and Ziff, M. (1986). *J. Immunol.* **137,** 2848.
Miossec, F., Cavender, D., and Ziff, M. (1986). *J. Immunol.* **136,** 2486.
Mitchell, R. L., Zokas, L., Shreiber, R. D., and Verma, I. M. (1985). *Cell* **40,** 209.

Mizel, S. B., Shirakawa, F., and Chedid, M. (1988). *Lymphokine Res.* **7**, 262.
Moncada, S., Gryglewski, R., Bunting, S., and Vane, J. R. (1976). *Nature (London)* **263**, 663.
Morrissey, J. H., Fakhari, H., and Edgington, T. S. (1987). *Cell* **50**, 129.
Muegge, K., Williams, T. M., Kant, J., Karin, M., Chiu, R., Schmidt, A., Siebenlist, U., Young, H. A., and Durum, Y. S. (1989). *Science* **246**, 249.
Müller, G., Behrens, J., Nussbaumer, U., Böhlen, P., and Birchmeier, W. (1987). *Proc. Natl. Acad. Sci. U.S.A.* **84**, 5600.
Müller, R., Bravo, R., Burchhardt, J., and Curran, T. (1984). *Nature (London)* **312**, 716.
Munker, R., Gasson, J., Ogawa, M., and Koeffler, H. P. (1986). *Nature (London)* **323**, 79.
Nachman, R. L., Hajjar, K. A., Silverstein, R. L., and Dinarello, C. A. (1986). *J. Exp. Med.* **163**, 1595.
Nagata, S., Tsuchiya, M., Asano, S., Kaziro, Y., Yamazaki, T., Yamamoto, O., Hirata, Y., Kubota, N., Oheda, M., Nomura, H., and Ono, M. (1986). *Nature (London)* **319**, 415.
Nawroth, P. P., and Stern, D. M. (1986). *J. Exp. Med.* **163**, 740.
Nawroth, P. P., Bank, I., Handley, D., Cassimeris, J., Chess, L., and Stern, D. (1986). *J. Exp. Med.* **163**, 1363.
Nishizuka, Y. (1988). *Nature (London)* **334**, 661.
Ny, T., Sawdey, M., Lawrence, D., Millan, J. L., and Loskutoff, D. J. (1986). *Proc. Natl. Acad. Sci. U.S.A.* **83**, 6776.
Palmer, D. G., Selvendran, Y., Allen, C., Revell, P. A., and Hogg, N. (1985). *Clin. Exp. Immunol.* **59**, 529.
Parslow, T. G., Blair, D. L., Murphy, W. J., and Granner, D. K. (1984). *Proc. Natl. Acad. Sci. U.S.A.* **81**, 2650.
Parslow, T. G., Blair, D. L., Murphy, W. J., and Granner, D. K. (1985). *Clin. Exp. Immunol.* **59**, 529.
Pfizenmaier, K., Scheurich, P., Schluter, C., and Kronke, M. (1987). *J. Immunol.* **138**, 975.
Philips, M., Juul, A. G., and Thorsen, S. (1984). *Biochim. Biophys. Acta* **802**, 99.
Pober, J. S., and Gimbrone, M. A., Jr. (1982). *Proc. Natl. Acad. Sci. U.S.A.* **79**, 6641.
Pober, J. S., Gimbrone, M. A., Jr., Cotran, R. S., Reiss, C. S., Burakoff, S. J., Fiers, W., and Ault, K. A. (1983). *J. Exp. Med.* **157**, 1339.
Pober, J. S., Bevilacqua, M. P., Mendrick, D. L., Lapierre, L. A., Fiers, W., and Gimbrone, M. A., Jr. (1986a). *J. Immunol.* **136**, 1680.
Pober, J. S., Gimbrone, M. A., Jr., Lapierre, L. A., Mendrick, D. L., Fiers, W., Rothlein, R., and Springer, T. A. (1986b). *J. Immunol.* **137**, 1893.
Pober, J. S., Lapierre, L. A., Stolpen, A. H., Brock, T. A., Springer, T. A., Fiers, W., Bevilacqua, M. P., Mendrick, D. L., and Gimbrone, M. A. (1987). *J. Immunol.* **138**, 3319.
Podor, T. J., Jirik, F. R., Loskutoff, D. J., Carson, D. A., and Martin, L. (1988). *Ann. N.Y. Acad. Sci.* **557**, 374.
Pohlman, T. H., Stanness, K. A., Beatty, P. G., Ochs, H. D., and Harlan, J. M. (1986). *J. Immunol.* **136**, 4548.
Poltorak, M., Sadoul, R., Keihauer, G., Landa, C., Fahrig, R., and Schachner, M. (1987). *J. Cell Biol.* **105**, 1893.
Price, T. H., Beatty, P. G., and Corpuz, S. R. (1987). *J. Immunol.* **139**, 939.
Quesenberry, P. J., and Gimbrone, M. A. (1980). *Blood* **56**, 1060.
Rappolee, D. A., Mark, D., Banda, M. J., and Werb, Z. (1988). *Science* **241**, 708.
Ratner, L., Josephs, S. F., Jarett, R., Reitz, M., and Wong-Staal, F. (1985). *Nucleic Acids Res.* **13**, 5007.
Ray, A., Tatter, S. B., May, L. T., and Sehgal, P. B. (1988a). *Proc. Natl. Acad. Sci. U.S.A.* **85**, 6701.
Ray, A., Tatter, S. B., Santhanam, U., Helfgott, D. C., May, L. T., and Sehgal, P. B. (1988b). *Ann. N.Y. Acad. Sci.* **557**, 353.
Reith, W. R., Satola, S., Sanchez, C. H., Amaldi, I., Lisowska-Grospierre, B., Griscelli, C., Hadam, M. R., and Mach, B. (1988). *Cell* **53**, 897.

Rosa, F., and Fellous, M. (1988). *J. Immunol.* **140,** 1660.
Rose, M. L., Coles, M. I., Griffin, R. J., Pomerance, A., and Yacoub, M. H. (1986). *Transplantation* **41,** 776.
Rosenberg, R. D., and Rosenberg, J. S. (1984). *J. Clin. Invest.* **74,** 1.
Rosenstreich, D. L., Tu, J. H., Kinkade, P., Maurer-Fogy, I., Kahn, J., Barton, R. W., and Farina, P. R. (1988). *J. Exp. Med.* **168,** 1767.
Rosoff, P. M., Savage, N., and Dinarello, C. A. (1988). *Cell* **54,** 73.
Ross, R., Raines, E. W., and Bowen-Pope, D. F. (1986). *Cell* **46,** 155.
Rothlein, R., Dustin, M. L., Marlin, S. D., and Springer, T. A. (1986). *J. Immunol.* **137,** 1270.
Rubin, L. A., Kurman, C. C., Fritz, M. E., Biddison, W. E., Boutin, B., Yarchoan, R., and Nelson, D. L. (1985). *J. Immunol.* **135,** 3172.
Ryseck, R.-P., Hirai, S. I., Yaniv, M., and Bravo, R. (1988). *Nature (London)* **334,** 716.
Saito, H., Maki, R. A., Clayton, L. K., and Tonegawa, S. (1983). *Proc. Natl. Acad. Sci. U.S.A.* **80,** 5520.
Sanchez-Madrid, F., Nagy, J. A., Robbins, E., Simon, P., and Springer, T. A. (1983). *J. Exp. Med.* **158,** 1785.
Sarkar, F. H., and Gupta, S. L. (1984). *Proc. Natl. Acad. Sci. U.S.A.* **81,** 5160.
Schall, T. J., Lewis, M., Koller, K. J., Lee, A., Rice, G. C., Wong, G. H. W., Gatanaga, T., Granger, G. A., Lentz, R., Raab, H., Kohr, W. J., and Goeddel, D. V. (1990). *Cell* **61,** 361.
Scheurich, P., Thoma, B., Uecer, U., and Pfizenmaier, K. (1987). *J. Immunol.* **138,** 975.
Schleef, R., Bevilacqua, M. P., Sawdey, M., Gimbrone, M. A., Jr., and Loskutoff, D. J. (1988). *J. Biol. Chem.* **263,** 5797.
Schröder, J.-M., Mrowietz, U., Morita, E., and Christophers, E. (1987). *J. Immunol.* **139,** 3474.
Seelentag, W. K., Mermod, J.-J., Montesano, R., and Vasslli, P. (1987). *EMBO J.* **6,** 2261.
Sehgal, P. B., and Sagar, A. D. (1980). *Nature (London)* **288,** 95.
Shalaby, M. R., Waage, A., and Espevik, T. (1989). *Cell. Immunol.* **121,** 372.
Shaw, S. (1987). *Immunol. Today* **8,** 1.
Shaw, G., and Kamen, R. (1986). *Cell* **46,** 659.
Sherman, P. A., Basta, P. V., and Ting, J. P.-Y. (1987). *Proc. Natl. Acad. Sci. U.S.A.* **84,** 4254.
Sherry, B., and Cerami, A. (1988). *J. Cell Biol.* **107,** 1269.
Shirakawa, F., Chedid, M., Suttles, J., Pollok, B. A., and Mizel, S. B. (1988). *Mol. Cell. Biol.* **9,** 959.
Sieff, C. A., Tsai, S., and Faller, D. V. (1987). *J. Clin. Invest.* **79,** 48.
Sieff, C. A., Niemeyer, C. M., Mentzer, S. J., and Faller, D. V. (1988). *Blood* **72,** 1316.
Siegelman, M. H., van de Rijin, M., and Weissman, I. L. (1989). *Science* **243,** 1165.
Simmons, D., Makgoba, M. W., and Seed, B. (1988). *Nature (London)* **331,** 624.
Sims, J. E., March, C. J., Cosman, D., Widmer, M. B., MacDonald, H. R., McMahan, J., Grubin, C. E., Wignall, J. M., Jackson, J. L., Call, S. M., Freiend, D., Alpert, A. R., Gillis, S., Urdal, D. L., and Dower, S. K. (1988). *Science* **241,** 585.
Sims, J. E., Acres, R. B., Grubin, C. E., McMahan, C. J., Wignall, J. M., March, C. J., and Dower, S. K. (1989). *Proc. Natl. Acad. Sci. U.S.A.* **86,** 8946.
Singer, I. I., Scott, S., Hall, G. L., Limjuco, G., Chin, J., and Schmidt, J. A. (1988). *J. Exp. Med.* **167,** 389.
Sironi, M., Breviario, F., Proserpio, P., Biondi, A., Vecchi, A., Damme, J. O., Dejan, A. E., and Mantovani, A. (1989). *J. Immunol.* **142,** 549.
Sisson, S. D., and Dinarello, C. A. (1988). *Blood* **72,** 1368.
Sitaras, N. M., Sariban, E., Pantazis, P., Zetter, B., and Antoniades, H. N. (1987). *J. Cell. Physiol.* **132,** 376.
Sive, H., and Roeder, R. G. (1986). *Proc. Natl. Acad. Sci. U.S.A.* **83,** 6382.
Smith, C. W., Marlin, S. D., Rothlein, R., Toman, C., and Anderson, D. (1989). *J. Clin. Invest.* **83,** 2008.
Starksen, N. F., Harsh, G. R., IV, Gibbs, V. C., and Williams, L. T. (1987). *J. Biol. Chem.* **262,** 14381.

Staunton, D. E., Marlin, S. D., Stratowa, C., Dustin, M. L., and Springer, T. A. (1988). *Cell* **52,** 925.
Staunton, D. E., Dustin, M. L., and Springer, T. A. (1989). *Nature (London)* **339,** 61.
Stenberg, P. E., McEver, R. P., Shuman, M. A., Jacques, Y. V., and Bainton, D. F. (1985). *J. Cell Biol.* **101,** 880.
Stern, D. M., Bank, I., Nawroth, P. P., Cassimeris, J., Kisiel, W., Fenton, J. W., Dinarello, C. A., Chess, L., and Jaffe, E. A. (1985a). *J. Exp. Med.* **162,** 1223.
Stern, D. M., Nawroth, P., Handley, D., and Kisiel, W. (1985b). *Proc. Natl. Acad. Sci. U.S.A.* **82,** 2523.
Stoolman, L. M. (1989). *Cell* **56,** 907.
Strieter, R. M., Kunkel, S. L., Showell, H. J., Remick, D. G., Phan, S. H., Ward, P. A., and Marks, R. M. (1989). *Science* **243,** 1467.
Stroobant, P., and Waterfield, M. D. (1984). *EMBO J.* **3,** 2963.
Sugiura, M., Inagami, T., and Kon, V. (1989). *Biochem. Biophys. Res. Commun.* **161,** 1220.
Suttles, J., Carruth, L. M., and Mizel, S. B. (1990). *J. Immunol.* **144,** 170.
Suzuki, H., Shibano, K., Okane, M., Kono, I., Matsui, Y., Yamane, K., and Kashiwagi, H. (1989a). *Am. J. Pathol.* **134,** 35.
Suzuki, H., Akama, T., Okane, M., Kono, I., Matsui, Y., Yamane, K., and Kashiwagi, H. (1989b). *Arthritis Rheum.* **32,** 1528.
Suzuki, H., Kamimura, J., Ayabe, T., and Kashiwagi, H. (1990). *J. Immunol.* **145,** 2140.
Takehara, K., LeRoy, E. C., and Grotendort, G. R. (1987). *Cell* **49,** 415.
Takuwa, N., Takuwa, Y., Yanagisawa, M., Yamashita, K., and Masaki, T. (1989). *J. Biol. Chem.* **284,** 7856.
Thieme, T. R., and Wagner, C. R. (1988). *Mol. Immunol.* **26,** 249.
Thieme, T. R., Hefeneider, S. H., Wagner, C. R., and Burger, D. R. (1987). *J. Immunol.* **139,** 1173.
Thornton, S., Mueller, S. N., and Levine, E. M. (1983). *Science* **222,** 623.
Tonnensen, M. G., Smedly, L. A., and Henson, P. M. (1984). *J. Clin. Invest.* **74,** 1581.
Tozzi, C. A., Poiani, G. J., Harangozo, M., Boyd, C. D., and Riley, D. J. (1989). *J. Clin. Invest.* **84,** 1005.
Trowsdale, J., Young, J. A. T., Kelly, A. P., Austin, P. J., Carson, S., Meunier, H., So, A., Erlich, H. A., Spielman, R. S., Bodmer, J., and Bodmer, W. F. (1985). *Immunol. Rev.* **85,** 5.
Tsujimoto, M., Yip, Y. K., and Vilcek, J. (1985). *Proc. Natl. Acad. Sci. U.S.A.* **82,** 7626.
Tsujimoto, M., Feinman, R., Kohase, M., and Vilcek, J. (1986). *Arch. Biochem. Biophys.* **246,** 563.
Tucker, R. F., Branum, G. L., Shipley, G. D., Ryan, R. J., and Moses, H. L. (1984). *Proc. Natl. Acad. Sci. U.S.A.* **81,** 6757.
Urdal, D. L., Call, S. M., Jackson, J. L., and Dower, S. K. (1988). *J. Biol. Chem.* **263,** 2870.
Van de Berg, E. A., Sprenger, E., Jaye, E., Burgess, W., and van Hinsbergh, V. W. M. (1987). *Thromb. Haemostasis* **58,** 15.
Wagner, C. R., Vetto, R. M., and Burger, D. R. (1985). *Cell. Immunol.* **93,** 91.
Walz, A., Peveri, P., Aschauer, H., and Baggiolini, M. (1987). *Biochem. Biophys. Res. Commun.* **149,** 755.
Warner, S. J. C., Auger, K. R., and Libby, P. (1987). *J. Immunol.* **139,** 1911.
Waterfield, M. D., Scrace, G. T., Whittle, N., Stroobant, P., Johnsson, A., Wasteson, A., Westermark, B., Heldin, C.-H., Huang, J. S., and Deuel, T. F. (1983). *Nature (London)* **304,** 35.
Weissenbach, J., Chernajovsky, Y., Zeevi, M., Shulman, L., Soreq, H., Nir, U., Wallach, D., Perricaudet, M., Tiollais, P., and Revel, M. (1980). *Proc. Natl. Acad. Sci. U.S.A.* **77,** 7152.
Wen, D., Rowland, A., and Derynck, R. (1989). *EMBO J.* **8,** 1761.
Wilcox, J. N., Smith, K. M., Williams, L. T., Schwartz, S. M., and Gordon, D. (1988). *J. Clin. Invest.* **82,** 1134.
Williams, A. F., and Barclay, A. N. (1988). *Annu. Rev. Immunol.* **6,** 381.
Wong, G. G., Witek, J. S., Temple, P. A., Wilkens, K. M., Leary, A. C., Luxenberg, D. P., Jones, S. S.,

Brown, E. L., Kay, R. M., Orr, E. C., Shoemaker, C., Golde, D. W., Kaufman, R. J., Hewick, R. M., Wang, E. A., and Clark, S. C. (1985). *Science* **228,** 810.
Wright, G. E., and Fozard, J. R. (1988). *Proc. Natl. Acad. Sci. U.S.A.* **155,** 201.
Wright, S. D., Rao, P. E., Van Vorrhis, W. C., Craigmyle, L. S., Iida, K., Talle, M. A., Westberg, E. F., Goldstein, G., and Silverstein, S. C. (1983). *Proc. Natl. Acad. Sci. U.S.A.* **80,** 5699.
Yanagisawa, M., and Masaki, T. (1989). *Trends Pharmacol. Sci.* **10,** 374.
Yanagisawa, M., Kurihara, H., Kimura, S., Tomobe, Y., Kobayashi, M., Mitui, Y., Yazaki, Y., Goto, K., and Masaki, T. (1988). *Nature (London)* **332,** 1.
Yoshimura, T., Matsushima, S., Tanaka, S., Robinson, E. A., Appella, E., Oppenheim, J. J., and Leonard, E. J. (1987). *Proc. Natl. Acad. Sci. U.S.A.* **84,** 9233.
Yoshizumi, M., Kurihara, H., Morita, T., Yamashita, T., Oh-hashi, Y., Sugiyama, T., Takaku, F., Yanagisawa, M., Masaki, T., and Yazaki, Y. (1990). *Biochem. Biophys. Res. Commun.* **166,** 324.
Zilberstein, A., Ruggieri, R., Korn, J. H., and Revel, W. (1986). *EMBO J.* **5,** 2529.
Zinkernagel, R. M., and Doherty, P. C. (1979). *Adv. Immunol.* **27,** 51.
Zsebo, K. M., Yuschenkoff, V., Schulter, S., Chong, D., McCall, E., Dinarello, C. A., Altrock, B., and Bagby, G. C. (1988). *Blood* **71,** 99.

Interphase Nucleolar Organizer Regions in Cancer Cells

MASSIMO DERENZINI* and DOMINIQUE PLOTON†

*Dipartimento di Patologia Sperimentale,
40126 Bologna, Italy
and
†Unité de Recherche INSERM 314,
51092 Reims, France

    I. Introduction

   II. Silver Staining Techniques for the Visualization of NORs
      A. Ammoniacal Silver Technique (Two Step)
      B. One-Step Silver Staining (70°C)
      C. One-Step Silver Staining (Room Temperature)

  III. General Factors Influencing the Specificity of the Silver Staining for NORs
      A. Fixatives
      B. pH
      C. Temperature and Time

  IV. Molecular Components Responsible for Silver Staining
      A. Silver Reactive Groups
      B. Identification of the Silver-Stained Proteins

   V. NORs Not Stained by the Ag-NOR Techniques

  VI. Localization of NORs in Interphase Nucleoli

 VII. Structure and Function of Interphase NORs
      A. Ribosomal Chromatin
      B. RNA Polymerase I and Topoisomerase I
      C. Ag-NOR Proteins

VIII. Nucleolar Morphology

  IX. Interphase NOR Distribution

   X. Distribution of Silver-Stained Interphase NORs in Neoplastic Cells

XI. Is the High Number of Interphase NORs a Peculiar Feature of Cancer Cells?

XII. Relationship between Interphase NOR Distribution and Neoplastic State of the Cell
   A. Interphase NOR Distribution and Ribosomal Transcriptional Activity
   B. Relationship between Metaphase and Interphase NORs
   C. Interphase NORs and Cell Duplication Rate

XIII. Structural Changes of Ribosomal Genes in Cells Stimulated to Proliferate
   References

I. Introduction

Nucleolar organizer regions (NORs) were first described by Heitz (1931) and by McClintock (1934) in plant cells, as chromatinic regions around which nucleoli reform during telophase. These regions, which are morphologically characterized by a low stainability, correspond to secondary constrictions of metaphase chromosomes of eukaryotic cells (Howell, 1982). In man, secondary constrictions are localized on short arms of chromosomes 13, 14, 15, 21, and 22 (Howell, 1982).

In situ hybridization experiments have demonstrated that NORs contain the ribosomal genes (Gall and Pardue, 1969, 1971). NORs are also characterized by the presence of proteins that are selectively stained by silver methods (Howell, 1982). During interphase, the nucleolus is the only site where both ribosomal genes and silver-stained proteins are located (Wachtler *et al.*, 1986). The evidence now available indicates that the fibrillar components of the nucleolus are the interphase counterpart of metaphase NORs (Hernandez-Verdun, 1983, 1986; Goessens, 1984). Recently, interphase NORs have become an object of attention for pathologists because their distribution in the nucleolus has been shown to constitute a useful tool for differentiating, at the optical level, malignant from benign lesions in histological and cytological routine preparations.

For a long time it has been known that abnormalities of the nucleolar morphology characterize neoplastic cells: hypertrophied and irregularly shaped nucleoli are frequently observed in cancer cells (Koller, 1963). However, these nucleolar morphological changes did not represent a reliable parameter for distinguishing malignant from the corresponding benign cells. Studies carried out in the past 10 years on the organization of the nucleolus and the relationship between its structural changes and functional activity have permitted a new objective parameter to be defined for the quantification of nucleolar abnormalities that characterize cancer cells.

This new parameter is represented by the quantitative evaluation of the distribution of interphase NORs in the nucleolus. A higher quantity of interphase NORs is generally observed in neoplastic cells than in the corresponding nonneoplastic cells.

The aim of the present article is to provide a comprehensive review of recent data about the structural–functional organization of interphase NORs, their importance in tumor pathology, and their relationship with the biological characteristics of cancer cells. We will first focus our attention on the technical points of the silver staining methods that have permitted the precise localization of NORs in the nucleolar components and their visualization and quantification in routine tumor histocytology.

II. Silver Staining Techniques for the Visualization of NORs

An extremely important property of NORs is their high affinity for silver (Fig. 1). Since 1975 (Goodpasture and Bloom, 1975), it has been known that this affinity is due to a protein component strictly localized at the same sites as NORs, visualized by *in situ* hybridization. Thus, silver staining immediately appeared as a very convenient and useful technique for localization of NORs. The finding that Ag staining may locate rRNA genes more easily than *in situ* hybridization enabled development of numerous applications of silver staining methods both on metaphase chromosomes and on interphase nucleoli (Howell, 1982; Babu and Verma, 1985).

Generally, silver staining techniques use two successive steps (La Velle, 1985), an impregnation phase with silver and a development phase with a developer. These two steps are very similar to photographic procedures in which a latent image (invisible image) is first obtained and is then transformed into a visible image by the action of a developer. In silver staining, impregnation results from the combination of silver ions with specific components, and if sufficient redox potential exists, very small cores of metallic silver appear in contact with molecules. During the second step, these tiny deposits of silver act as cores for subsequent growth of silver deposits due to the action of a reducing agent present in the developing solution. Thus most of the NOR silver methods use two steps: an impregnation step with $AgNO_3$ and a development step with a reducing agent such as ammonia or formic acid. However, techniques in which impregnation and development are performed simultaneously have also been devised in order to control better the silver deposit growth phase (Howell and Black, 1980).

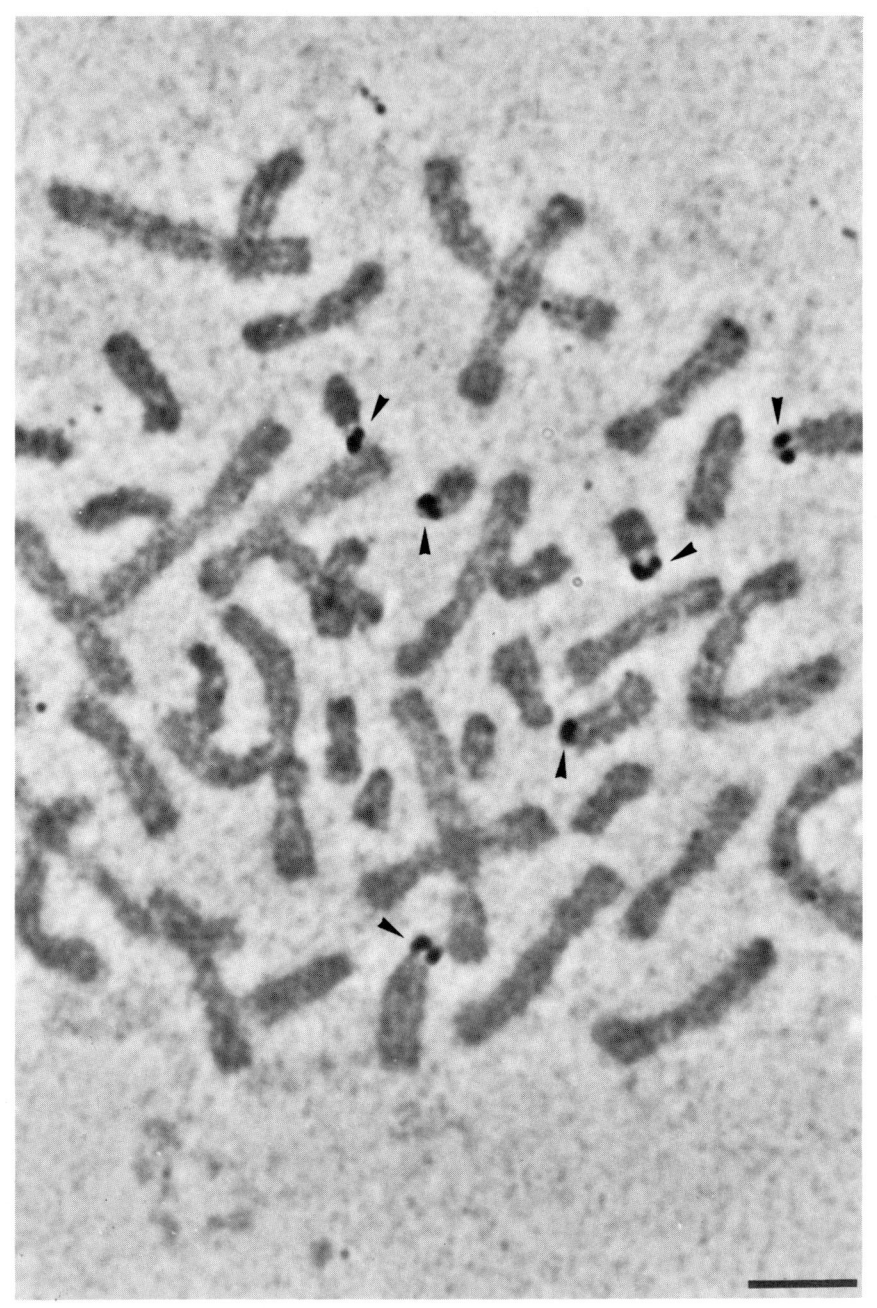

FIG. 1. Metaphasic plate of human chromosomes stained with the one-step silver staining method. No counterstaining. Phase contrast. Six acrocentric chromosomes show silver granules (arrowheads). Bar = 4 μm.

Several methods were published in the past; we will focus our attention on the more recent, specific, and frequently employed techniques. These techniques differ from each other in reliability, specificity, rapidity, and simplicity. However, their results are very similar: they consist of dots of metallic silver localized on the secondary constriction of human acrocentric chromosomes

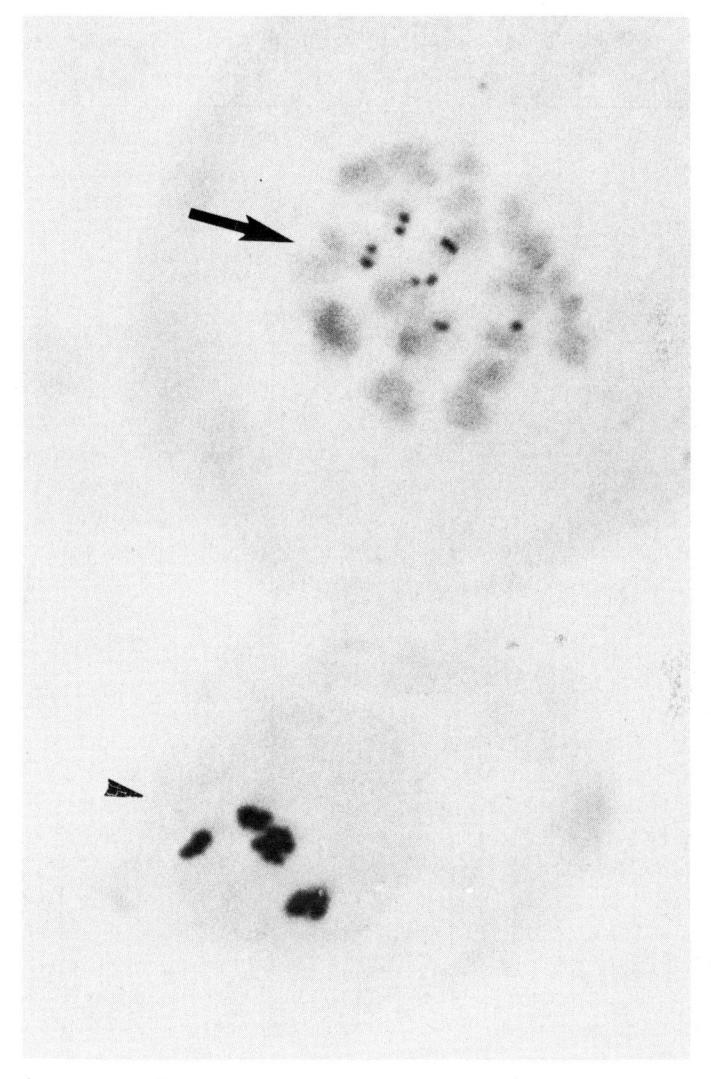

FIG. 2. Silver staining of NORs in mitotic chromosomes (arrow) and interphase nucleoli in two neuroblastoma cells cultured *in vitro* (arrowhead) (×3000).

and within interphase nucleoli (Fig. 2). The NORs stained with any of these methods are called "Ag-NORs" (Howell, 1982).

A. Ammoniacal Silver Technique (Two Step)

This technique (Goodpasture and Bloom, 1975) is a two-step staining procedure. The first step involves impregnation of cells or chromosomes with an aqueous silver solution during exposure under a photoflood light. The second step involves development with a mixture of ammoniacal silver and formalin ion at pH 6, at room temperature, within a few minutes. Development is monitored under a light microscope and is stopped by rinsing in water.

B. One-Step Silver Staining (70°C)

This very simple and reliable technique (Howell and Black, 1980) was developed in order to overcome some drawbacks of the technique of Goodpasture and Bloom (1975), i.e., nonspecific precipitation of silver, instability of solutions (thus limiting standardization), and irregular staining on the slide. The principle of the one-step procedure is the use of a protective colloidal developer, which limits instability of the solution and nonspecific staining. As stated by Howell and Black (1980), the main feature of this technique is that "the procedure has been standardized for the first time."

C. One-Step Silver Staining (Room Temperature)

In the method by Howell and Black (1980), the staining reaction is carried out at 70°C. Under these conditions, even if the NORs are very rapidly stained (2 minutes), the background also increases very rapidly and monitoring the development is very difficult. In order to avoid unspecific silver precipitates and to control the staining reaction better, Ploton et al. (1982, 1986) modified the original procedure of Howell and Black (1980) by lowering the temperature of the staining solution to room temperature (20–25°C) and by increasing the staining time to 14–20 minutes. A rinse in 5% thiosulfate was recommended to wash out free silver ions at the end of the staining reaction. This improved staining procedure was shown to be very useful for the visualization of NORs in sections of routinely fixed and paraffin-embedded samples (Ploton et al., 1986). This procedure is now the one most frequently used, and details of the staining technique are given in Table I.

TABLE I

PRACTICAL PROCEDURE FOR SILVER STAINING WITH THE ONE-STEP METHOD[a]

1. **Primary fixation of specimens**[b]
   Smears, chromosomes, etc.: cells are smeared and air dried.
   Paraffin sections (4 μm thick) of tissues are fixed with formaldehyde, alcohol, Bouin's fluid, etc., and are dewaxed in several baths of xylene and passed through 100% ethanol.
   Semi-thin sections of Epon- or Lowicryl-embedded cells and tissues are deplasticized with KOH or water, respectively.
   Cells and tissues for EM studies are fixed 10 minutes in 2% glutaaraldehyde in 0.1 M PBS and are then rinsed three times in PBS.
2. **Secondary fixation of specimens**
   After the first fixation, all specimens are postfixed 10 minutes in Clarke's solution [ethanol or methanol (100%) and glacial acetic acid, 3 : 1].
3. **Preparation of the silver staining solution**
   Two solutions are needed: the first one is a 2% gelatin solution dissolved in ultrapure water to which formic acid is then added to make a 1% solution; the second one is a 50% silver nitrate solution in ultrapure water.
   Staining solution is extemporaneously obtained by rapidly mixing one part gelatin solution with two parts silver nitrate solution.
4. **Staining**
   On slides:
   Staining solution (~0.3 ml) is poured on the slide. Staining takes 10 to 20 minutes at room temperature, depending on the desired intensity of the reaction. Even with longer times, no background is seen. Although protection from light is not necessary, it is better to avoid direct sunlight during the staining. After staining, the solution is poured off and the slide is washed in several baths of ultrapure water, is placed for 10 minutes in a 5% thiosulfate solution, is washed again in several baths of water, then is dehydrated and mounted.
   For tissues:
   Fragments of tissues are put into small Petri dishes, in which 1 ml of staining solution is poured. After 10 to 20 minutes, fragments are taken off, are put in several baths of ultrapure water, are placed for 10 minutes in a 5% thiosulfate solution, are washed again in water, then are dehydrated and Epon embedded.

[a] The method is described by Ploton *et al.* (1982, 1986).
[b] Abbreviations: EM, electron microscopic; PBS, phosphate-buffered saline.

III. General Factors Influencing the Specificity of the Silver Stain for NORs

A. FIXATIVES

As different types of proteins may bind silver, during fixation it is necessary to solubilize any protein that could induce nonspecific staining. In this respect a step using a mixture of acetic acid and methanol may be extremely important to avoid nonspecific staining (Hernandez-Verdun *et al.*, 1980b).

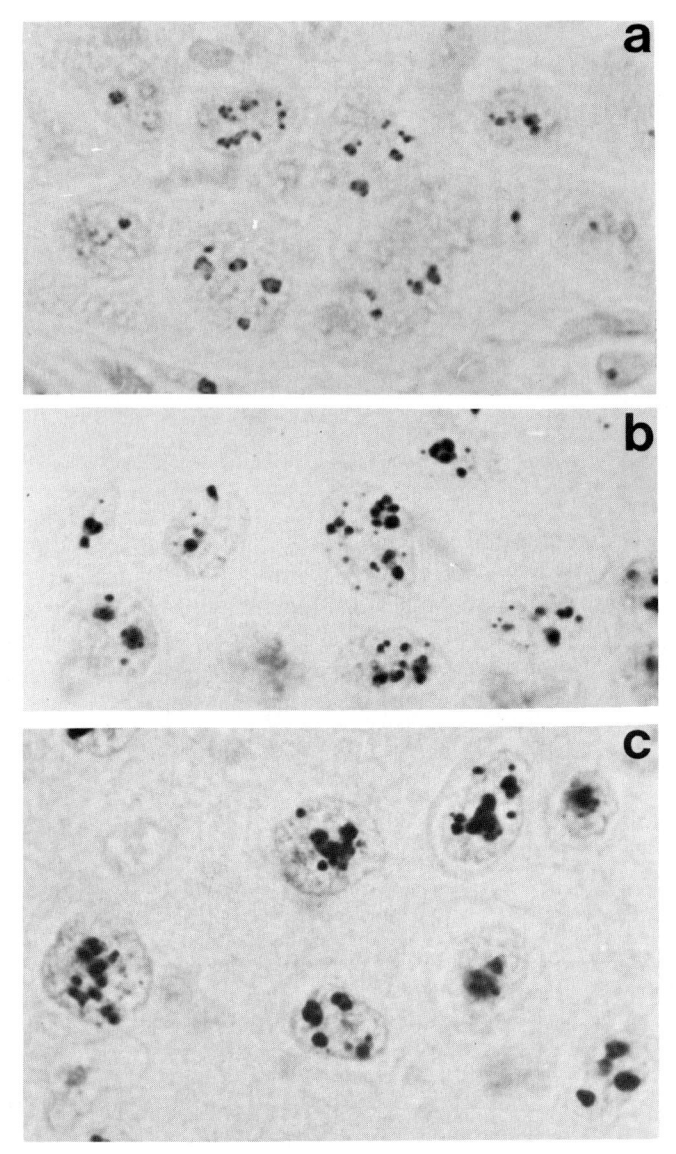

FIG. 3. Silver staining of Ag-NOR proteins (Ploton et al., 1986) of sections from lung carcinoma fixed with formalin (a), ethanol (b) and Clarke's fluid (c). Interphase NORs are much better visualized in b and c than in a (×2000).

Thus formaldehyde fixation alone gives nonspecific staining, but use of acetic acid alone abolishes Ag staining because of solubilization of Ag-NOR proteins (Hubbell, 1985). Treatment of formaldehyde- or glutaraldehyde-fixed cells or tissues with Clarke's fluid (methanol : acetic acid 3 : 1) permits specific staining of Ag-NORs for ultrastructural examination (Hernandez-Verdun *et al.*, 1980b; Pebusque *et al.*, 1981; Ploton *et al.*, 1982).

Derenzini *et al.* (1988b) found that at the light microscopic level, the best visualization of NORs in tissue sections was obtained if samples were fixed with ethanol only or Clarke's fluid only. Formalin or Bouin's fluid gave rise to a lower and less specific stainability of NORs (Fig. 3).

B. pH

Lomholt and Toft (1987) reported the effect of pH variations between 6.5 and 12 on the staining of acrocentric chromosomes. They showed that at pH 3.5, 90% of the cells in mitosis displayed normal NOR staining; between pH 6.5 and 10, no staining occurs; between pH 10.5 and 11.6, only 10% of the cells in mitosis are stained; and at pH 11.5 and 11.8, NOR staining is similar to that at pH 3.5. At some unfavorable pH values, G and T banding could also be obtained. This work clearly demonstrates the great importance of pH during silver staining and also confirms that at two very different pH values (3.5 and 11.7) the same results may be obtained by the one-step technique of Howell and Black (1980) and the ammonical silver technique according to Goodpasture and Bloom (1975).

C. Temperature and Time

The choice of a given temperature and time depends on the desired speed of development and the acceptable level of background. These two parameters are strictly related to each other. The higher the temperature, the shorter the time necessary to obtain selective NOR staining. Even if an optimal fixation has been employed, if the staining reaction is prolonged beyond the time for the selective staining of NORs, other cell structures are progressively stained. Therefore, staining procedures that are carried out at low temperatures (e.g., according to Ploton *et al.*, 1986) are preferable.

IV. Molecular Components Responsible for Silver Staining

A. Silver Reactive Groups

Howell *et al.* (1975), Buys and Osinga (1980), and Schwarzacher *et al.* (1978) demonstrated that RNase or trichloroacetic acid (TCA) extraction or

HCl treatment causes no reduction of Ag staining. In contrast, treatment with trypsin abolishes the Ag reaction: this demonstrates that Ag-stainable material is probably an acidic protein (or nonhistone protein).

Contradictory results have been obtained about the exact nature of silver-reactive groups within proteins. Buys and Osinga (1980) demonstrated accumulation of protein-bound sulfhydryl and disulfide groups at the level of NORs. De Capoa et al. (1982) showed that only sulfhydryl groups interact with silver. However, Hubbell (1985) showed that sulfhydryl groups, disulfide bridges, methionine, and lysine are not responsible for Ag staining. In the same work, it was demonstrated that dephosphorylation with alkaline phosphatase decreased silver staining. These findings were confirmed by Satoh and Busch (1981), who showed that serine- and threonine-bound phosphate groups of phosphoproteins are responsible for silver staining. On the other hand, it was suggested (Clavaguera et al., 1983, 1984) that silver stainability of proteins could be questionable because DNA, RNA, histones, nonhistones, and high-mobility group proteins seem to bind silver with some affinity. These authors suggested that silver staining could indeed be related to various decondensation states of chromatin. In the same way, Haaf et al. (1984) showed that experimentally undercondensed heterochromatic regions were silver positive and that nonhistone proteins were the origin of this "nonspecific" staining.

B. Identification of the Silver-Stained Proteins

As some of the molecules responsible for Ag staining seemed to be proteins, several groups have tried to isolate nucleolar proteins and stain them with silver on gel electrophoresis. Thus, several putative candidates for silver stainability were proposed: (1) a "Ag-NOR protein" (Hubbell et al., 1979); (2) the large subunit of RNA polymerase I (Williams et al., 1982); B_{23} and C_{23} proteins (Busch et al., 1982), and (4) C_{23} (or nucleolin) only (Ochs and Busch, 1984).

Although the demonstration of C_{23} protein as a silver-staining protein seemed convincing (Ochs and Busch, 1984), one recent paper (Biggiogera et al., 1989) on immunolocalization of C_{23} protein demonstrated that this protein is not localized within nucleolar structures, which are, however, very reactive with silver. This work suggests that another molecule could be responsible for silver staining.

Finally, work by Dhar et al. (1987) shed some light on the problem by demonstrating that human rRNA gene fragments amplified in hamster cells are transcribed by RNA polymerase II only and that they are not silver stained. This important work is further proof that silver staining is neither due to rRNA genes nor to rRNA transcripts, but that staining is very probably due to a molecule of the machinery needed for transcription of rRNA genes by RNA polymerase I.

V. NORs Not Stained by the Ag-NOR Techniques

There is evidence that, as far as human beings are concerned, not all the metaphase NORs detected by *in situ* hybridization are stained with silver. Whereas *in situ* hybridization detects all the NORs located in the secondary constrictions on the short arms of chromosome pairs 13, 14, 15, 21, and 22 (Henderson *et al.*, 1972; Evans *et al.*, 1974), the silver staining techniques reveal only three to nine NORs (Varley, 1977). The positivity of NORs to silver staining has been related to the transcriptional activity of the ribosomal cistrons (Schmiady *et al.*, 1979; Angelier *et al.*, 1982; Morton *et al.*, 1983; Hubbell, 1985; Ferraro and Prantera, 1988). There is some evidence that the Ag-NOR methods stain those metaphase NORs that had been actively transcribing during the preceding interphase (Miller *et al.*, 1976). Because the silver staining methods do not actually stain ribosomal genes but in fact stain the acidic proteins associated with ribosomal genes, during interphase the Ag-NOR proteins are located exclusively in transcriptionally active NORs.

During interphase only the portion of ribosomal genes associated with the Ag-NOR proteins is transcriptionally active, as has been very elegantly demonstrated by Wachtler *et al.* (1986) in a study on the position of ribosomal genes in interphase nuclei. The authors, using a nonautoradiographic method that permits the use of fluorochrome-labeled antibodies for a very high resolution of the labeled structures, observed that in human resting lymphocytes several agglomerates of ribosomal DNA were scattered over the whole nuclear area. Only ribosomal genes located in the nucleolus (which is the site of ribosomal biogenesis) were, on the contrary, stained by silver.

VI. Localization of NORs in Interphase Nucleoli

The Ag-NOR staining techniques, commonly employed in cytogenetics to visualize NOR-bearing chromosomes, were rapidly adapted for electron microscopic identification of the nucleolar structures, where NORs are located during interphase.

At the ultrastructural level, five main components are systematically recognized in thin sections routinely stained with uranium and lead salts (see reviews by Goessens, 1984; Hernandez-Verdun, 1986) (Fig. 4). The fibrillar centers (FCs), which are spherical structures of different sizes with a very low

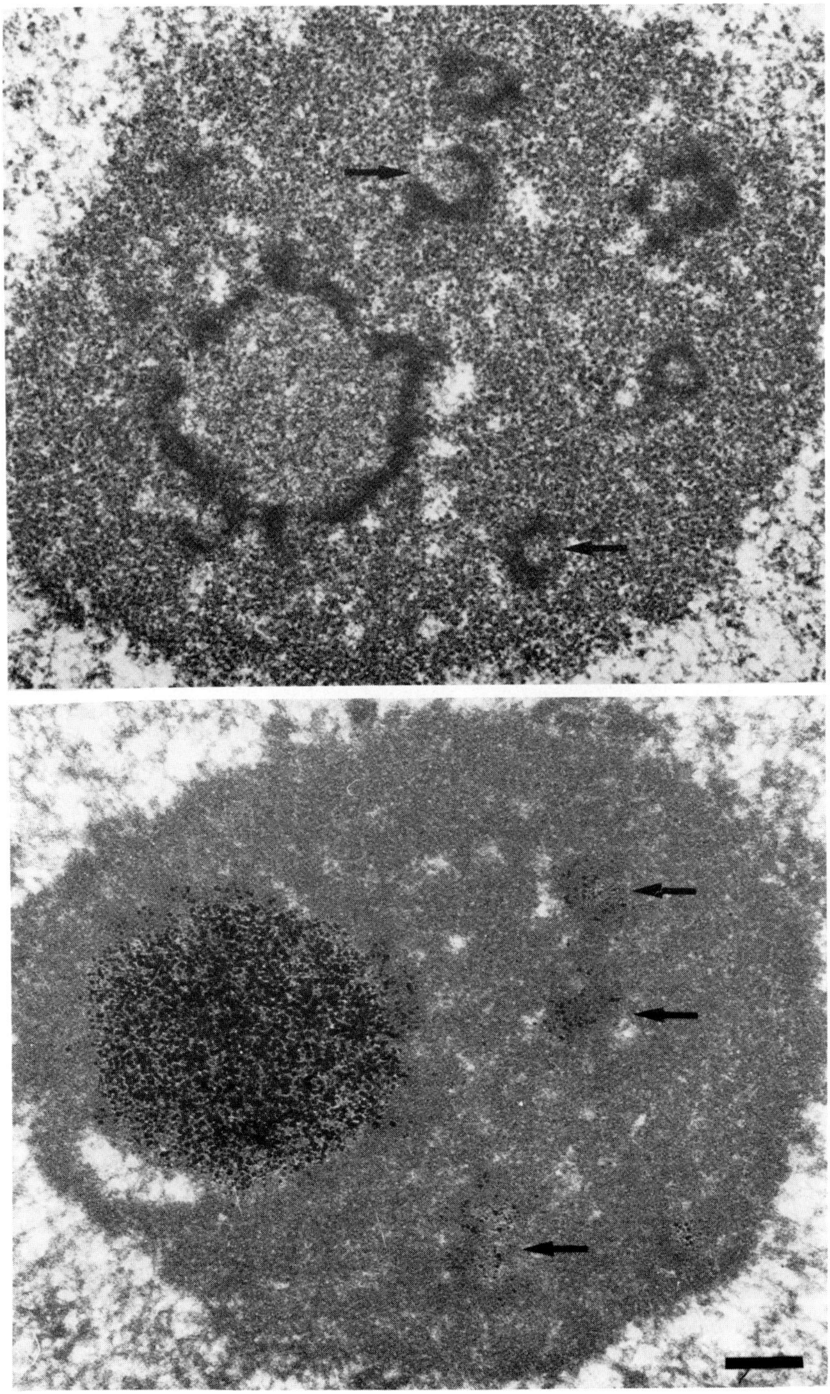

shape in which one gene (trunk of the tree) is transcribed by a great number of RNA polymerase I molecules at the same time. The branches of the tree represent rRNA precursors at different steps of elongation. These rRNA molecules are rapidly associated with ribosomal proteins and constitute fibrillar ribonucleoprotein complexes (Hadjiolov, 1985). There is evidence that actively transcribed ribosomal genes and the nontranscribed spacers interspaced between them have, in spread preparations, an extended nonnucleosomal configuration. Long-term inactivated ribosomal chromatin exhibits, on the other hand, a nucleosomal structure indistinguishable from that of the bulk of inactive chromatin (Scheer and Zentgraf, 1982).

Definition of the structural organization of ribosomal chromatin present in interphase NORs has been achieved using the Feulgen-like osmium–ammine reaction (Cogliati and Gautier, 1973) as an ultrastructural DNA tracer *in situ* (Derenzini *et al.*, 1981b). By means of this technique, the nucleosomal organization of transcriptionally inactive chromatin, as defined by morphological, biochemical, and physical studies carried out on *in vitro* chromatin (Kornberg, 1977; Finch *et al.*, 1977; Chambon, 1978), has been repeatedly shown in the compact chromatin *in situ*. In thin sections in which only DNA was rendered electron opaque by osmium–ammine, the nucleosomes appeared as roundish units with a diameter of ~11 nm, constituted by an intensely stained DNA ring, encircling an unstained, proteinaceous, inner core (Derenzini *et al.*, 1981a,b, 1983a). After the selective DNA staining, three levels of chromatin organization were observed to characterize intranuclear chromatin of mammalian cells: (1) highly compact clumps; (2) fibers with a thickness ranging from 11 to 30 nm, and (3) loose agglomerates of extended DNA filaments with a thickness of 2–3 nm. Both the clumps and fibers of chromatin had a nucleosomal organization that, on the contrary, was always absent in the loose agglomerates. These latter structures have been observed to be peculiar to the intranucleolar chromatin (Derenzini *et al.*, 1982) and the distribution has been found to be superimposable on that of the fibrillar centers and the dense fibrillar component (Derenzini *et al.*, 1983b, 1987a) (Figs. 9 and 10). The location of these completely extended, nonnucleosomal DNA filaments in the confines of interphase NORs has also been demonstrated by the fact that in cells selectively stained for the Ag-NOR proteins and DNA, silver deposits had the same distribution as that of DNA filaments (Hernandez-Verdun *et al.*, 1982) (Figs. 11 and 12).

The observation that DNA of interphasic NORs has a completely extended nonnucleosomal configuration has stimulated investigations to define the histone complement of this type of DNA. Using the acrolein–silver–methenamine technique to reveal histones in nucleoli of human lymphocytes (Derenzini *et al.*, 1985) and in a human tumor cell line (TG cells) (Derenzini *et al.*, 1987a), histones were not detected in the fibrillar center nor in the

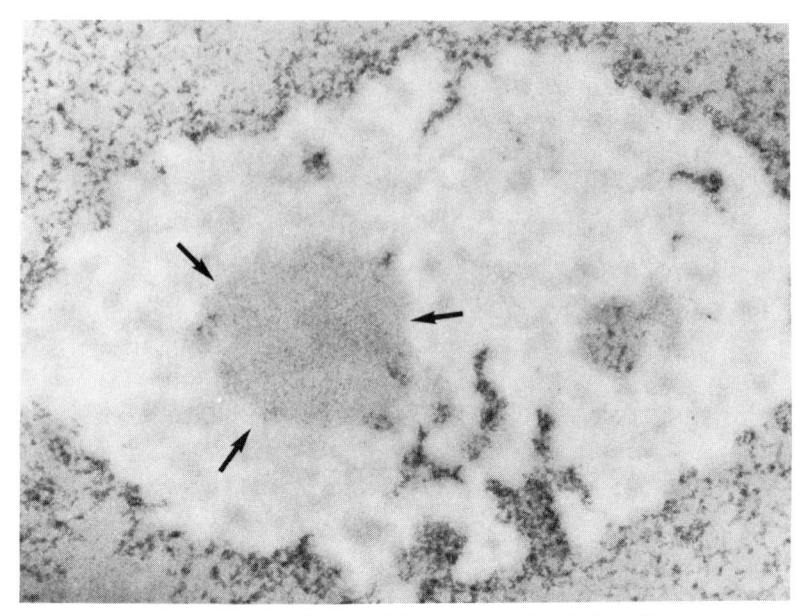

FIG. 9. TG cell nucleolus selectively stained for DNA with the Feulgen-like osmium–ammine reaction. In the nucleolar body only the DNA-containing structures are rendered electron opaque. Arrows indicate a large agglomerate of highly dispersed DNA structures, with the same location as that of the large fibrillar centers shown in Figs. 7 and 8 (×30,000). [Reproduced with permission from Derenzini et al. (1983a).]

dense fibrillar component. The same results were obtained in an immunocytochemical study, at the ultrastructural level, using purified antibodies linked to colloidal gold or to protein A/colloidal gold to reveal histone distribution in the nucleolus (Derenzini et al., 1985). Thiry and Muller (1989) produced immunocytochemical results indicating a very slight histone immunolabeling exclusively at the periphery of the fibrillar centers of Erhlich tumor cell nucleoli.

Taken together, these data indicate that if histones are present in the ribosomal chromatin of interphase NORs they are in a very low quantity and are not uniformly distributed on the ribosomal chromatin.

B. RNA Polymerase I and Topoisomerase I

RNA polymerase I is an enzyme that selectively transcribes ribosomal genes. Using various immunolabeling techniques, Scheer and Rose (1984) and Scheer and Raska (1987) have demonstrated that RNA polymerase I is

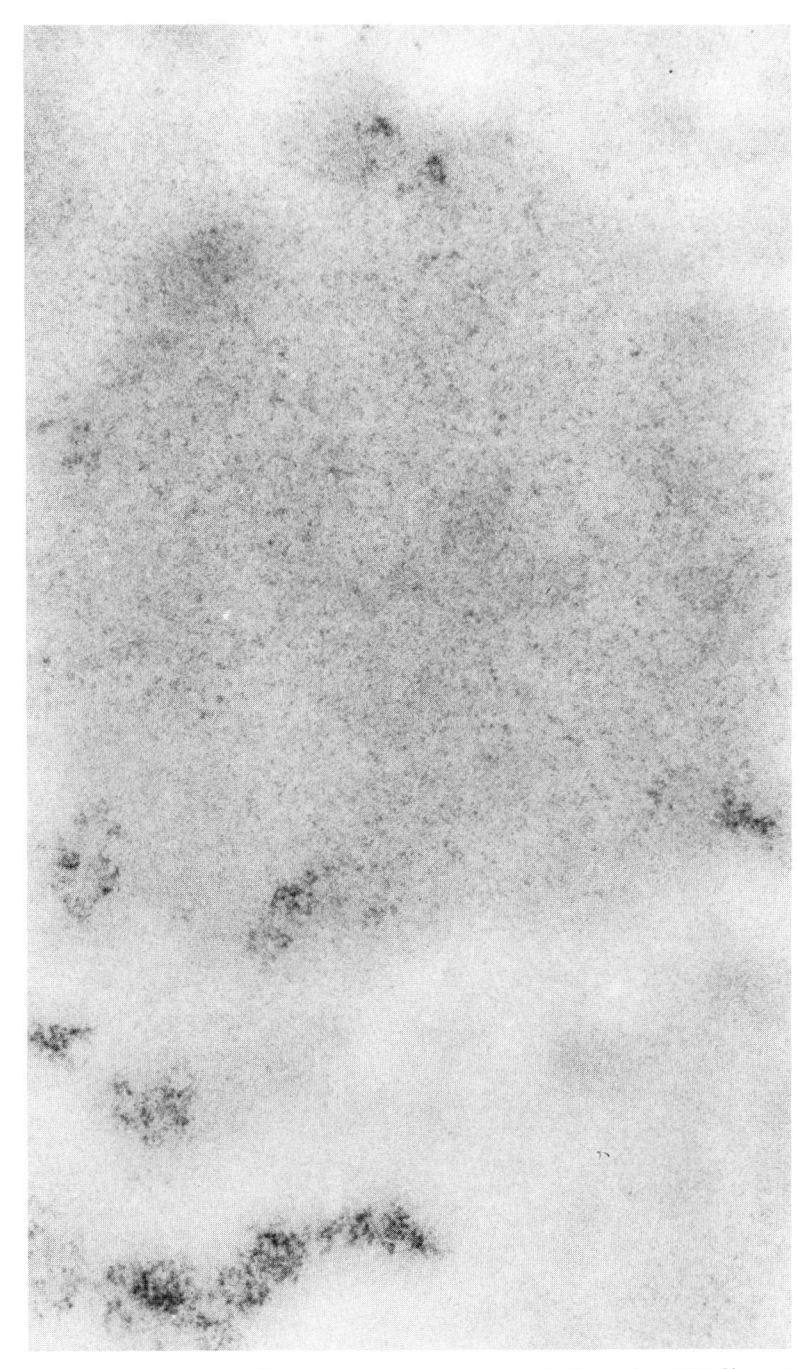

FIG. 10. Detail of Fig. 9. The loose agglomerate is composed of very thin DNA filaments, 2–3 nm thick (×150,000). [Reproduced with permission from Derenzini et al. (1983a).]

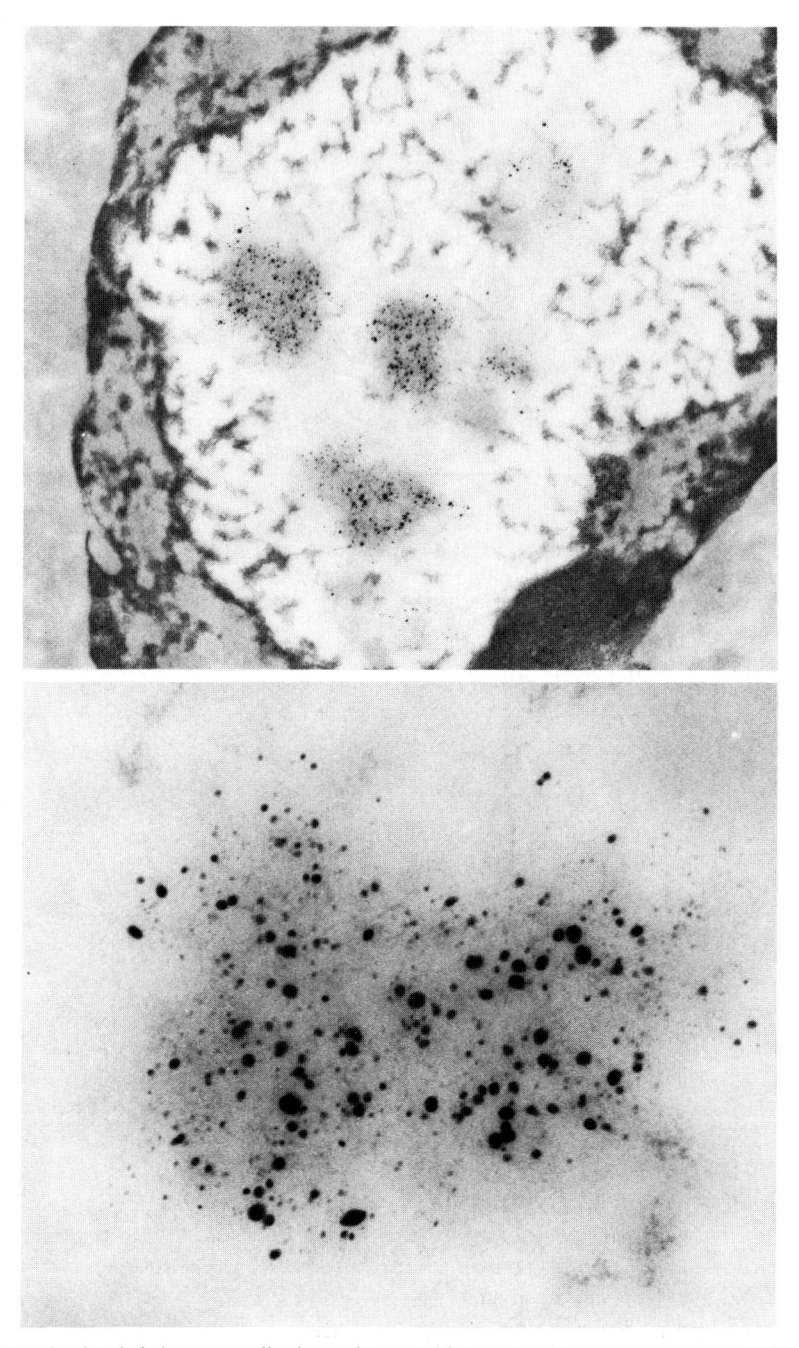

FIG. 11 (top). Ehrlich tumor cell selectively stained for DNA and Ag-NOR proteins. The clusters of silver granules appear not to be associated with fibers and clumps of compact chromatin in the nucleolar body (×30,000).

FIG. 12 (bottom). Detail of Fig. 11, showing the presence of DNA filaments, 2–3 nm thick, among the silver granules (×150,000).

located in the fibrillar centers but not in the dense fibrillar component. More recently, Raska et al. (1989) found that the dense fibrillar component was a site of RNA polymerase I localization, even if the immunogold labeling was less than that of the fibrillar centers.

Topoisomerase I activity is necessary for the ribosomal transcriptional processes (Brill et al., 1987; Zhang et al., 1988) and topoisomerase I molecules are associated with ribosomal genes that are actively transcribing (Zhang et al., 1988). The precise localization of topoisomerase I molecules has been obtained, using immunogold labeling at the ultrastructural level, by Raska et al. (1989), who showed that the dense fibrillar component was the site of the main accumulation of the gold particles.

It therefore appears that, according to the bulk of the autoradiographic studies showing [^{3}H]uridine localization in the dense fibrillar component (reviewed by Fakan, 1978), the ribosomal transcriptional process does not occur throughout the whole interphase NOR but at periphery, in the zone that corresponds to the dense fibrillar component. The presence of RNA polymerase I molecules in the central portion of interphase NORs, which correspond to the fibrillar center, does not mean that these molecules are in fact actively transcribing, because they are also found in metaphase NORs (Scheer and Rose, 1984; Matsui and Sandberg, 1985) and, in interphase nucleoli, after D-galactosamine-induced inhibition of ribosomal transcription (Hadjiolova et al., 1986).

These observations imply that a portion of ribosomal chromatin in interphase NORs is transcriptionally inactive, independently of its completely extended configuration.

C. The Ag-NOR Proteins

As reported in Section IV,B, the Ag-NOR proteins represent a set of acidic proteins that are selectively located in the NORs. Their identification and characterization are currently under investigation. Nevertheless, many data indicate the C_{23} protein (Jordan, 1987) is the main silver-stained protein of the nucleolus. From a functional point of view, it has been suggested that the Ag-NOR proteins might be involved in assembling and processing pre-rRNA (Lischwe et al., 1979), and nucleolin has been shown to be associated with nascent pre-rRNA (Herrera and Olson, 1986). It has also been proposed that nucleolin might control the rate of ribosomal gene transcription by modification of the phosphorylated state (Lapeyre et al., 1987).

On the other hand, some data indicate that some of the Ag-NOR proteins are not linked to an effective synthesis of rRNA. The Ag-NOR proteins are associated with metaphase ribosomal genes that are transcriptionally inactive. Furthermore, after 95% inhibition of rRNA synthesis by D-galactomsamine

(Gajdardjieva et al., 1982), silver-stained proteins were present in rat hepatocyte nucleolar fibrillar components devoid of growth-arrested pre-rRNA chains.

The Ag-NOR proteins are constantly distributed on the same sites where the completely extended, nonnucleosomal chromatin is present even after physiological (during metaphase) or drug-induced (actinomycin-D) inhibition of rRNA synthesis (Hernandez-Verdun and Derenzini, 1983; Hernandez-Verdun et al., 1984). Moreover, the Ag-NOR proteins are not randomly distributed in interphase NORs. They are in fact structured in a threadlike configuration that can be completely superimposed on the structural organization of the nonnucleosomal filaments (Derenzini et al., 1987a). The distribution of these Ag-NOR proteins and their constant association with the nonnucleosomal chromatin of NORs strongly suggest that these proteins might have a structural function. Indeed, it has been demonstrated that nucleolin induces chromatin decondensation by binding to histone H1 (Erard et al., 1988).

It appears that the constant extended configuration of NOR ribosomal chromatin, independent of a current transcriptional activity, may be due to the association with nucleolin or to other still uncharacterized Ag-NOR proteins.

In conclusion, interphase NOR chromatin has the same structural organization, independently of its transcriptional activity. Transcriptionally inactive interphase NORs, for example those of human circulating lymphocytes, are nevertheless structurally ready for transcription. The constant extended configuration of interphase NOR ribosomal chromatin greatly simplifies the control of rRNA synthesis because the first step of gene activation, the nucleosomal DNA unwinding, is already performed. As already stated, this peculiar mechanism of control of gene activity appears, from a teleological point of view, reasonable, because ribosomal genes, in contrast to the other genes, are expressed in all cells of a given organism, independently of any cell specialization (Derenzini et al., 1987a).

VIII. Nucleolar Morphology

The structural organization of the nucleolar components is highly variable, depending on the cell type and, for a given cell, on its functional activity. Three kinds of nucleoli have been described regarding the distribution of the nucleolar components (see reviews by Goessens, 1984; Hernandez-Verdun, 1986):

1. The ring-shaped nucleoli, characterized by a solitary large fibrillar center surrounded by a ribonucleoprotein rim of fibrils and granules.

2. The nucleolonema-structured nucleoli in which the fibrillar and granular ribonucleoprotein components constitute interwoven threads, whereas numerous fibrillar centers, very small in size, are scattered throughout the nucleolar body.

3. The compact nucleoli in which fibrils and granules are separated and the granular component predominates in the nucleolar body; the fibrillar centers are few and large, surrounded by a circular rim of dense firbillar component, which is completely surrounded by the granular component.

The different intranucleolar distributions of the ribonucleoprotein components and the changes in their relative proportion have been considered to be a consequence of different rates of ribosomal RNA synthesis and processing (Goessens, 1984; Hernandez-Verdun, 1986). However, in a study carried out on regenerating rat hepatocytes (characterized by a nucleolonema ribonucleoprotein organization) and an established tumor cell line (TG cells, characterized by a compact ribonucleoprotein distribution), it was found that the two cell types were very similar from the biochemical point of view of nuclear activity, both types of cells being active in synthesizing DNA and RNA. As far as ribosomal RNA synthesis was concerned, the radioactivity in pre-rRNA species appeared to be the same in both types of cells, showing similar rates of transcriptional activity and of pre-rRNA processing (Derenzini *et al.*, 1983b). In that case, therefore, the different nucleolar ribonucleoprotein distribution could not be explained by a different pattern of rRNA synthesis. On the other hand, the two cell types exhibited a completely different distribution of interphase NOR extended ribosomal chromatin. In the case of regenerating hepatocytes, the extended ribosomal chromatin formed numerous and small agglomerates, whereas in TG cells it constituted few and large agglomerates. Because ribosomal RNA synthesis takes place at the periphery of the agglomerates of ribosomal chromatin (see Section VI), the resultant distribution pattern of ribonucleoprotein components is necessarily influenced by the spatial distribution of ribosomal chromatin in the nucleolar body. In the case of nucleoli with a nucleolonema configuration, the rings of dense fibrillar component located at the periphery of the numerous agglomerates of ribosomal chromatin, as a consequence of the proximity of the agglomerates, come in contact with each other, thus giving rise to continuous cordlike structures. In the case of compact nucleoli, the rims of the dense fibrillar component, as a consequence of the low number of and large size of ribosomal chromatin agglomerates, were well separated from each other, never assuming the cordlike organization characteristic of the nucleolonema. The relationship between the extended ribosomal chromatin distribution and nucleolar morphology was also demonstrated in human resting lymphocytes stimulated to proliferate by phytohemagglutinin (Derenzini *et al.*, 1987b). The progressive changes of the nucleolar morphology appeared in

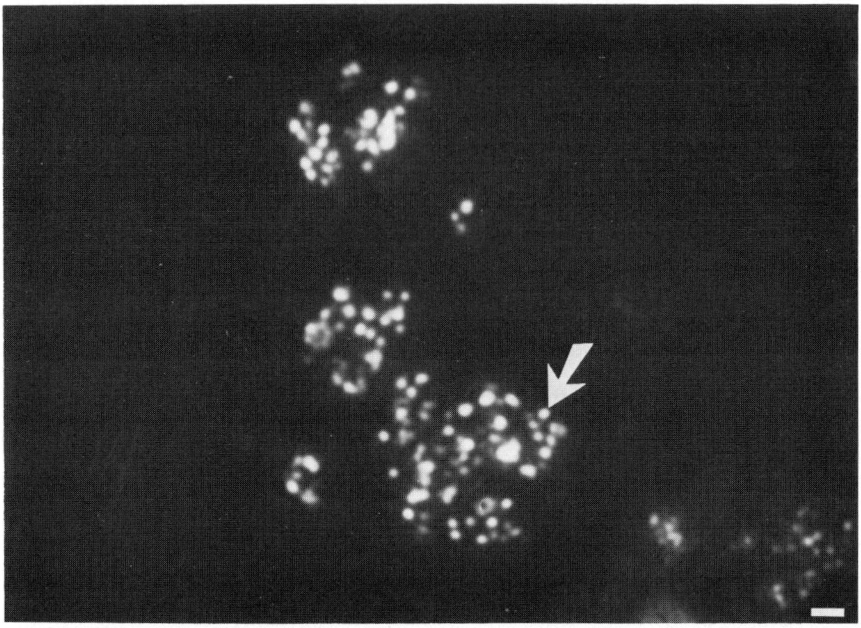

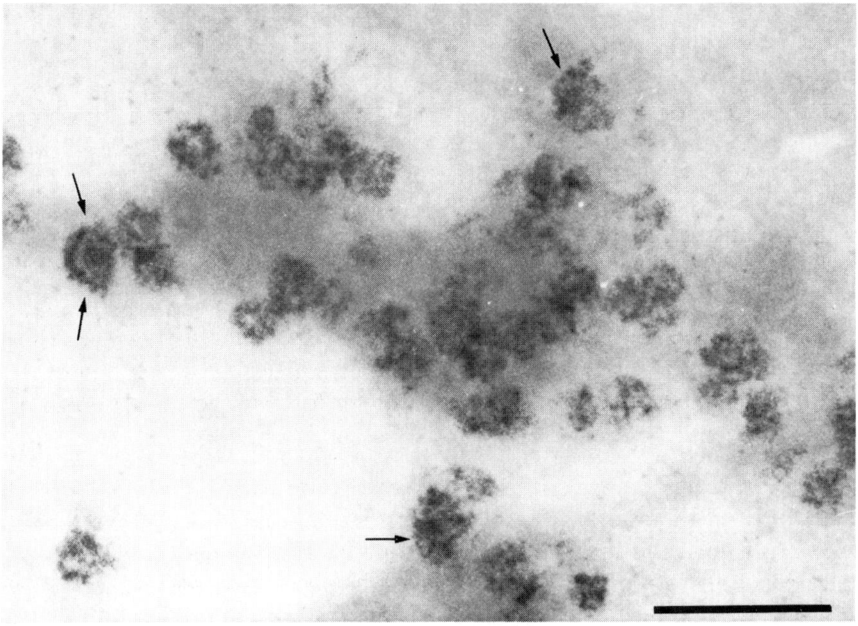

fact to be strictly correlated to the distributional changes of the extended ribosomal chromatin.

Since the extended ribosomal chromatin is uniformly distributed in the interphase NORs, these results led to the conclusion that the different nucleolar morphological patterns can be distinguished from each other on the basis of the different distributions of the interphase NORs.

IX. Interphase NOR Distribution

At the end of the last century, Pianese (1896) found that unusually large vacuolated and irregularly shaped nucleoli characterized numerous human tumors. Since that time, a series of light microscopy works have been published (see the review by Busch and Smetana, 1970) that consider these nucleolar changes to be important cytological parameters for the diagnosis of malignancy. However, electron microscopy investigations, focused on the structural organization of the nucleolar components, failed to reveal any pathognomonic changes in cancer cell nucleoli. No peculiar feature distinguishes, for example, a hypertrophied cancer cell nucleolus from that of nonmalignant, rapidly growing cells of embryonic, regenerating, or glandular tissues (Bernhard and Granboulan, 1968). Nevertheless, independently of these ultrastructural data, the nucleolar morphology has maintained a certain importance for the diagnosis of malignancy. The possibility of estimating the differences of the nucleolar morphology in an objective and reliable manner, such as by measuring the size and number of the interphase NORs, has raised new interest in the evaluation of the nucleolus for the cytologic diagnosis of malignancy.

The interphase NOR distribution was evaluated in an electron microscopy study carried out on eight cases of benign nevi and eight cases of malignant melanomas. It was observed that NOR distribution was quite different in benign and malignant nucleoli. Benign nevocytes had two to three prominent interphase NORs, whereas malignant cell nucleoli exhibited numerous and small interphase NORs. The evaluation of interphase NOR distribution was therefore proposed as a diagnostic parameter for distinguishing benign nevi

---

FIG. 13 (top). Silver-stained cells (K-562 cells) observed with reflected light. Arrow denotes argyrophilic granules. Bar = 1 μm.

FIG. 14 (bottom). Silver-stained K-562 cells seen with a high-voltage electron microscope within a 2-μm-thick section. The argyrophilic components appear as roundish structures of about 0.5 μm composed of one center (fibrillar center) and with surrounding loops of dense fibrillar component (arrows). These roundish structures correspond well with argyrophilic granules observed at the optical level (Fig. 13, arrow). Bar = 1 μm.

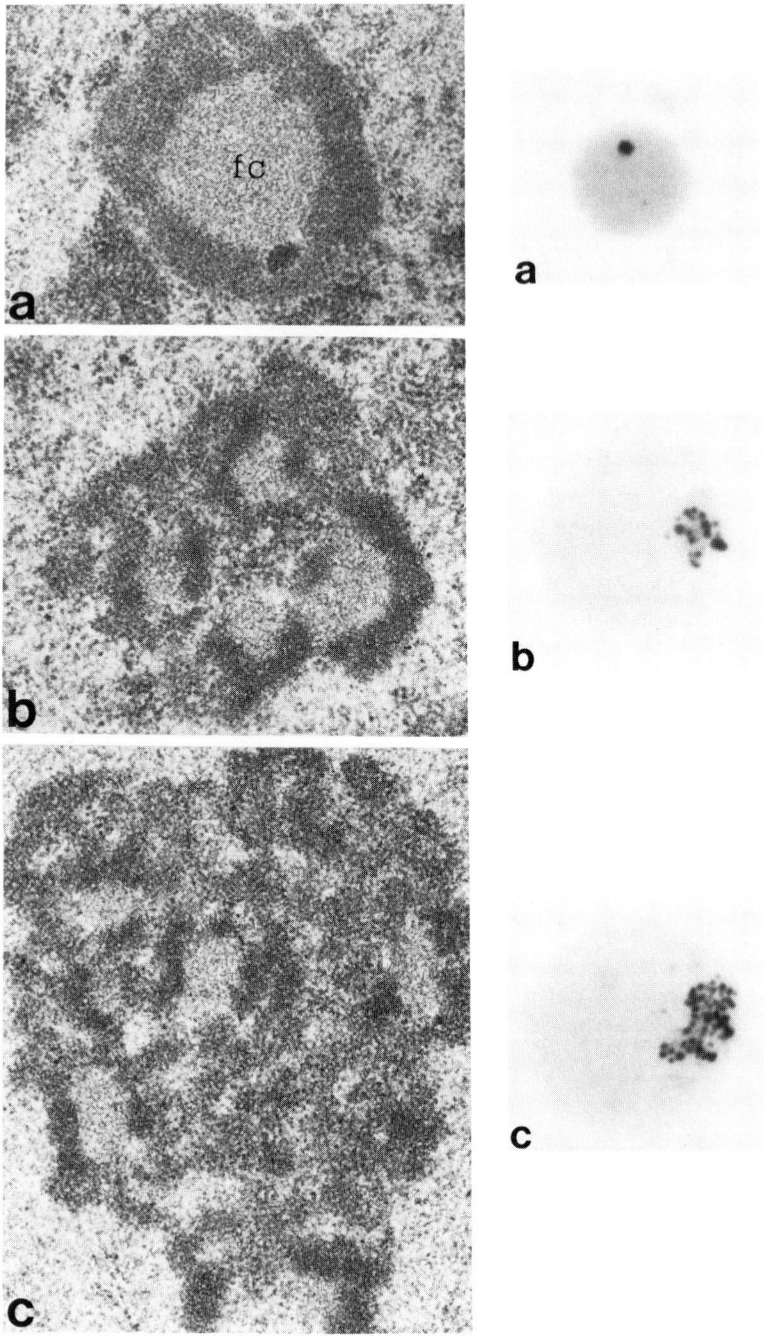
fc
a
b
c
a
b
c

from malignant melanomas at the ultrastructural level (Derenzini et al., 1986).

However, the parameter relative to interphase NOR distribution is of little value in routine histocytopathological diagnoses of tumor lesions, in which electron microscopy is not mandatorily utilized. In fact, electron microscopy is time consuming and permits only limited observations; to obtain valuable information on interphase NOR distribution patterns in neoplastic nucleoli, the largest possible number of tumor cells must be screened. As previously mentioned (Section II,C), in 1986, Ploton and co-workers applied the one-step silver method for staining Ag-NOR proteins and succeeded in visualizing interphase NORs at the light microscopic level in cytological and histological routine samples. In the preparations stained according to the procedure used by Ploton et al. (1986), the interphase NORs appear as well-defined black dots. Each black dot corresponds to one interphase NOR as visualized at the electron microscopic level (Figs. 13 and 14). The changes in nucleolar shape and size can therefore be easily recognized and quantified by a simple evaluation of the number and distribution of silver-stained dots (Figs. 15 and 16).

In the first application of this silver staining method for the diagnostic detection of interphase NORs, paraffin-embedded human prostatic cancer cells were shown to be characterized by many silver-stained nucleolar dots, whereas hyperplastic gland cells exhibited markedly fewer silver-stained dots. The application of this silver staining technique to routinely processed human neoplastic tissues was recommended to study interphase NOR distribution in relation to grading cancer cells and/or evaluating the differentiation state of cancer cells *in situ* (Ploton et al., 1986).

X. Distribution of Silver-Stained Interphase NORs in Neoplastic Cells

The possibility of using the silver staining technique for proteins of interphase NORs as a tool to obtain quantifiable information on the structural organization of nucleoli had been immediately positively considered by pathologists for application in routine histocytology of tumor diagnosis. In this context, the first application of silver-stained interphase NOR counting in a

---

FIG. 15 (left). Ultrastructural aspects of control (a) and phytohemagglutinin-stimulated human lymphocytes (b and c). Note the different nucleolar morphology as a consequence of the different distributions of the interphase NORs [fibrillar centers (fc) plus dense fibrillar component] (×37,000). [Reproduced with permission from Derenzini et al. (1987b).]

FIG. 16 (right). Smeared preparations of the lymphocyte samples shown in Fig. 15. Silver staining for the Ag-NOR proteins (Ploton *et al.*, 1986) (×30,000).

series of cases large enough to be clearly significant was carried out by Crocker and Skilbeck (1987) on cutaneous melanotic lesions. The authors found that the number of interphase NORs of lentigo maligna, superficial spreading melanoma, and melanocarcinoma greatly exceeded that of a variety of benign melanotic lesions (7.9 versus 1.21 interphase NORs per nucleus). Many subsequent studies of the distribution of interphase NORs have been performed (see Table II) in different types of tumor tissues and have

TABLE II

Tumor Lesions in which Interphasic Ag-NOR Evaluation Has Been Shown to Be Useful for the Diagnosis of Malignancy

Type of tumor	Interphasic Ag-NOR evaluation	Number of cases examined	Reference
Lymphomas	Number counted	100	Crocker and Nar (1987)
Melanocytic lesions	Number counted	50	Crocker and Skilbeck (1987)
Small cell tumor of childhood	Number counted	50	Egan et al. (1987)
Non-Hodgkin's lymphomas	Number counted	20	Crocker et al. (1988)
Breast lesions	Number counted	46	Smith and Crocker (1988)
Neuroblastomas	Number counted	20	Egan et al. (1988c)
Liver lesions	Number counted	54	Crocker and McGovern (1988)
Cervical lesions	Number counted	24	Rowlands (1988)
Salivary gland lesions	Number counted	35	Morgan et al. (1988)
Melanocytic lesions	Number counted	45	Fallowfield et al. (1988)
Intestinal lesions	Number counted	25	Derenzini et al. (1988a)
Cervical lesions	Number counted	50	Egan et al. (1988a)
Nose papillomas	Number counted	19	Egan and Ramsden (1988)
Pleural effusions	Number counted	45	Ayres et al. (1988)
Breast lesions	Number counted	214	Giri et al. (1989b)
Human effusions	Morphometric analysis	30	Derenzini et al. (1989a)
Rhabdomyoblastic lesions	Number counted	15	Eusebi et al. (1989)
Melanocytic lesions	Number counted	78	Leong and Gilham (1989)
Breast lesions	Number counted	149	Raymond and Leong (1989)
Bladder tumors	Number counted	39	Ooms and Veldhuizen (1989)
Breast lesions	Number counted	25	Giri et al. (1989a)
Leukemic bone marrows	Morphometric analysis	10	Arden et al. (1989)
Melanocytic lesions	Number counted	33	Fallowfield and Cook (1989)
Myogenic tumors of the stomach	Number counted	26	Sinn et al. (1989)
Epithelial lesions of the stomach	Number counted	45	Suarez et al. (1989)
Endometrial lesions	Number counted	62	Wilkinson et al. (1990)

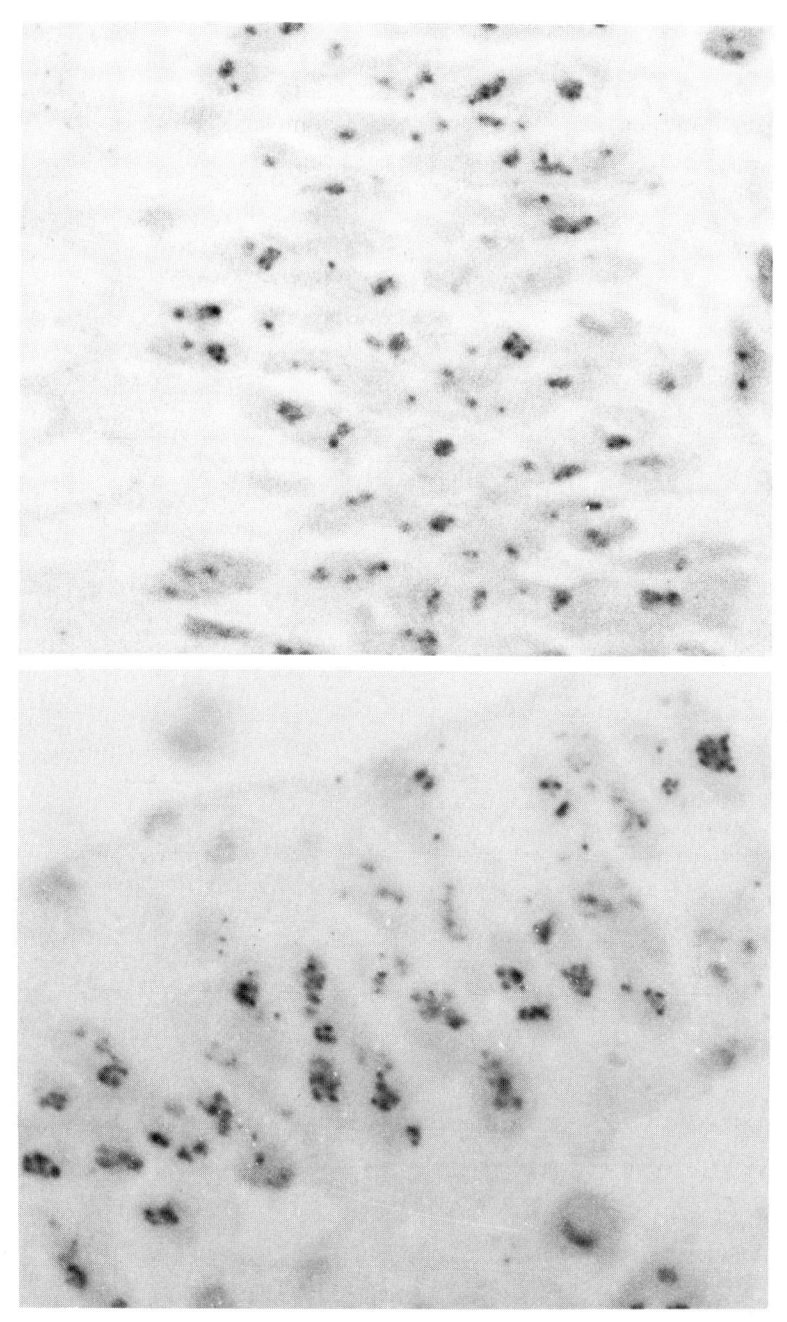

FIG. 17 (top). Paraffin-embedded section of a polyp from human colon, stained for the Ag-NOR proteins (×1500).

FIG. 18 (bottom). Paraffin-embedded section of human colon adenocarcinoma, stained for the Ag-NOR proteins; note the greater number of silver-stained interphase NORs as compared to the polyp nuclei in Fig. 17 (×1500).

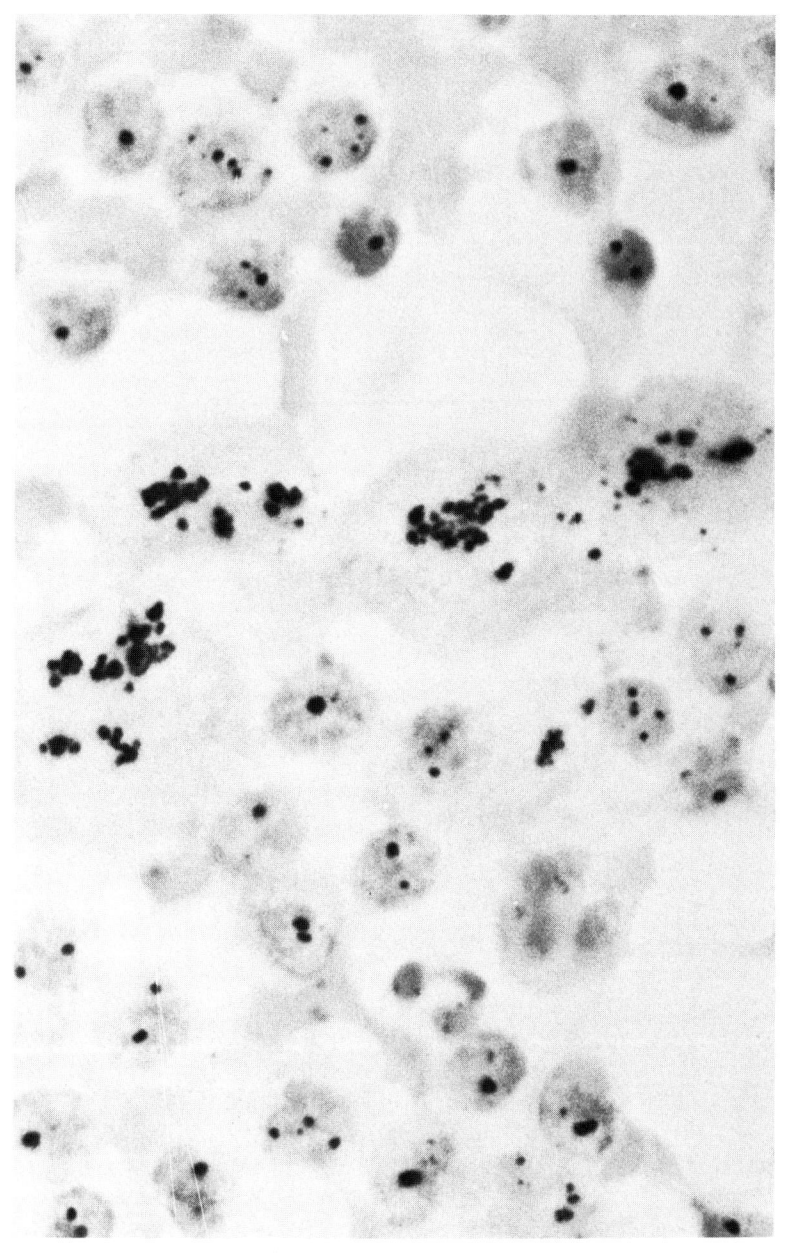

FIG. 19. Adenocarcinomatous effusion. Four neoplastic cells can be easily distinguished from the reactive nonneoplastic cells on the basis of the silver-stained interphase NOR number (×2500).

shown that malignant cells were characterized by a higher number of interphase NORs than the corresponding normal or hyperplastic cells (see Table II) (Figs. 17 and 18). Evaluation of the number of interphase NORs has therefore been regarded as a new tool that can be used quantitatively or semiquantitatively to help pathologists in the diagnosis of malignancy (Anonymous, 1987).

Apart from clear-cut benign and malignant tumors (for which silver staining is obviously of very little value for the experienced pathologist), evaluation of silver-stained interphase NOR distribution has proved to be useful for defining the nature of lesions such as florid dysplasia, in which the diagnosis of malignancy is frequently difficult on purely morphologic grounds. In a study carried out on benign intradermal nevi, compound nevi with no evidence of melanocyte dysplasia, malignant melanomas, and compound nevi exhibiting moderate to severe melanocytic dysplasia, Fallowfield *et al.* (1988) found a highly significant difference in the numbers of silver-stained NORs in benign nevus cells and atypical melanocytes and in malignant melanocytes. Furthermore, another well-known diagnostic problem has been tackled with the help of silver-stained NOR evaluation, i.e., the distinction, in human pleural effusions, between neoplastic (both metastatic carcinoma and mesothelioma) cells and reactive mesothelial cells (Fig. 19). In this case, instead of measurement of the NOR number, the mean areas occupied by silver-stained NORs were measured by densitometric analysis using an automated image analyzer. This objective and reliable method for statistically evaluating interphase NOR distribution clearly showed that cancer cells contained a greater number of silver-stained NORs than did mesothelial reactive cells (Derenzini *et al.*, 1989a).

XI. Is the High Number of Interphase NORs a Peculiar Feature of Cancer Cells?

The results reported in the preceding paragraph on the distribution of interphase NORs in neoplastic cells would lead to the enthusiastic conclusion that a malignant cell might be distinguished from the corresponding benign cell on the basis of a higher quantity of silver-stained interphase NORs. However, just after the promulgation by *Lancet* of the usefulness of interphase silver-stained NOR counting for the diagnosis of malignancy, the limits of this method for its universal application in tumor pathology began to be stressed. Preliminary observations on the interphase distribution of silver-stained NORs in breast tumor lesions have in fact demonstrated that no clear-cut separation exists between the interphase NOR values of benign and some malignant breast tumors (Derenzini *et al.*, 1987c). Detailed studies on inter-

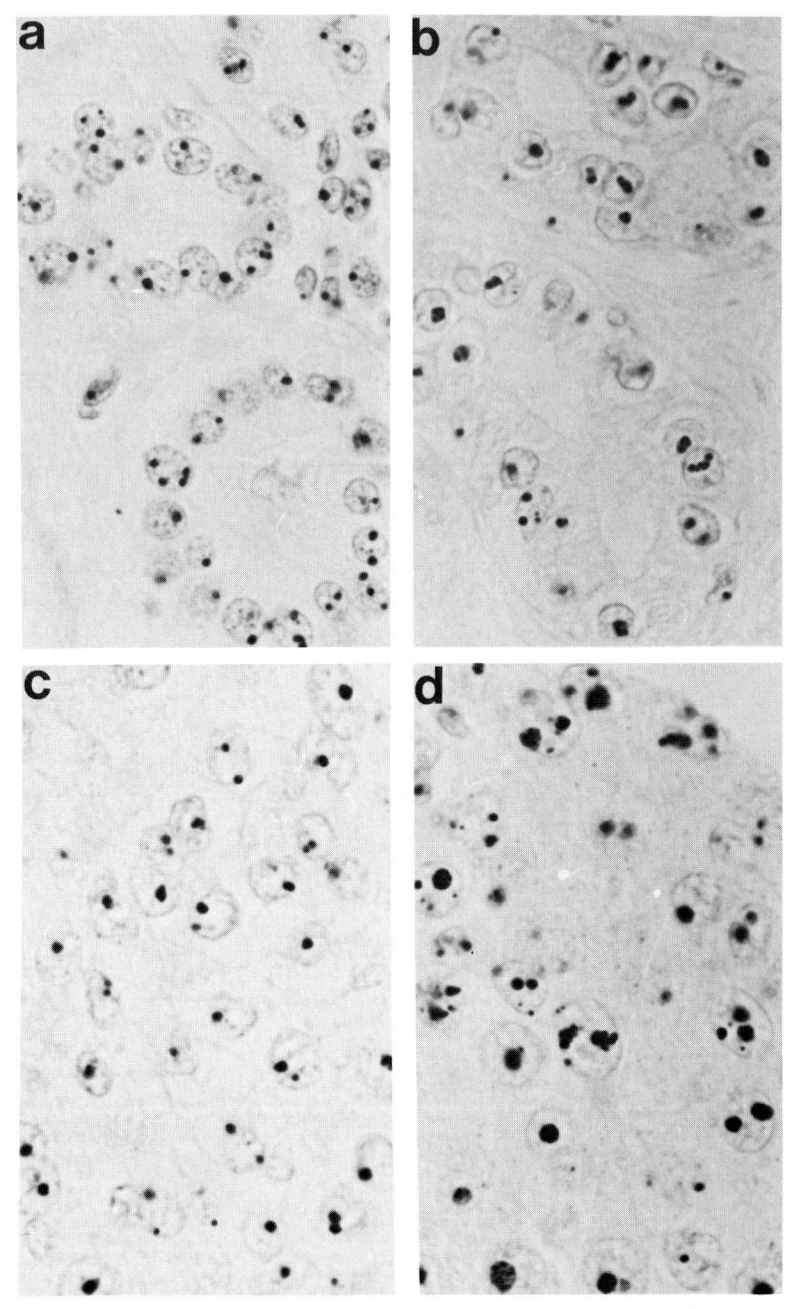

FIG. 20. Interphase silver-stained NOR distribution in paraffin-embedded samples of human breast. (a) Normal, (b) adenoma, (c) grade I, and (d) grade III ductal infiltrating carcinoma. No differences in Ag-NOR amounts are detectable in grade I carcinoma and normal or adenomatous cells (×1500).

phase NOR distribution in tumor lesions of the breast subsequently clearly showed that the silver-stained NOR value cannot be considered as a parameter of absolute diagnostic value (Fig. 20). Giri *et al.* (1989b) examined 214 benign and malignant breast lesions by counting the number of silver-stained interphase NORs. They found that if the mean of interphase NOR counts of all benign and malignant lesions were considered, a significative difference existed. However, if the number of Ag-NORs in each case was measured, the counts in 25–30% of carcinomas overlapped those of benign lesions. Practically, the same results have been obtained when the Ag-NOR quantity was measured in benign and malignant lesions of the breast using an automated image analyzer to make a morphometric evaluation of stained areas (Derenzini *et al.*, 1990a). About 30% of the lower values of malignant lesions in fact overlapped those of benign lesions. Also, thyroid tumor interphase Ag-NOR counting did not permit differentiation of benign from malignant tumors (Nairn *et al.*, 1988); only a very limited number of anaplastic cancers exhibited Ag-NOR counts significantly higher than those of benign tumors.

From these data it can be argued that caution must be used in employing the distribution of silver-stained interphase NORs as a parameter for the cytohistological diagnosis of malignancy, even if in many types of tumors the Ag-NOR counting method has been demonstrated to be of actual diagnostic value. The quantitative evaluation of interphase NORs appears therefore to represent a useful parameter in addition to the other methods for the diagnosis of malignancy. Only in some cases, e.g., pleural effusions, can Ag-NOR evaluation can be regarded as a cytological parameter sufficient to enable the precise identification of cancer cells.

XII. Relationship between Interphase NOR Distribution and Neoplastic State of the Cell

The observation that cancer cells generally have more interphase silver-stained NORs than do the corresponding hyperplastic and normal cells, apart from having an immediate and important impact on tumor pathology diagnosis, has also stimulated investigations on the biological role of these nucleolar components in the cancer cell.

As previously stressed (Section VII), the nucleolus must be considered as a morphological–functional unit in which ribosomal genes, located in the interphase NORs, are engaged in ribosomal biogenesis. According to available evidence, the nucleolar morphology, and therefore the distribution of interphase NORs, changes by varying the ribosomal transcriptional activity (Goessens, 1984; Hernandez-Verdun, 1986). Therefore, the higher number of interphase NORs in cancer cells might simply reflect a higher level of rRNA synthesis, which frequently characterizes these cells as compared to normal cells. Another change that might occur in neoplastic cells, which can determine the modification of the nucleolar distribution of interphase NORs, is the variation in the number of acrocentric chromosomes carrying the NORs. Because hyperdiploidy is the most frequent change in chromosome number, the high quantity of interphase NORs might be a consequence of a higher number, compared to normal cells, of metaphase NORs in neoplastic cells. Finally, the altered NOR distribution observed in cancer cells might be related to their continuous dividing state.

We will consider separately the relationship between the interphase NOR distribution and these three different morphofunctional characteristics of neoplastic cells.

A. Interphase NOR Distribution and Ribosomal Transcriptional Activity

Support that a strict relationship exists between the interphase NOR number and ribosomal transcriptional activity has been provided by the following observations. During the cell cycle, when ribosomal biogenesis begins in the late telophase, only one fibrillar center with the closely associated dense fibrillar component (interphase NOR) is present in the nucleolus. With the progression of the cell cycle, ribosomal transcriptional activity increases and interphase NORs become more numerous (Goessens and Lepoint, 1974; Hernandez-Verdun *et al.*, 1980a). In human fibroblasts cultured *in vitro*, the number of interphase NORs per nucleolus decreases from the exponential phase of the growth to the confluent phase. Inhibition of rRNA synthesis by actinomycin D treatment induced an even more pronounced reduction of interphase NOR number (Jordan and McGovern, 1981). In human circulating lymphocytes a solitary interphase NOR characterizes the nucleolus in which ribosomal biogenesis is negligible. After stimulation by phytohemagglutinin (PHA), lymphocytes enter the cell cycle and ribosomal transcriptional activity is strongly enhanced. During the course of PHA stimulation, the number of interphase NORs progressively increases (Arrighi *et al.*, 1980; Derenzini *et al.*, 1987b). This increase in the number of interphase NORs is not related to the duplication of ribosomal genes, because it also occurs before DNA synthesis begins (Derenzini *et al.*, 1987b). In resting rat hepatocytes the number of interphase NORs (visualized by silver staining) was found to be approximately four per nucleolus. In rat hepatocytes induced to duplicate by partial hepatectomy, there were approximately 15 interphase NORs per nucleolus 18 hours after the operation (Busch *et al.*, 1979).

During differentiation and progressive inactivation of transcriptional activity, which occurs in epithelial cells of the small intestine during cellular chromosome number demonstrated about 30 Ag-NORs. Therefore, it is reasonable to suppose that the increased number of interphase silver-stained NORs in cancer cells might be due to the increased number of acrocentric chromosomes carrying them.

To verify this supposition, a quantitative study has been carried out on the relationship between the number of Ag-NOR metaphase chromosomes and interphase Ag-NORs in two neuroblastoma cell lines, CHP 212 and HTB 10 (Derenzini *et al.*, 1989b). The results indicate that the mean number of Ag-NOR-bearing chromosomes is very similar in both types of cells (5.5 versus 5.1), whereas the number of interphase Ag-NORs was found to be quite different in the two cell lines, being more than double in CHP 212 cells compared to HTB 10 cells (52.3 versus 23.0 interphase NORs). Because not all of the NORs of metaphase chromosomes can be visualized by silver staining (Miller *et al.*, 1976) and because ribosomal genes might not be localized exclusively on the acrocentric chromosomes, a consequence of structural alterations in tumor cell chromosomes (Trent *et al.*, 1981), in the same study the possibility was also considered that the greater number of interphase Ag-NORs detected in CHP 212 cells might be related to a greater quantity of ribosomal DNA, without changes of chromosome number. Measurements of the actual quantity of ribosomal sequences in the two neuroblastoma cell lines by hybridization with radiolabeled rDNA, showing no significant difference in rDNA content in the two cell lines, demonstrated that this was not the case. These data, therefore, indicated that no direct relationship exists between the quantitative changes of interphase Ag-NORs and the number of metaphase chromosomes carrying ribosomal genes in cancer cells.

C. Interphase NORs and Cell Duplication Rate

Cell proliferation is one of the most important characteristics of cancer tissue. As the cell enters the mitotic cycle, marked changes in the nucleolar structural organization are induced (Derenzini *et al.*, 1987b). A progressive increase in the nucleolar size with an increase in the numbers of interphase NORs occurs from G_1 to S phase (Hubbell *et al.*, 1980). The continuously dividing state of the cancer cells might therefore be responsible for the higher number of interphase NORs compared to normal and hyperplastic cells. Several lines of evidence indicate that this is in fact the case. In neuroblastoma cells cultured *in vitro*, serum deprivation caused a progressive reduction of proliferation activity as measured by [^{3}H]thymidine incorporation (Derenzini *et al.*, 1989b). Quantitative analysis of the silver-stained interphase NORs showed a progressive reduction of the nucleolar silver-stained structures in serum-deprived cells. If serum was again added to cells at various times after serum deprivation, cell proliferation was stimulated again up to the control level, with a parallel quantitative increase of silver-stained interphase NORs. Moreover, in a study carried out on 13 different neuroblastoma cell lines, the quantity of silver-stained nucleolar structures measured by means of an atuomated image analyzer was strictly proportional to the proliferative activity of the cells (Fig. 21). Cell lines with a difference of only 4 hours doubling time were characterized by a statistical difference in interphase Ag-NOR quantity (Trerè et al., 1989).

The relationship between the quantity of interphase silver-stained NORs and cell proliferation activity was also demonstrated by comparing data on interphase NOR values and cell kinetics obtained using either DNA flow cytometry or Ki-67 immunoreactivity. Crocker et al. (1988) showed that in a series of 20 non-Hodgkin's lymphomas, the number of silver-stained interphase NORs permitted low- and high-grade histological types to be clearly discriminated. Comparison with DNA flow cytometry data obtained on paraffin-embedded samples of the same lymphomas indicated the presence of a linear correlation between the mean numbers of interphase Ag-NORs and the

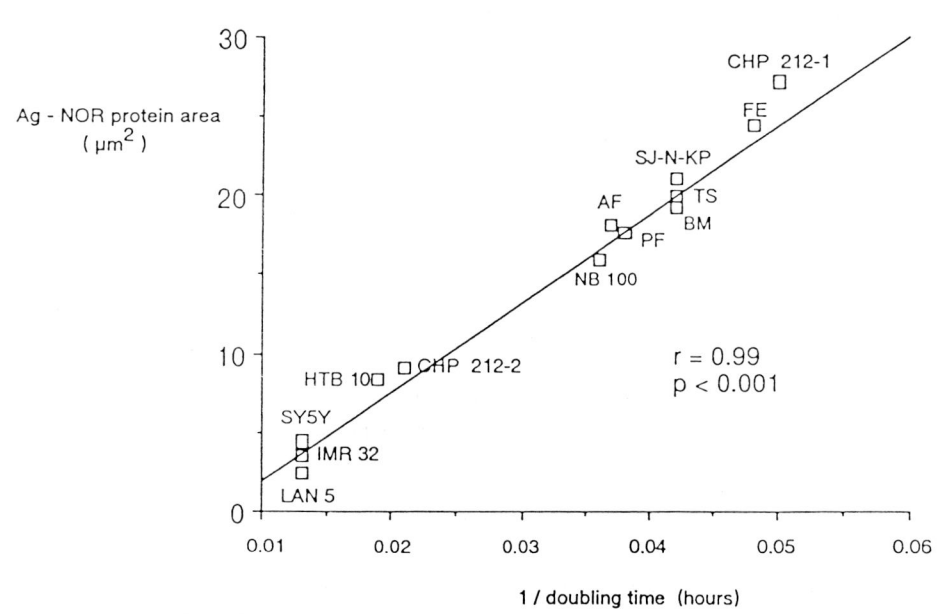

FIG. 21. Correlation between Ag-NOR protein quantity and doubling time in 13 neuroblastoma cell lines.

percentage of S-phase cells for each case. A less clear relationship between cell growth fractions, as evaluated by DNA flow cytometry, and interphase Ag-NOR counts was observed in breast carcinomas (Giri et al., 1989b). Tumors having more than three interphase Ag-NORs per nucleus had growth phase fractions (S + G_2 + M%) of 19.15 ± 12.31%, whereas those with less than three interphase Ag-NORs had a mean value of 13.94 ± 5.55%. However, as was pointed out by the authors, although the measurement gave rise to a positive trend, the values were not statistically significant.

A comparison of interphase NOR distribution and immunoreactivity to Ki-67 antibody was performed on non-Hodgkin's lymphomas (Hall et al., 1988) and breast carcinomas (Dervan et al., 1989). Ki-67 is a monoclonal antibody for a nuclear antigen that is present only in proliferating cells in the G_1, S, M, and G_2 phases of the cell cycle (Gerdes et al., 1984; Schwarting et al., 1986). It does not react with cells in the G_0 phase. Therefore, the percentage of Ki-67 positivity indicates the proportion of tumor cells that entered the mitotic cycle. Examining 80 cases of non-Hodgkin's lymphomas for Ki-67 immunoreactivity and for interphase Ag-NOR distribution, Hall et al. (1988) observed that the proportion of tumor cells with nuclear positivity to Ki-67 antibody and the mean number of interphase Ag-NORs were linearly related. A highly significant correlation between nucleolar Ag-NOR and Ki-67 scores was also observed in 27 benign breast lesions and 70 breast carcinomas (Dervan et al., 1989). Epithelial benign lesions contained a mean of 2.65–6.8 Ag-NORs per cell, whereas malignant cells contained 4.6–26.9 Ag-NORs. In benign tissues, Ki-67 scores ranged from 0 to 4% and in malignant tumors, from 3 to 98%. In a study confined to malignant breast tumors, a positive relationship between the mean number of nucleolar Ag-NORs per nucleus and tumor growth fraction, as determined by Ki-67 immunostaining, was also reported (Raymond and Leong, 1989).

The strict correlation between the quantity of interphase Ag-NORs and the cell duplication rate has recently been demonstrated to be valid, even when different cancer cell lines were considered (Derenzini et al., 1990b). The proliferative activity of 12 neoplastic cell lines from different human cancers (neuroblastomas, colon, and breast adenocarcinomas; cervical, tubal, and laryngeal carcinomas) was measured by [^{3}H]thymidine incorporation, whereas interphase Ag-NOR quantities were measured using the automated image analyzer. A linear relationship was found for these two parameters independently of the type of cancer cell.

These data indicate that the quantity of interphase Ag-NORs is only strictly related to the duplication rate and, therefore, the evaluation of this quantity may represent a very promising method for determining the proliferative activity of neoplastic tissues in routine histopathology.

XIII. Structural Changes of Ribosomal Genes in Cells Stimulated to Proliferate

Wachtler *et al.* (1986), in a comparative study on the distribution of ribosomal genes visualized either by silver staining for Ag-NOR proteins or by *in situ* hybridization, demonstrated that in resting lymphocytes the ribosomal genes associated with the Ag-NOR proteins in the nucleolus were part of ribosomal genes that, as revealed by *in situ* hybridization, were also distributed in the nucleoplasmic space. After phytohemagglutinin stimulation, a progressive increase of the nucleolar silver-stained structures occurs; this is paralleled by a progressive reduction of the extranucleolar ribosomal genes, which, in fact, tend to collect in the nucleolar body. These distributional changes in ribosomal genes take place before DNA synthesis begins. In the same work, by considering the intensity of the fluorescence signals of ribosomal genes revealed by *in situ* hybridization, as an indicator of the structure of ribosomal genes, the authors suggested that the extranucleolar ribosomal genes are in a highly condensed state, whereas, after migration into the nucleolus, they assume a decondensed state. These observations were consistent with the ultrastructural results showing that, in thin sections selectively stained for DNA with the Feulgen-like osmium–ammine reaction, all the extranucleolar chromatin of resting lymphocytes was in a highly compact configuration. Only ribosomal chromatin located in interphase NORs was in an extended configuration (Derenzini *et al.*, 1987b). Following 20 hours of stimulation by phytohemagglutinin, when DNA synthesis had not yet begun, the quantity of interphase NORs with extended ribosomal chromatin was greatly increased. The same events have been observed to occur during the G_1 phase in rat hepatocytes stimulated to proliferate by partial hepatectomy (Pession *et al.*, 1989). It is worth noting that in both cases the increase in amounts of ribosomal chromatin with extended configurations in the nucleolus paralleled the increase in Ag-NOR protein quantity. As was previously stressed (see Section VII,A), the Ag-NOR proteins are always associated with ribosomal chromatin with extended configurations. The increase in the quantity of Ag-NOR protein that occurs during G_1 might therefore be related to the progressive decondensation of highly condensed ribosomal genes that migrate from the nucleoplasmic space into the nucleolus. The decondensation of all ribosomal genes during G_1 would be a necessary step for gene duplication during the following S phase. Indeed, in a study carried out on synchronized HeLa cells to evaluate the quantitative changes in the Ag-NOR proteins during the cell cycle, Hubbell *et al.* (1980) found that the Ag-NOR protein quantity progressively increased during G_1 and then remained constant up to the late G_2.

These observations might also suggest the reason for the positive relationship that exists between interphase silver-stained NORs and the cell duplication rate. In fact, in rapidly proliferating cells, a higher percentage of cells is in S and G_2 phases than is seen in slowly dividing cells. Therefore, because the higher values of Ag-NOR proteins were found in nucleoli from the late G_1 to the late G_2 phase, the very rapidly proliferating cells will be characterized by a higher quantity of nucleolar Ag-NOR proteins.

Acknowledgments

Thanks are due to Professor P. Jeannesson for kindly providing HL-60, K-562, and Friend cell lines. Dominique Ploton would like to thank Mrs. M. Menager for excellent technical work and for help in the preparation of the manuscript. Mrs. A. Quiqueret and Miss C. Champion are thanked for their typing assistance. The authors are most grateful to Dr. Christine M. Betts for kindly correcting the manuscript.

The work from Massimo Derenzini's laboratory was supported by grants from M.P.I. (Rome) and A.I.R.C. (Milan).

References

Altmann, G. G., and Leblond, C. P. (1982). *J. Cell Sci.* **56,** 83.
Angelier, N., Hernandez-Verdun, D., and Bouteille, M. (1982). *Chromosoma (Berlin)* **86,** 661.
Anonymous (1987). *Lancet* **1,** 1413.
Arden, K. C., Bucana, C. D., Johnston, D. A., and Pathak, S. (1989). *Int. J. Cancer* **43,** 395.
Arrighi, F. E., Lau, Y. F., and Spallone, A. (1980). *Cytogenet. Cell Genet.* **26,** 244.
Arroua, M. L., Hartung, M., Devictor, M., Berge-Lefranc, J. L., and Stahl, A. (1982). *Biol. Cell.* **44,** 337.
Ayres, J. G., Crocker, J. G., and Skilbeck, N. Q. (1988). *Thorax* **43,** 366.
Babu, K. A., and Verma, R. S. (1985). *Int. Rev. Cytol.* **94,** 151.
Bernhard, W., and Granboulan, N. (1968). *In* "The Nucleus" (A. J. Dalton and F. Haguenau, eds.), pp. 81–149. Academic Press, New York.
Biggiogera, M., Fakan, S., Kaufmann, S. H., Black, A., Shaper, J. H., and Busch, H. (1989). *J. Histochem. Cytochem.* **37,** 1371.
Bourgeois, C. A., Hernandez-Verdun, D., Hubert, J., and Bouteille, M. (1979). *Exp. Cell Res.* **123,** 449.
Brill, S. J., Di Nardo, S., Voelkel-Meiman, K., and Sternglanz, R. (1987). *Nature (London)* **326,** 414.
Busch, H., and Smetana, K. (1970). *In* "The Nucleolus," pp. 448–471. Academic Press, New York.
Busch, H., Daskal, Y., Gyorkey, F., and Smetana, K. (1979). *Cancer Res.* **39,** 857.
Busch, H., Lischwe, M. A., Michalik, J., Chan, P. K., and Busch, R. K. (1982). *In* "The Nucleolus" (E. G. Jordan and C. A. Cullis, eds.). Cambridge Univ. Press, London.
Buys, C. H. C. M., and Osinga, J. (1980). *Chromosoma (Berlin)* **77,** 1.
Chambon, P. (1978). *Cold Spring Harbor Symp. Quant. Biol.* **42,** 1209.
Clavaguera, A., Querol, E., Coll, D., Genesca, J., and Egozcue, J. (1983). *Cell. Mol. Biol.* **29,** 255.
Clavaguera, A., Querol, E., Coll, D., and Egozcue, J. (1984). *Cell. Mol. Biol.* **30,** 175.
Cogliati, R., and Gautier, A. (1973). *C. R. Hebd. Seances Acad. Sci. Ser. D* **276,** 3041.
Crocker, J., and McGovern, J. (1988). *J. Clin. Pathol.* **41,** 1044.

Crocker, J., and Nar, P. (1987). *J. Pathol.* **151,** 111.
Crocker, J., and Skilbeck, N. (1987). *J. Clin. Pathol.* **40,** 885.
Crocker, J., Macartney, J. C., and Smith, P. J. (1988). *J. Pathol.* **154,** 151.
De Capoa, A., Ferraro, M., Lavia, P., Pelliccia, F., and Finazzi-Agrò, A. (1982). *J. Histochem. Cytochem.* **30,** 908.
Derenzini, M., Hernandez-Verdun, D., and Bouteille, M. (1981a). *Biol. Cell.* **41,** 161.
Derenzini, M., Viron, A., and Puvion-Dutilleul, F. (1981b). *J. Ultrastruct. Res.* **80,** 133.
Derenzini, M., Hernandez-Verdun, D., and Bouteille, M. (1982). *Exp. Cell Res.* **141,** 463.
Derenzini, M., Hernandez-Verdun, D., Pession, A., and Novello, F. (1983a). *J. Ultrastruct. Res.* **84,** 161.
Derenzini, M., Hernandez-Verdun, D., and Bouteille, M. (1983b). *J. Cell Sci.* **61,** 137.
Derenzini, M., Pession, A., Betts-Eusebi, C. M., and Novello, F. (1983c). *Exp. Cell Res.* **145,** 127.
Derenzini, M., Pession, A., Licastro, F., and Novello, F. (1985). *Exp. Cell Res.* **157,** 50.
Derenzini, M., Betts, C. M., Ceccarelli, C., and Eusebi, V. (1986). *Virchows Arch. B* **52,** 343.
Derenzini, M., Hernandez-Verdun, D., Farabegoli, F., Pession, A., and Novello, F. (1987a). *Chromosoma (Berlin)* **95,** 63.
Derenzini, M., Farabegoli, F., Pession, A., and Novello, F. (1987b). *Exp. Cell Res.* **170,** 31.
Derenzini, M., Betts, C. M., and Eusebi, V. (1987c). *Lancet* **8853,** 286.
Derenzini, M., Romagnoli, T., Mingazzini, P., and Marinozzi, V. (1988a). *Virchows Arch. B* **54,** 334.
Derenzini, M., Romagnoli, T., Ceccarelli, C., and Eusebi, V. (1988b). *J. Histochem. Cytochem.* **36,** 1453.
Derenzini, M., Nardi, F., Farabegoli, F., Ottinetti, A., Roncaroli, F., and Bussolati, G. (1989a). *Acta Cytol.* **33,** 491.
Derenzini, M., Pession, A., Farabegoli, F., Trerè, D., Badiali, M., and Dehan, P. (1989b). *Am. J. Pathol.* **134,** 925.
Derenzini, M., Betts, C. M., Trerè, D., Mambelli, V., Millis, R. R., Cancellieri, A., and Eusebi, V. (1990a). *Ultrastruct. Pathol.* **14,** 233.
Derenzini, M., Pession, A., and Trerè, D. (1990b). *Lab. Invest.* **63,** 137.
Dervan, P. A., Gilmartin, L. G., Loftus, B. M., and Carney, D. N. (1989). *Am. J. Clin. Pathol.* **92,** 401.
Dhar, V. N., Miller, D. A., Kulkarni, A. B., and Miller, O. J. (1987). *Mol. Cell. Biol.* **7,** 1289.
Egan, M., and Ramsden, J. C. (1988). *Histopathology* **13,** 579.
Egan, M. J., Raafat, F., Crocker, J., and Smith, K. (1987). *J. Pathol.* **153,** 275.
Egan, M., Freeth, M., and Crocker, J. (1988a). *Histopathology* **13,** 561.
Egan, M. J., Raafat, F., Crocker, J., and Smith, K. (1988b). *J. Clin. Pathol.* **41,** 31.
Egan, M., Raafat, F., Crocker, J., and William, D. (1988c). *J. Clin. Pathol.* **41,** 527.
Erard, M. S., Belenguer, P., Caizergues-Ferrer, M., Pantaloni, A., and Amalric, F. (1988). *Eur. J. Biochem.* **175,** 525.
Eusebi, V., Ceccarelli, C., Cancellieri, A., and Derenzini, M. (1989). *Tumori* **75,** 4.
Evans, H. J., Buckland, R. A., and Pardue, M. L. (1974). *Chromosoma (Berlin)* **48,** 405.
Fallowfield, M. E., and Cook, M. G. (1989). *Histopathology* **14,** 299.
Fallowfield, M. E., Dodson, A. R., and Cook, M. G. (1988). *Histopathology* **13,** 95.
Fakan, S. (1978). *In* "The Cell Nucleus" (H. Busch, ed.), Vol. V, pp. 3–53. Academic Press, New York.
Ferraro, M., and Prantera, G. (1988). *Cytogenet. Cell Genet.* **47,** 58.
Finch, J. J., Lutter, L. C., Rhodes, D., Brown, R. S., Rushton, B., Levitt, M., and Klug, A. (1977). *Nature (London)* **269,** 29.
Friedlander, M. L., Hedley, D. W., and Taylor, W. (1984). *J. Clin. Pathol.* **37,** 961.
Gajdardjieva, K. G., Markov, D. V., Dimova, R. N., Kermekchiev, M. B., Todorov, I. T., Dabeva, M. D., and Hadjiolov, A. A. (1982). *Exp. Cell Res.* **140,** 95.
Gall, J. G., and Pardue, M. L. (1969). *Proc. Natl. Acad. Sci. U.S.A.* **63,** 378.

Gall, J. G., and Pardue, M. L. (1971). *In* "Methods in Enzymology" (L. Grossman and K. Moldave, eds.), Vol. 21, pp. 470–480. Academic Press, New York.
Gerdes, J., Lemke, H., Baisch, H., Wacker, H. H., Schwab, U., and Stein, H. (1984). *J. Immunol.* **133,** 1710.
Giri, D. D., Dundas, S. A., Sanderson, P. R., and Howat, A. J. (1989a). *Acta Cytol.* **33,** 173.
Giri, D. D., Nottingham, J. F., Lawry, J., Dundas, S. A. C., and Underwood, J. C. E. (1989b). *J. Pathol.* **157,** 307.
Goessens, G. (1984). *Int. Rev. Cytol.* **87,** 107.
Goessens, G., and Lepoint, A. (1974). *Exp. Cell Res.* **87,** 63.
Goodpasture, C., and Bloom, S. E. (1975). *Chromosoma (Berlin)* **53,** 37.
Haaf, T., Weis, H., Schindler, D., and Schmid, M. (1984). *Chromosoma (Berlin)* **90,** 149.
Hadjiolov, A. A. (1985). *Cell Biol. Monogr.* **12,** 1.
Hadjiolova, K., Rose, K., and Scheer, V. (1986). *Exp. Cell Res.* **165,** 481.
Hall, P. A., Awatts, J. C., and Stansfeld, A. G. (1988). *Histopathology* **12,** 373.
Heitz, E. (1931). *Planta* **12,** 774.
Henderson, A. S., Warburton, D., and Atwood, K. C. (1972). *Proc. Natl. Acad. Sci. U.S.A.* **69,** 3394.
Hernandez-Verdun, D. (1983). *Biol. Cell.* **49,** 191.
Hernandez-Verdun, D. (1986). *Methods Achiev. Exp. Pathol.* **12,** 26.
Hernandez-Verdun, D., and Derenzini, M. (1983). *Eur. J. Cell Biol.* **31,** 360.
Hernandez-Verdun, D., Hubert, J., Bourgeois, C. A., and Bouteille, M. (1978). *C. R. Hebd. Seances Acad. Sci. Ser. D* **287,** 1421.
Hernandez-Verdun, D., Hubert, J., Bourgeois, C. A., and Bouteille, M. (1979). *Exp. Cell Res.* **123,** 449.
Hernandez-Verdun, D., Bourgeois, C. A., and Bouteille, M. (1980a). *Biol. Cell.* **37,** 1.
Hernandez-Verdun, D., Hubert, J., Bourgeois, C. A., and Bouteille, M. (1980b). *Chromosoma (Berlin)* **79,** 349.
Hernandez-Verdun, D., Derenzini, M., and Bouteille, M. (1982). *Chromosoma (Berlin)* **85,** 461.
Hernandez-Verdun, D., Derenzini, M., and Bouteille, M. (1984). *J. Ultrastruct. Res.* **88,** 55.
Herrera, A. H., and Olson, M. O. J. (1986). *Biochemistry* **25,** 6258.
Howell, W. M. (1982). *In* "The Cell Nucleus" (H. Busch and L. Rothblum, eds.), Vol. IX, pp. 89–142. Academic Press, New York.
Howell, W. M., and Black, D. A. (1980). *Experientia* **36,** 1014.
Howell, W. M. Denton, T. E., and Diamond, J. R. (1975). *Experientia* **31,** 260.
Hubbell, H. R. (1985). *Stain Technol.* **60,** 285.
Hubbell, H. R., and Hsu, T. C. (1977). *Cytogenet. Cell Genet.* **19,** 185.
Hubbell, H. R., Rothblum, L. I., and Hsu, T. C. (1979). *Cell Biol. Int. Rep.* **3,** 615.
Hubbell, H. R., Lau, Y. F., Brown, R. L., and Hsu, T. C. (1980). *Exp. Cell Res.* **129,** 139.
Jordan, E. G. (1987). *Nature (London)* **29,** 489.
Jordan, E. G., and McGovern, J. H. (1981). *J. Cell Sci.* **52,** 373.
Koller, P. C. (1963). *Exp. Cell Res., Suppl.* **9,** 3.
Kornberg, R. D. (1977). *Annu. Rev. Biochem.* **46,** 931.
Lapeyre, B., Bourbon, H., and Amalric, F. (1987). *Proc. Natl. Acad. Sci. U.S.A.* **84,** 1472.
La Velle, A. (1985). *Stain Technol.* **60,** 271.
Leong, A. S., and Gilham, P. (1989). *Hum. Pathol.* **20,** 257.
Lischwe, M. A., Smetana, K., Olson, M. O. J., and Busch, H. (1979). *Life Sci.* **25,** 701.
Lomholt, B. E., and Toft, J. M. (1987). *Stain Technol.* **62,** 101.
Matsui, S., and Sandberg, A. A. (1985). *Chromosoma (Berlin)* **92,** 1.
McClintock, B. (1934). *Z. Zellforsch. Mikrosk. Anat.* **21,** 294.
Miller, O. L., and Bakken, A. H. (1972). *Acta Endocrinol. (Copenhagen), Suppl.* **168,** 155.
Miller, O. L., and Beatty, B. R. (1969). *Science* **164,** 955.

Miller, D. A., Dev, V. G., Tantravahi, R., and Miller, O. J. (1976). *Exp. Cell Res.* **101,** 235.
Mirre, C., and Knibiehler, R. (1982). *J. Cell Sci.* **55,** 247.
Mirre, C., and Stahl, A. (1978). *J. Ultrastruct. Res.* **64,** 377.
Mirre, C., and Stahl, A. (1981). *J. Cell Sci.* **48,** 105.
Morgan, D. W., Crocker, J., Watts, A., and Shenoi, P. M. (1988). *Histopathology* **13,** 553.
Morton, C. C., Brown, J. A., Holmes, W. M., Nance, W. E., and Wolf, B. (1983). *Exp. Cell Res.* **145,** 405.
Nairn, E. R., Crocker, J., and McGovern, J. (1988). *J. Clin. Pathol.* **41,** 1136.
Ochs, R. L., and Busch, H. (1984). *Exp. Cell Res.* **152,** 260.
Ooms, E. C., and Veldhuizen, R. W. (1989). *Virchows Arch. A: Pathol. Anat. Histol.* **414,** 365.
Pebusque, M. J., Vio, M., and Seite, R. (1981). *Biol. Cell.* **40,** 151.
Pession, A., Trerè, D., Farabegoli, F., Novello, F., Romagnoli, T., and Derenzini, M. (1989). *Proc. Nuclear Workshop, 11th* p. 141.
Pianese, G. (1896). *Beitr. Pathol. Anat. Allg. Pathol.* **142** (Suppl. 1), 1.
Ploton, D., Bobichon, H., and Adnet, J. J. (1982). *Biol. Cell.* **43,** 229.
Ploton, D., Menager, M., Jeannesson, P., Himber, G., Pigeon, F., and Adnet, J. J. (1986). *Histochem. J.* **18,** 5.
Raska, I., Reimer, G., Jarnik, M., Kostrouch, Z., and Raska, K. (1989). *Biol. Cell.* **65,** 79.
Raymond, W. A., and Leong, A. S. (1989). *Hum. Pathol.* **20,** 741.
Rowlands, D. C. (1988). *J. Clin. Pathol.* **41,** 1200.
Satoh, K., and Busch, H. (1981). *Cell Biol. Int. Rep.* **5,** 857.
Scheer, U., and Raska, I. (1987). *Chromosomes Today* **9,** 284.
Scheer, U., and Rose, K. M. (1984). *Proc. Natl. Acad. Sci. U.S.A.* **81,** 1431.
Scheer, U., and Zentgraf, H. (1982). *In* "The Cell Nucleus" (H. Busch and L. Rothblum, eds.), Vol. XI, pp. 143–176. Academic Press, New York.
Schmiady, H., Münke, M., and Sperling, K. (1979). *Exp. Cell Res.* **121,** 425.
Schwarting, R., Gerdes, J., Niehus, J., Jaeschke, L., and Stein, H. (1986). *J. Immunol. Methods* **90,** 65.
Schwarzacher, H. G., Mikelsaar, A. V., and Schnedl, W. (1978). *Cytogenet. Cell Genet.* **20,** 24.
Sinn, H. P., Lebert, T., Kandetski, C., and Waldherr, R. (1989). *Virchows Arch. A: Pathol. Anat. Histol.* **415,** 317.
Smith, P. J., and Crocker, J. (1988). *Histopathology* **12,** 113.
Suarez, V., Newman, J., Hiley, C., Crocker, J., and Collins, M. (1989). *Histopathology* **14,** 61.
Thiry, M. (1988). *Exp. Cell Res.* **179,** 204.
Thiry, M., and Muller, S. (1989). *J. Histochem. Cytochem.* **37,** 853.
Thiry, M., and Thiry-Blaise, L. (1989). *Eur. J. Cell Biol.* **50,** 235.
Thiry, M., Scheer, U., and Goessens, G. (1988). *Biol. Cell.* **63,** 27.
Trent, J. M., Carlin, D. A., and Davis, J. R. (1981). *Cytogenet. Cell Genet.* **30,** 31.
Trerè, D., Pession, A., and Derenzini, M. (1989). *Exp. Cell Res.* **184,** 131.
Vagner-Capodano, A. M., Henderson, A. S., Lissitzky, S., and Stahl, A. (1984). *Biol. Cell.* **51,** 11.
Varley, J. M. (1977). *Chromosoma (Berlin)* **61,** 207.
Wachtler, F., Hopman, A. H. N., Wiegant, J., and Schwarzacher, H. G. (1986). *Exp. Cell Res.* **167,** 227.
Wachtler, F., Hartung, M., Devictor, M., Weigant, J., Stahl, A., and Schwarzacher, H. G. (1989). *Exp. Cell Res.* **184,** 61.
Wilkinson, N., Buckley, C. H., Chawner, L., and Fox, H. (1990). *Int. J. Gynecol. Pathol.* **9,** 55.
Williams, M. A., Kleinschmidt, J. A., Krohne, G., and Franke, W. W. (1982). *Exp. Cell Res.* **137,** 341.
Zatsepina, O., Hozak, P., Babadjanyan, D., and Chentson, Y. (1988). *Biol. Cell.* **62,** 211.
Zhang, H., Wang, J. C., and Liu, F. L. (1988). *Proc. Natl. Acad. Sci. U.S.A.* **85,** 1060.

Antineutrophil Cytoplasmic Autoantibodies: Disease Associations, Molecular Biology, and Pathophysiology

J. CHARLES JENNETTE,* LINDA A. CHARLES,* and RONALD J. FALK†

*Department of Pathology and †Department of Medicine
University of North Carolina
Chapel Hill, North Carolina 27599*

I. Introduction

II. Clinical and Pathologic Spectrum of ANCA-Associated Diseases
   A. Basic ANCA-Associated Pathologic Lesion
   B. ANCA-Associated Systemic Vasculitis
   C. ANCA-Associated Glomerulonephritis
   D. A Unifying Concept for ANCA-Associated Diseases

III. Elucidation of ANCA Antigen Specificity
   A. C-ANCA versus P-ANCA
   B. Cell Specificity
   C. Organelle Specificity
   D. Molecular Specificity

IV. Pathogenetic Potential of ANCAs
   A. Accessibility of ANCA Antigens
   B. ANCA-Induced Respiratory Burst
   C. ANCA-Induced Degranulation
   D. Putative Pathogenesis of ANCA-Induced Diseases

V. Conclusion
   References

I. Introduction

Antineutrophil cytoplasmic autoantibodies (ANCAs) are found in the circulation of patients with necrotizing inflammatory injury to vessels, including Wegener's granulomatosis, polyarteritis nodosa, and idiopathic crescentic glomerulonephritis. ANCAs have specificity for proteins in the cytoplasmic granules of neutrophils and the lysosomes of monocytes. There are multiple ANCA types with different specificities, e.g., ANCAs specific for myeloperoxidase (MPO-ANCA) and ANCAs specific for proteinase 3 (PR3-ANCA) (Jennette et al., 1989; Jennette and Falk, 1990b). The most commonly used method for detecting ANCAs is indirect immunofluorescence microscopy using alcohol-fixed neutrophils as substrate, although enzyme-linked immunosorbent assays (ELISAs) using neutrophil subcellular fractions or purified proteins are also used. Two major patterns of ANCA staining are observed by immunofluorescence microscopy (Fig. 1). ANCAs specific for granule proteins (e.g., PR3) that remain in granules after alcohol fixation produce cytoplasmic neutrophil staining (C-ANCA), whereas ANCAs specific for granule proteins (e.g., MPO) that diffuse from granules and artifactually bind to nuclei after alcohol fixation produce perinuclear staining (P-ANCA).

ANCAs were first reported in 1982 by Davies et al. in eight patients with segmental necrotizing glomerulonephritis and systemic vasculitis, five of whom had evidence for pulmonary disease. This observation was confirmed shortly thereafter by Hall et al. (1984) in four patients with pulmonary disease, three of whom had focal necrotizing glomerulonephritis, two had skin vasculitis, and two had gastrointestinal disease. In 1985, a collaborative group in Europe independently reported the presence of ANCAs in patients

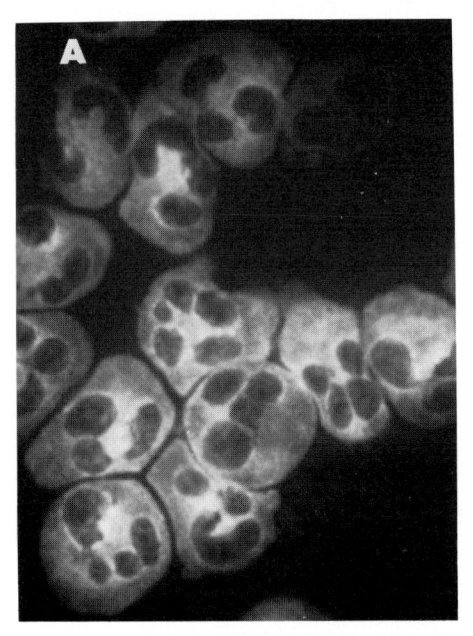

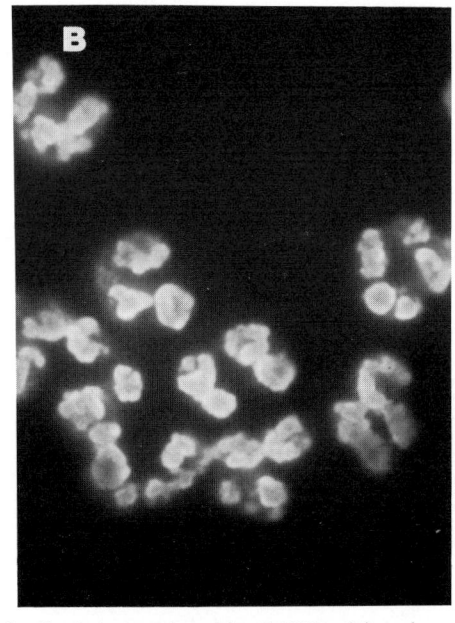

FIG. 1. Indirect immunofluorescence micrograph of staining produced by C-ANCAs (A) and P-ANCAs (B) using alcohol-fixed normal human neutrophils as substrate and fluoresceinated antihuman IgG as secondary antibody. [From Jennette and Falk (1990b) with permission.]

with active Wegener's granulomatosis (van der Woude et al., 1985). Subsequent publications reported ANCAs in patients with polyarteritis nodosa (Savage et al., 1987; Venning et al., 1987; Falk and Jennette, 1988; Wathen and Harrison, 1987), Churg–Strauss allergic granulomatosis (Wathen and Harrison, 1987), and idiopathic crescentic glomerulonephritis (Falk and Jennette, 1988; Walters et al., 1988; Cohen Tervaert et al., 1990).

Although the clinical manifestations of ANCA-associated disease are extremely varied among patients because of different organ system distributions of vascular injury, the basic pathologic lesion is very similar (Jennette et al., 1989). By light microscopy, this ANCA-associated lesion is characterized by vascular necrosis accompanied by leukocyte infiltration. By immunohistology, the lesion has no or only scanty evidence for immunoglobulin deposition, therefore being distinct from inflammatory vascular lesions that are caused by immune complexes or antibasement membrane antibodies, which are characterized, respectively, by granular or linear immunostaining for immunoglobulin.

Thus the pathogenesis of ANCA-associated disease cannot be attributed to immune complexes or antibasement membrane antibodies. Evidence is now emerging suggesting that ANCA-associated vascular injury is mediated by ANCA-induced neutrophil and monocyte activation (Falk et al., 1990a). Such ANCA-induced activation may require synergistic priming of leukocytes, for example, by cytokines released during viral infections.

II. Clinical and Pathologic Spectrum of ANCA-Associated Diseases

Patients with ANCA-associated diseases can present with a broad range of clinical manifestations dependent upon the distribution of vascular lesions (Jennette et al., 1989; Jennette and Falk, 1990b). Respiratory tract and renal tissues are most often affected; therefore, symptoms and signs of sinus, lung, and kidney disease are frequent in patients with ANCAs. As will be discussed later, the clinicopathologic characteristics of disease correlate to a degree with ANCA specificity, e.g., C-ANCA with PR3 specificity is most common in patients with Wegener's granulomatosis and P-ANCA with MPO specificity is most common in patients with idiopathic crescentic glomerulonephritis (Jennette et al., 1989; Jennette and Falk, 1990b).

A. BASIC ANCA-ASSOCIATED PATHOLOGIC LESION

The most ubiquitous pathologic lesion in ANCA-associated diseases is necrotizing inflammation of vessels (Jennette et al., 1989). Virtually any type of blood vessel other than the aorta and large veins can be affected, including capillaries, venules, small veins, arterioles, small arteries, and medium-sized (i.e., main visceral) arteries. The lesions in larger arteries may in fact arise from mural microvascular injury (i.e., injury arising in the vasa vasora).

1. *Light Microscopy*

By light microscopy, the necrosis is characterized by the presence of deeply acidophilic fibrinoid material mixed with and/or surrounded by leukocytes (Fig. 2). Either neutrophils or mononuclear phagocytes can predominate in the infiltrates, often with a component of leukocytoclasia. The most distinctive form of ANCA-associated necrotizing inflammation is a destructive form of granulomatous inflammation that occurs in the subset of patients with Wegener's granulomatosis (Fig. 3). Some of the time the vasocentric nature of the granulomatous inflammation is apparent, but at other times it is not. In these instances the lesion appears to be welling out of the interstitium, but, even here, the lesion may have begun in a small interstitial vessel that has been destroyed by the necrosis and is thus no longer visible.

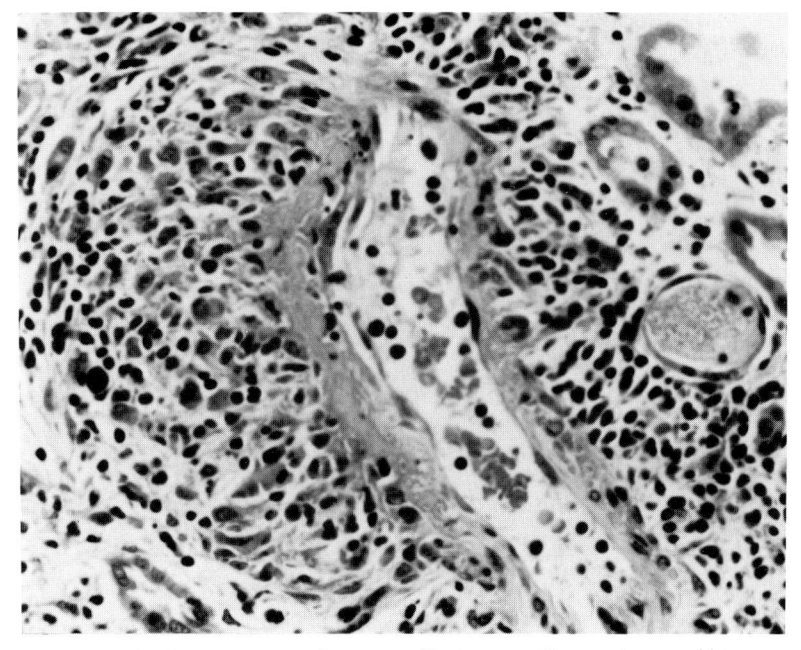

FIG. 2. Micrograph of ANCA-associated arteritis affecting a small artery in a renal biopsy specimen (hematoxylin and eosin stain). [From Jennette and Falk (1990b) with permission.]

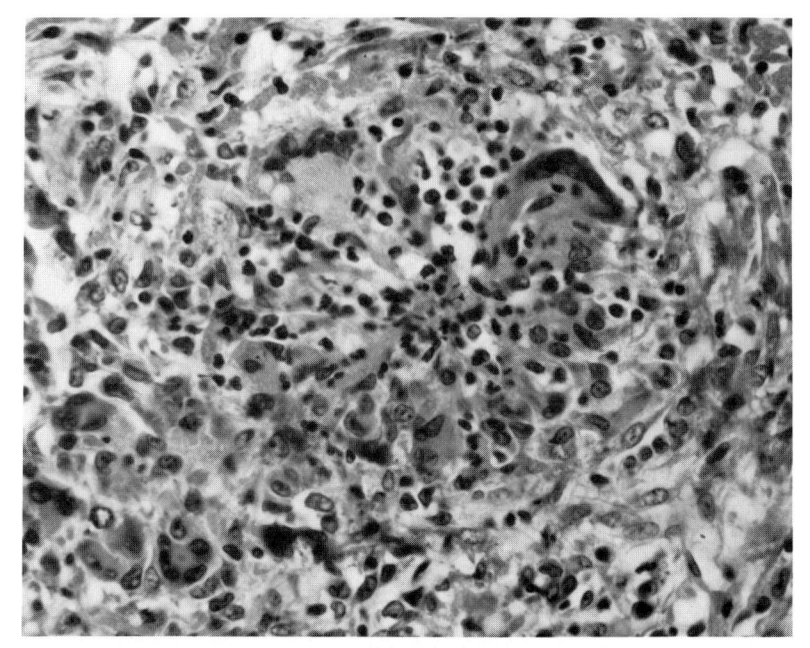

Fig. 3. Micrograph of necrotizing granulomatous pulmonary inflammation in a patient with Wegener's granulomatosis (hematoxylin and eosin stain).

2. *Immunofluorescence Microscopy*

Necrotizing vascular inflammation can be caused by more than one immunopathogenic mechanism. This varied pathogenesis is indicated by different patterns of immunoglobulin deposition, as demonstrated by direct immunohistology, e.g., immunofluorescence microscopy. For example, necrotizing alveolar capillary lesions and crescentic glomerulonephritis can both be categorized into immune complex-mediated lesions characterized by granular immunostaining for immunoglobulins, antibasement membrane antibody-mediated injury characterized by linear immunostaining for immunoglobulins, or "pauci-immune" injury characterized by a paucity of immunostaining for immunoglobulins. The ANCA-associated vascular injury usually falls into the latter category (Jennette *et al.,* 1989; Jennette and Falk, 1990b). However, a minority of patients with ANCA-associated disease will have relatively well-defined vascular granular immunostaining for immunoglobulins, and a few will have linear staining indicative of antibasement membrane antibody-mediated injury. The latter patients will have concurrent ANCAs and antibasement membrane antibodies in their serum. Therefore, in a minority of patients, there may be concurrent vascular injury by more than one immunopathogenic mechanism.

B. ANCA-Associated Systemic Vasculitis

Most patients with ANCAs have clinical and pathologic evidence for vasculitis in multiple organ systems. The distribution and histologic features of the systemic vasculitis are used to categorize patients into recognized clinicopathologic syndromes, including Wegener's granulomatosis, polyarteritis nodosa, and Churg–Strauss allergic granulomatosis; however, some patients are difficult to classify because of overlapping or vague disease manifestations. In addition, the clinicopathologic expressions of systemic vasculitis are somewhat different in patients with C-ANCAs compared to those with P-ANCAs (Jennette and Falk, 1990b) (Fig. 4).

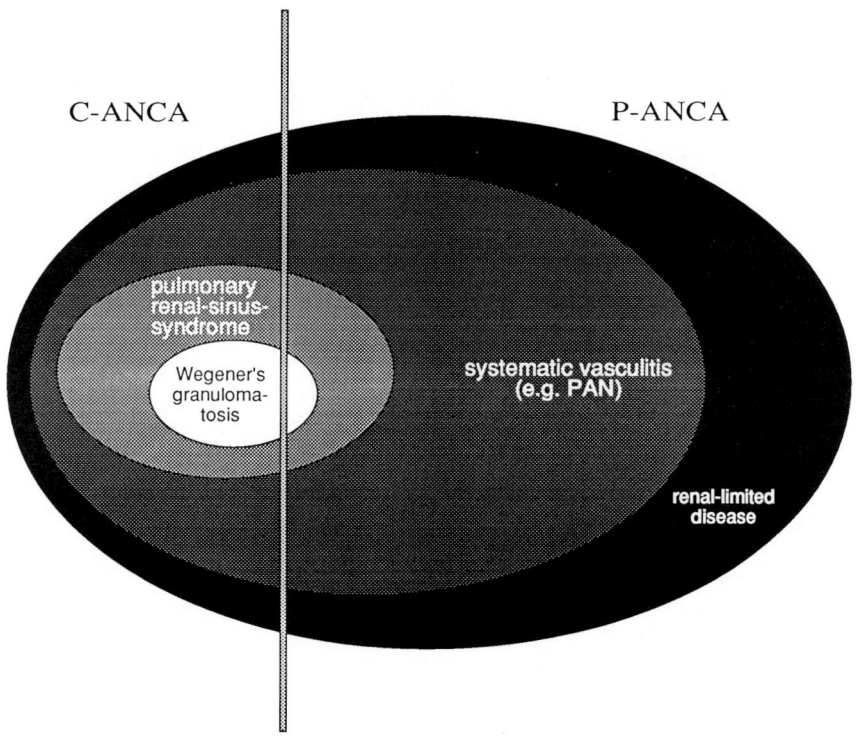

FIG. 4. Diagrammatic representation of the distribution of vascular diseases in patients with C-ANCAs and P-ANCAs. [From Jennette and Falk (1990b) with permission.]

The frequency with which ANCAs are detected, and the titer, are affected by disease activity. In patients with diseases that are known to be associated with ANCAs, patients with active disease have higher frequency ANCA detection than do patients with inactive disease. In general, in a patient with documented ANCA-positive disease, the ANCA titer decreases with treatment and resolution of disease manifestations, and increases with subsequent exacerbations. However, we have observed a minority of patients who have maintained high ANCA titers in the face of resolution of disease manifestations, as well as patients with quiescent disease who have had marked rises in ANCA titer without evidence for disease recrudescence. These exceptions to a correlation between ANCA titer and disease activity might be explained by the hypothesis that ANCAs are necessary but not sufficient factors in the induction of ANCA-associated disease (see Section IV,D).

1. Wegener's Granulomatosis

Klinger (1931) and Wegener (1939) first recognized Wegener's granulomatosis, but Godman and Churg set forth the definition of the disease that has been most widely used (Godman and Churg, 1954). They defined Wegener's granulomatosis as the concurrence of upper and/or lower respiratory tract granulomatous inflammation, systemic necrotizing arteritis, and focal glomerulonephritis (Godman and Churg, 1954). A major subsequent modification of this definition allowed for limited forms of Wegener's granulomatosis, e.g., patients with injury confined to the respiratory tract (Carrington and Liebow, 1966; Deremee et al., 1976). As will be discussed later, the absolute prerequisite for identifying granulomatous inflammation in order to make a diagnosis of Wegener's granulomatosis is being questioned by some. Interest in and a need for reconsidering the definition of Wegener's granulomatosis have been stimulated in part by the discovery of ANCAs that have shown the close relatedness to Wegener's granulomatosis of pulmonary vasculitis without granulomatous inflammation (Jennette et al., 1989; Jennette and Falk, 1990b).

The collaborative study in Europe led to the first report of the very high frequency of ANCAs in patients with active Wegener's granulomatosis (van der Woude et al., 1985). This study reported ANCAs in 25 of 27 patients with active Wegener's granulomatosis and in 4 of 32 patients with inactive Wegener's granulomatosis.

An analysis of C-ANCA in a large series of patients with Wegener's granulomatosis was reported by Nolle et al. (1989). In patients with generalized Wegener's granulomatosis, by indirect immunofluorescence microscopy, C-ANCAs were detected in 88 of 92 patients (96%) with active disease, in 84 of 119 patients (71%) during partial remission, and in 11 of 27 patients (41%)

either the C-ANCA or the P-ANCA can be present. To show the relatedness of these processes, one approach would be to call all ANCA-associated pulmonary–renal–sinus syndromes "Wegener's vasculitis," and to reserve the term Wegener's granulomatosis for cases with granulomatous inflammation.

2. *Polyarteritis Nodosa*

In 1866 Kussmaul and Maier described a systemic disease characterized by vascular inflammation that affected vessels ranging in size from main visceral arteries to microscopic vessels, including glomeruli. This disease is now called polyarteritis nodosa, and has a varied clinical presentation dependent upon the organ distribution of vasculitis.

In a sense, all forms of necrotizing systemic arteritis can be considered variants of polyarteritis nodosa. In fact, Wegener's granulomatosis and Churg–Strauss allergic granulomatosis both were originally considered to be variants of polyarteritis nodosa (Godman and Churg, 1954; Churg and Strauss, 1951). Wegener's granulomatosis has the features of polyarteritis nodosa with the addition of a granulomatous component to the inflammation; Churg–Strauss allergic granulomatosis appears to be an altered form of polyarteritis nodosa or Wegener's granulomatosis occurring in patients with asthma and characterized pathologically by eosinophilia in the tissues and blood.

Given these overlapping pathologic features, it is not surprising that polyarteritis nodosa (especially so-called "microscopic" polyarteritis nodosa), Wegener's granulomatosis, and Churg–Strauss allergic granulomatosis share a serologic marker (i.e., ANCA), which may be a common pathogenetic factor.

Polyarteritis nodosa, however, appears to be a structural phenotype of vascular injury that can be mediated by more than one pathogenetic process. In most patients with polyarteritis nodosa, the arteritis is not associated with immune deposits, and these patients have a high frequency of ANCAs (with P-ANCAs about as frequent as C-ANCAs) (Jennette *et al.*, 1989). A small minority of patients with polyarteritis nodosa have vascular deposits of immune complexes, and the vascular inflammation in these patients appears to be mediated by these deposits.

C. ANCA-Associated Glomerulonephritis

As already noted, some patients with ANCAs have renal-limited disease (Fig. 4). The most ubiquitous renal lesion in such patients is glomerulonephritis with segmental necrosis (Fig. 6) and crescent formation, although necrotizing arteritis and necrotizing medullary peritubular capillaritis also occur (Jennette *et al.,* 1989; Jennette and Falk, 1990b).

Crescentic glomerulonephritis is traditionally categorized on the basis of immunohistology into antiglomerular basement membrane antibody-medi-

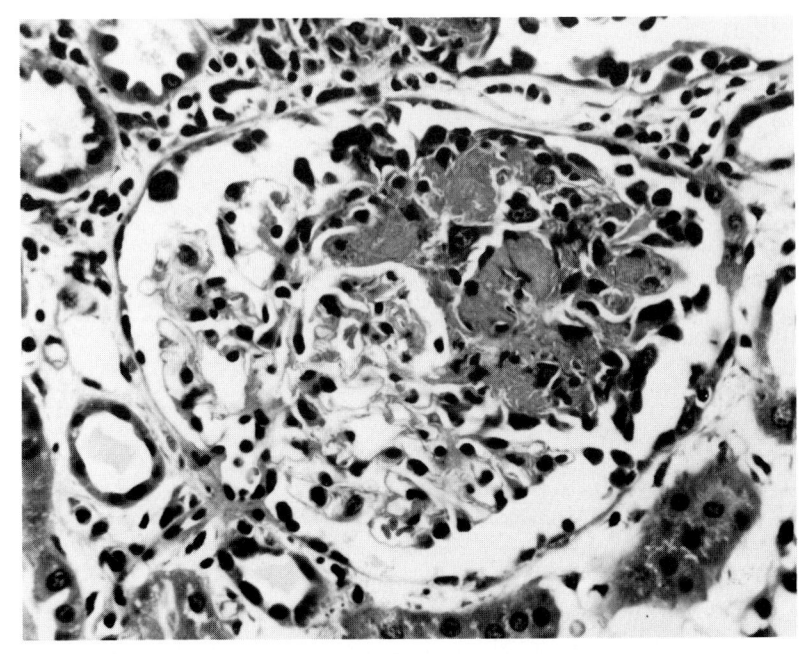

FIG. 6. Micrograph of ANCA-associated segmental necrotizing glomerulonephritis (hematoxylin and eosin stain). [From Jennette et al. (1989) with permission.]

ated disease (characterized by linear glomerular capillary immunostaining for immunoglobulins), immune complex-mediated disease (characterized by granular glomerular immunostaining for immunoglobulins), and idiopathic disease (characterized by a paucity of immunostaining for immunoglobulins). The last category is strongly associated with ANCAs (Fig. 7), although a few patients in the other two categories will have ANCAs (Jennette et al., 1989; Jennette and Falk, 1990b). Therefore, ANCAs are a useful serologic marker for categorizing crescentic (i.e., rapidly progressive) glomerulonephritis (Jennette and Falk, 1990a) (Fig. 8). The form of immune complex-mediated glomerulonephritis with which ANCAs are observed most often is lupus glomerulonephritis, wherein some patients will have P-ANCAs, including MPO-ANCAs and elastase-ANCAs (Jennette et al., 1989; Jennette and Falk, 1990b).

D. A Unifying Concept for ANCA-Associated Diseases

In patients with ANCA-associated diseases, the vascular lesions in different vessels (e.g., glomerular and alveolar capillaries, arterioles, venules, veins, and arteries) and different tissues (e.g., kidney, lung, skin, muscle, and

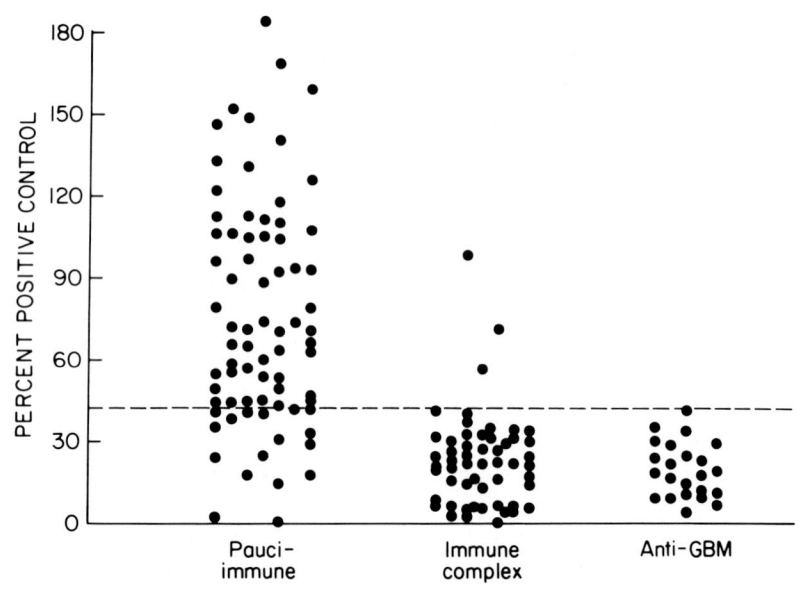

FIG. 7. Detection of ANCA activity using an ELISA with nitrogen bomb cavitate of neutrophils as substrate. Results are expressed as a percentage of a positive control specimen. The dashed line is the mean plus two standard deviations for normal control sera. Note the frequent positive values in sera from patients with pauci-immune necrotizing and crescentic glomerulonephritis, compared to the predominantly negative values in patients with nonlupus immune complex-mediated or antibasement membrane antibody-mediated crescentic glomerulonephritis. [From Jennette et al. (1989) with permission.]

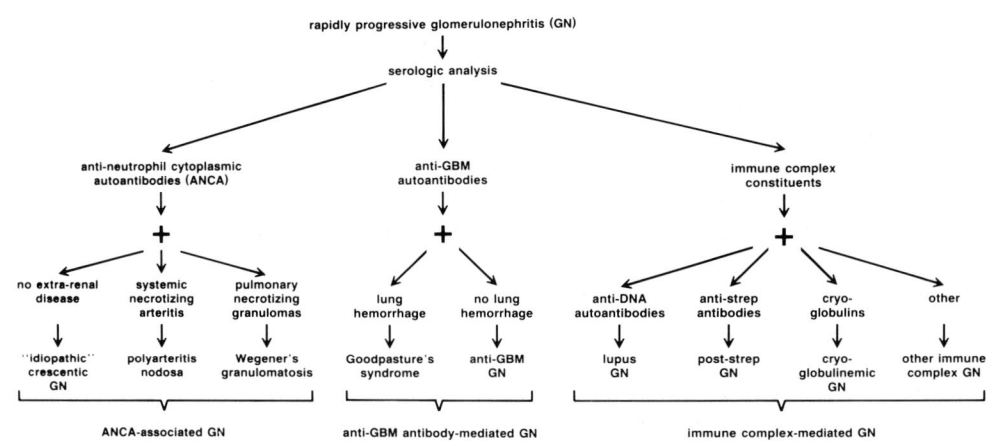

FIG. 8. Algorithm for classifying rapidly progressive (i.e., crescentic) glomerulonephritis based on serologic analysis and disease distribution. [From Jennette and Falk (1990a) with permission.]

nerves) have very similar necrotizing features by light microscopy and are typically pauci-immune by immunohistology. In addition, the glomerulonephritis in patients with ANCA-associated renal-limited disease (i.e., idiopathic crescentic glomerulonephritis) is identical to that in patients with ANCA-associated systemic necrotizing vasculitis (e.g., Wegener's granulomatosis and polyarteritis nodosa). Therefore, it is reasonable to suggest that Wegener's granulomatosis, polyarteritis nodosa, and idiopathic crescentic glomerulonephritis are pathogenetically related processes, and that the shared serologic marker (ANCA) is in fact a shared pathogenetic factor. As will be discussed in Section IV, there is evidence that both C-ANCAs and P-ANCAs are capable of activating neutrophils and monocytes to release injurious products that would be capable of causing vascular necrosis.

III. Elucidation of ANCA Antigen Specificity

In order to understand the pathobiology of ANCA, the antigen specificity of ANCA must be known at both the cellular and molecular level. The former has been determined by immunofluorescence microscopy, and the latter, primarily by ELISA, radioimmunoassay (RIA), and Western blot analysis using neutrophil subcellular fractions and purified molecules as antigen.

A. C-ANCA versus P-ANCA

As mentioned in Section I, by indirect immunofluorescence microscopy using alcohol-fixed neutrophils as substrate, two major patterns of ANCA staining occur, i.e., C-ANCA and P-ANCA patterns (Fig. 1). However, when formalin-fixed neutrophils are used as substrate, both C-ANCAs and P-ANCAs produce identical diffuse granular cytoplasmic staining (Charles et al., 1989). The distribution of P-ANCA staining on alcohol-fixed neutrophils is an artifact caused by the diffusion of soluble nucleophilic ANCA antigens from the cytoplasm to the nucleus during preparation of the substrate (Charles et al., 1989). Formalin fixation immobilizes the P-ANCA antigens by covalent cross-linking and thus preserves the *in vivo* cytoplasmic distribution of antigens. In fact, the C-ANCA pattern on alcohol-fixed cells is also artifactually distorted in that there is central accentuation of staining (Fig. 1A) that does not occur on formalin-fixed cells.

Even though the P-ANCA staining pattern is an artifact of neutrophil alcohol fixation that can be corrected by formalin fixation, it is a useful tool for distinguishing between two categories of ANCAs that have different molecular specificities, and, as noted in Section II, somewhat different disease associations.

B. Cell Specificity

Indirect immunofluorescence microscopy of blood cells has demonstrated that ANCAs react with neutrophils and monocytes, but not with lymphocytes or eosinophils (although there may be rare ANCAs that react with eosinophils). The reactivity with both neutrophils and monocytes is not surprising given the very close lineal relationship between these cells, which is closer than that between eosinophils and neutrophils. ANCAs do not react with tissue cells, including endothelial cells. ANCA antigens are present in the HL-60 myeloid cell line, which has differentiation features common to both neutrophils and monocytes (Charles *et al.*, 1989) (Fig. 9).

When alcohol-fixed monocytes are used as substrate for indirect immunofluorescence microscopy, C-ANCAs produce cytoplasmic staining that is accentuated in the concavity of the nucleus, and P-ANCAs produce perinuclear

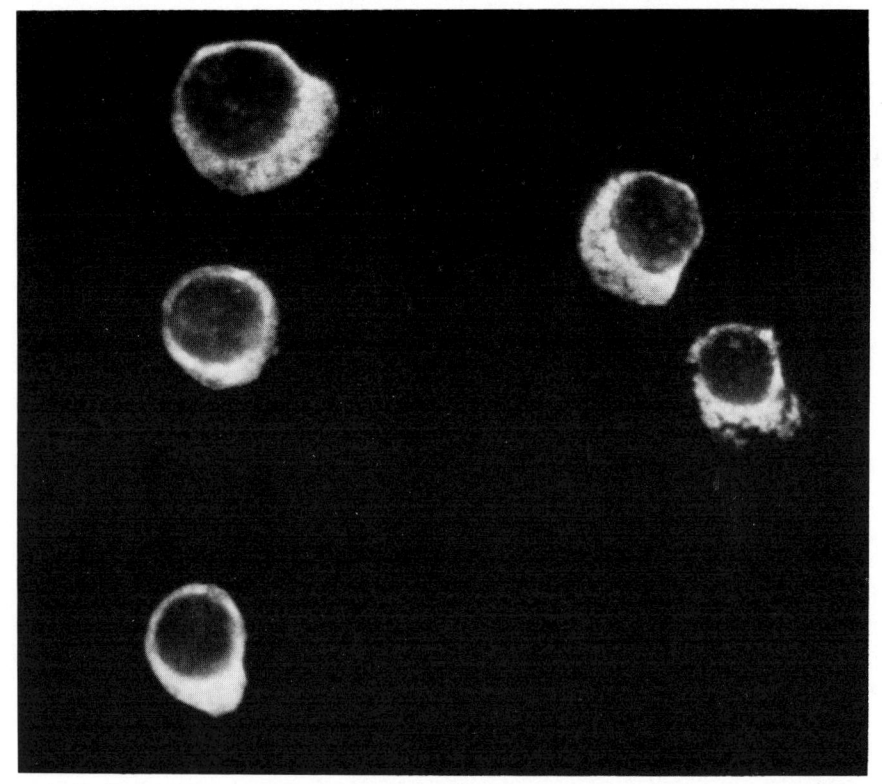

FIG. 9. Indirect immunofluorescence micrograph of staining produced by a C-ANCA serum using alcohol-fixed HL-60 cells as substrate and fluoresceinated antihuman IgG as secondary antibody.

or nuclear staining. Although monocytes contain ANCA antigens, differentiated macrophages do not. We have shown that when monocytes are cultured *in vitro,* ANCA antigens disappear as the cells mature into macrophages (Charles *et al.,* 1990a). This loss of ANCA antigens coincides with the loss of myeloperoxidase-positive lysosomes from monocytes as they transform into macrophages, which have myeloperoxidase-negative lysosomes. The absence of ANCA antigens in macrophages was confirmed by demonstrating the nonreactivity of pulmonary lavage macrophages with ANCAs (Charles *et al.,* 1990a).

C. ORGANELLE SPECIFICITY

The location of ANCA antigens within cytoplasmic organelles has been determined by immunoassay analysis of ANCA reactivity with subcellular fractions and by immunoelectron microscopy.

Using subcellular fractions of neutrophil cytoplasm, we demonstrated that ANCAs react with constituents of primary (i.e., azurophilic) granules (Falk and Jennette, 1988). Neutrophils were disrupted by nitrogen cavitation, and cytoplasmic constituents were fractionated by density gradient separation into an α fraction containing predominantly primary (azurophilic) granules, a β fraction containing predominantly secondary (specific) granules, and a γ fraction containing predominantly plasma membranes. ANCAs reacted selectively with the primary α granule fraction (Fig. 10). Using a similar approach, Goldschmeding *et al.* (1989a) also observed ANCA reactivity with the primary granule fraction.

Calafat *et al.* used immunoelectron microscopy to localize ANCA antigens in neutrophil and monocyte organelles (Calafat *et al.,* 1990). They observed binding of ANCAs to primary (azurophilic) granules in neutrophils and peroxidase-positive lysosomes in monocytes.

There are two types of lysosomes in mononuclear phagocytes, MPO-positive lysosomes and MPO-negative lysosomes. ANCA antigens are within the MPO-positive lysosomes only (Goldschmeding *et al.,* 1989a; Calafat *et al.,* 1990). The ANCA antigen-containing lysosomes of monocytes are exocytosed during monocyte activation (Goldschmeding *et al.,* 1989a). ANCA antigen-negative lysosomes are the only lysosomes of macrophages. These two types of mononuclear phagocyte lysosomes reflect two major stages of mononuclear phagocyte function. During initial activation, monocytes carry out functions that are very analogous to those of neutrophils, e.g., release of reactive oxygen radicals and lysosomal enzymes into phagocytic vacuoles or into the extracellular fluid (during "sloppy or frustrated phagocytosis"). Thereafter, monocytes differentiate into macrophages, which have very different functions compared to neutrophils. If ANCAs are able to activate ANCA-positive

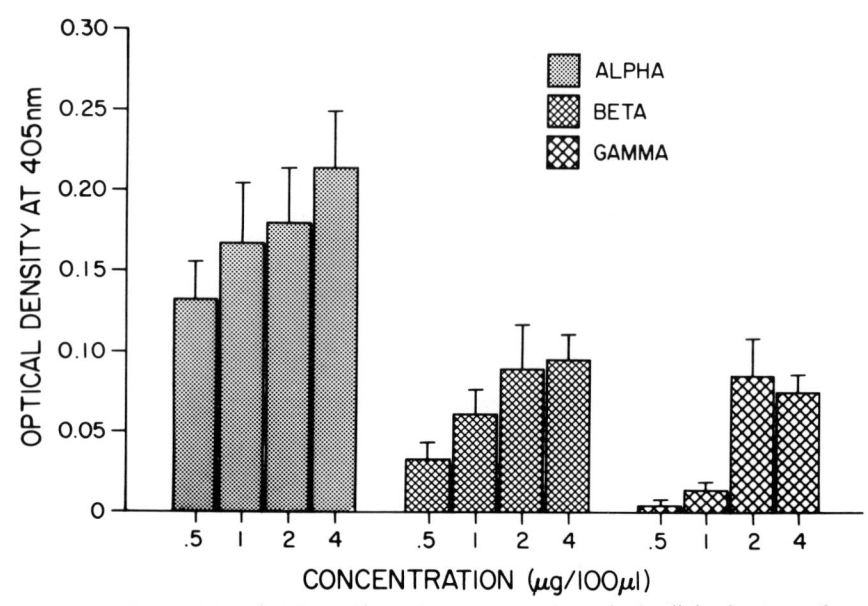

FIG. 10. ELISA reactivity of ANCAs with varying concentrations of subcellular fractions of neutrophil cytoplasm. The α fraction contains predominantly primary granule constituents, the β fraction contains predominantly secondary granule constituents, and the γ fraction contains predominantly plasma membranes. [From Falk and Jennette (1988) with permission.]

cells, as will be indicated in Section IV, then the target cells of ANCA activation are neutrophils and monocytes, which would produce very similar effects in tissues.

To date, the only exception to a primary granule location for vasculitis-associated ANCAs is the relatively rare occurrence of ANCAs specific for lactoferrin, which is a secondary granule protein.

D. MOLECULAR SPECIFICITY

The molecular specificities of ANCAs have been determined by specific immunoassays using purified neutrophil proteins as target antigens. Such studies have shown that there are multiple types of ANCAs with different specificities. Most patients have ANCAs of only one specificity, but some patients have multiple ANCA types with different specificities.

1. *MPO-ANCAs*

The first ANCA specificity that was recognized is for MPO (Falk and Jennette, 1988). MPO-ANCAs are the most common form of P-ANCAs in patients with systemic necrotizing vasculitis or idiopathic crescentic glomerulonephritis (Jennette et al., 1989; Jennette and Falk, 1990b).

Using two different ELISA assays with purified MPO as antigen, we demonstrated that some ANCAs have reactivity with MPO (Falk and Jennette, 1988) (Figs. 11 and 12). We also noted that MPO-ANCAs produce a P-ANCA rather than a C-ANCA staining pattern by indirect immunofluorescence microscopy (Falk and Jennette, 1988; Jennette et al., 1989) (Fig. 11). When MPO-ANCAs are the only ANCAs in a serum sample, the resultant P-ANCA staining can be blocked by monoclonal anti-MPO antibodies (Jennette et al., 1990). The specificity of some P-ANCAs for MPO has also been documented by Goldschmeding and associates (Cohen Tervaert et al., 1990; Goldschmeding et al., 1989b).

ANCAs specific for neutrophil MPO do not react with eosinophil peroxidase. This is not surprising, because neutrophil MPO and eosinophil peroxidase are the products of different genes.

2. Other P-ANCAs

Heterologous antibodies against many neutrophil proteins will cause perinuclear staining of alcohol-fixed neutrophils, including antibodies against primary granule constituents (e.g., MPO and elastase), and antibodies against secondary granule constituents (e.g., lactoferrin). Human ANCAs with

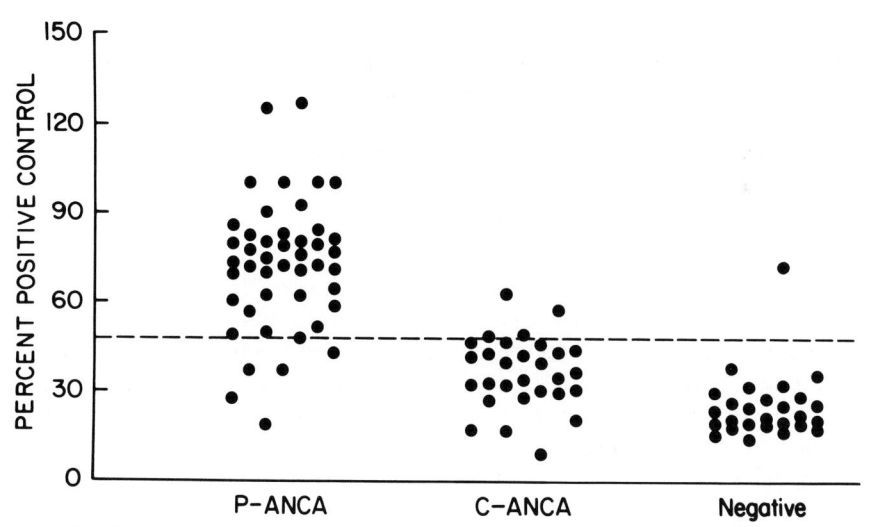

FIG. 11. ELISA reactivity of P-ANCA-positive, C-ANCA-positive, and ANCA-negative sera with purified MPO expressed as a percentage of a positive control serum. The dashed line represents the mean plus two standard deviations for negative control sera. [From Jennette et al. (1989) with permission.]

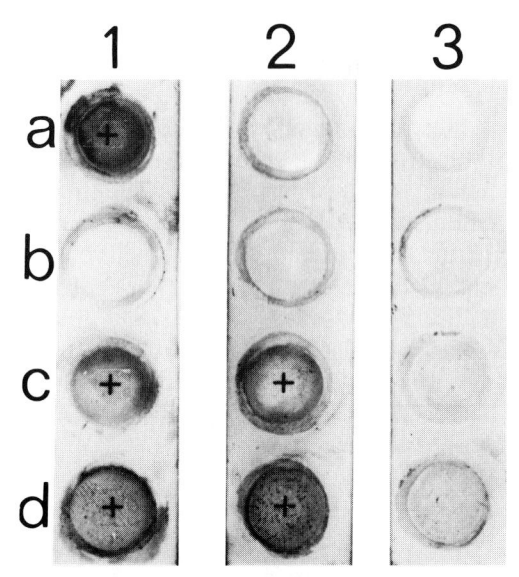

FIG. 12. Dot blot ELISA results for a P-ANCA serum (column 1), lupus serum (column 2), and normal control serum (column 3) reacted with purified MPO (row a), alkaline phosphatase (row b), the α fraction (i.e., primary granules) of neutrophils (row c), and neutrophil nitrogen cavitate (row d). Only the P-ANCA serum reacts with MPO, but the lupus serum does have reactivity with some component of the α fraction of neutrophils. [From Falk and Jennette (1988) with permission.]

each of these specificities have been identified, although, in our experience, ANCAs specific for elastase and lactoferrin are rare compared with MPO-ANCAs in patients with pauci-immune vasculitis and glomerulonephritis. We have observed the highest frequency of elastase-ANCAs in patients with systemic lupus erythematosus (unpublished observations).

P-ANCAs also occur in patients with a few nonvasculitic diseases, e.g., Felty's syndrome and inflammatory bowel disease. These P-ANCAs have specificities that differ from those in patients with vasculitis or glomerulonephritis. For example, the P-ANCAs in patients with ulcerative colitis do not react with MPO or elastase (Falk et al., 1990b).

3. PR3-ANCAs

A number of investigators have demonstrated reactivity of C-ANCAs with a 29-kDa neutrophil cytoplasmic protein that is a diisopropylfluorophosphate-binding elastinolytic serine proteinase (Goldschmeding et al., 1989a; Niles et al., 1989; Ludemann et al., 1990). These investigators suggested that this protein might be proteinase 3 because of the biochemical similarities between the 29-kDa C-ANCA antigen and the described features of PR3 (Kao et al., 1988). We confirmed this suspicion by demonstrating that some C-ANCAs are specific for purified PR3 (Fig. 13) (Jennette et al., 1990). We also demonstrated that the C-ANCA neutrophil staining pattern produced by PR3-ANCAs could be blocked by monoclonal anti-PR3 antibodies (Jennette et al., 1990).

4. *Other C-ANCAs*

Not all C-ANCAs are specific for PR3 (Falk et al., 1990c). When C-ANCAs are assayed by Western blot analysis, those that react with the 29-kDa fraction of neutrophil cytoplasmic constituents have specificity for PR3, but there are other C-ANCAs that do not react with the 29-kDa fraction, but do show reactivity with other Western blot bands. Some patients will have ANCAs of only one specificity, but others will have multiple ANCA types.

By Western blot analysis, some C-ANCAs that do not react with the 29-kDa PR3 band do react with a 57-kDa band (Falk et al., 1990c). By ELISA, these C-ANCAs have reactivity with a purified 57-kDa cationic protein (CAP57), which is a constituent of neutrophil primary granules. In addition, the C-ANCA staining caused by the CAP57-reactive ANCAs can be blocked by murine monoclonal anti-CAP57 antibodies.

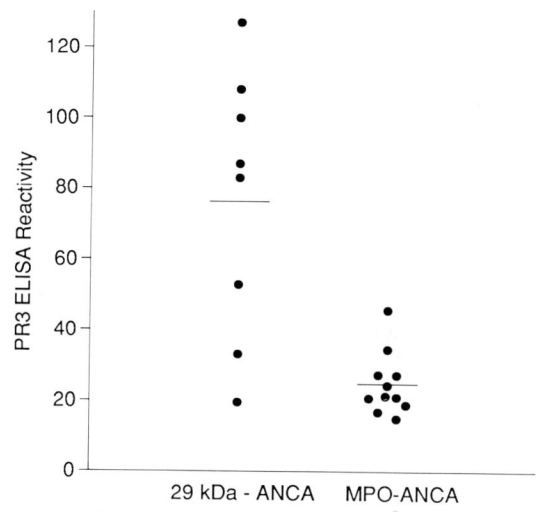

FIG. 13. ELISA reactivity of ANCA-positive sera with purified PR3 expressed as a percentage of the positive control serum (the horizontal bar indicates the mean reactivity). Sera that reacted with a 29-kDa fraction of neutrophil cytoplasm had higher PR3 reactivity than did MPO-ANCA-positive sera. [From Jennette et al. (1990) with permission.]

IV. Pathogenetic Potential of ANCAs

As noted in Section II, the vasculitis and glomerulonephritis associated with ANCAs are characterized by little or no localization of immunoglobulins or complement in vessel walls. Therefore, the vascular injury cannot be readily attributed to initiation of inflammation by immune complex deposition or *in situ* formation in vessel walls, or by antibody attachment to structures in vessel walls (e.g., antibasement membrane antibodies). We propose that ANCAs can activate neutrophils and monocytes, and that these ANCA-activated neutrophils and monocytes then mediate the necrotizing vascular injury of ANCA-associated diseases.

A. Accessibility of ANCA Antigens

In order for ANCA to have a specific effect on neutrophils and monocytes, ANCA must be able to interact with ANCA antigens; but, in unactivated neutrophils and monocytes, ANCA antigens are within cytoplasmic granules, not on the cell surface. During inflammatory diseases, neutrophils and monocytes become "primed," i.e., there is an up-regulation of their readiness to participate in inflammatory events, including the release of small amounts of granule and lysosome contents at the cell surface.

We have documented this release of ANCA antigens at the cell surface *in vitro* (Falk *et al.*, 1990a). When neutrophils are exposed to small amounts of priming factors, such as cytokines [e.g., tumor necrosis factor (TNF), which is released by leukocytes during inflammatory processes such as viral infections] or formyl peptides [e.g., N-formyl-L-Met-L-Leu-L-Phe (FMLP), which is an analog of products release by bacteria during infection], ANCA antigens appear at the cell surface. This phenomenon has been demonstrated by flow cytometry (Falk *et al.*, 1990a). After varying intervals of exposure to priming agents, viable neutrophils in suspension were fixed with paraformaldehyde, which immobilized any ANCA antigens at the cell surface and impermeabilized the cells. Flow cytometry using fluoresceinated ANCA IgG, as well as fluoresceinated heterologous antibodies specific for primary granule constituents, demonstrated that ANCA antigens were released at the cell surface during priming. Using FMLP ($10^{-7} M$), the ANCA antigen MPO was expressed on neutrophil cell surfaces after 30 seconds, with maximum effect at 1–2 minutes. After incubation for 5 minutes with 2 ng/ml TNF, MPO was expressed on the membrane (Fig. 14), with maximum effect at 30 minutes. Therefore, during priming, small amounts of ANCA antigens are released at the cell surface and are available to interact with ANCAs in the plasma and interstitial fluid.

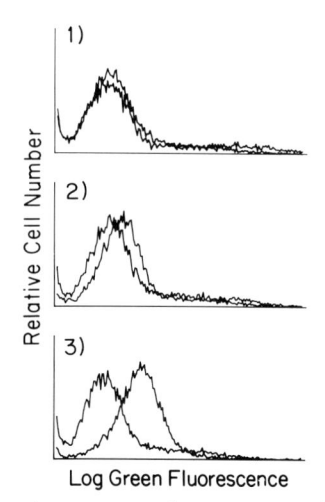

FIG. 14. Flow cytometric data demonstrating the expression of MPO at the surface of neutrophils after 2 minutes (1), 5 minutes (2), and 30 minutes (3) of exposure to TNF. Control cells with no primary antibody are on the left in each panel. [From Falk et al. (1990a) with permission.]

B. ANCA-Induced Respiratory Burst

The two major processes that neutrophils and monocytes carry out that produce acute injury to invading microorganisms or tissues are a respiratory burst and degranulation (i.e., release of granule/lysosome contents into phagocytic vacuoles or the extracellular fluid). The respiratory burst generates reactive oxygen species, e.g., superoxide, and, with the help of MPO, hypochlorous acid and resultant chloramines. These products of the respiratory burst are toxic and therefore cause damage when released into tissues adjacent to neutrophils and monocytes.

Using two different assay systems, we have observed that ANCA IgG can cause neutrophils to undergo a respiratory burst with the release of reactive oxygen species into the extracellular fluid (Falk et al., 1990a).

1. Chemiluminescence Assay

Release of reactive oxygen species (ROS), as measured by luminol-enhanced chemiluminescence, occurred when neutrophils were incubated with 13 ANCA-positive sera as compared to 5 normal sera (35.7×10^3 cpm ± 28.6 versus 2.2×10^3 cpm ± 2, respectively) (Falk et al., 1990a) (Fig. 15). Purified IgG gave similar results (28.8×10^3 cpm ± 27.2 versus 4.5×10^3 cpm ± 4.3, respectively). Both C-ANCA and P-ANCA IgG induced release of ROS (Figs. 15 and 16). Catalase diminished the production of ANCA-induced

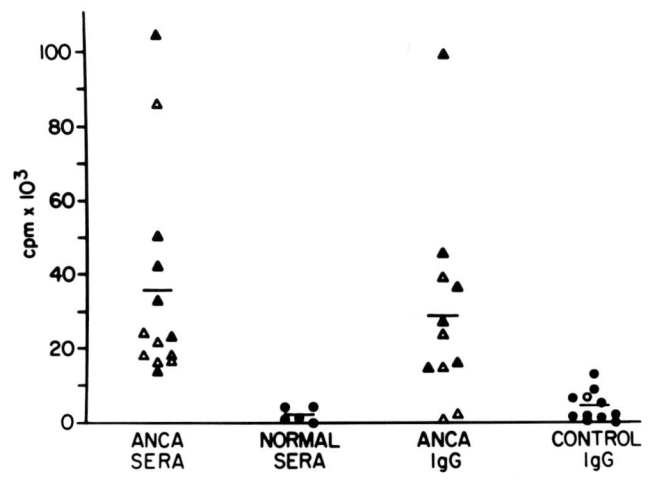

FIG. 15. ANCA-induced respiratory burst as measured by chemiluminescence. Among the ANCA sera and isolated IgG groups, the solid triangles represent MPO-ANCAs (i.e., P-ANCAs) and the open triangles represent C-ANCAs. Among the control IgG group, the solid circles represent normal controls and the open circles represent ANCA-negative diseased controls. [From Falk *et al.* (1990a) with permission.]

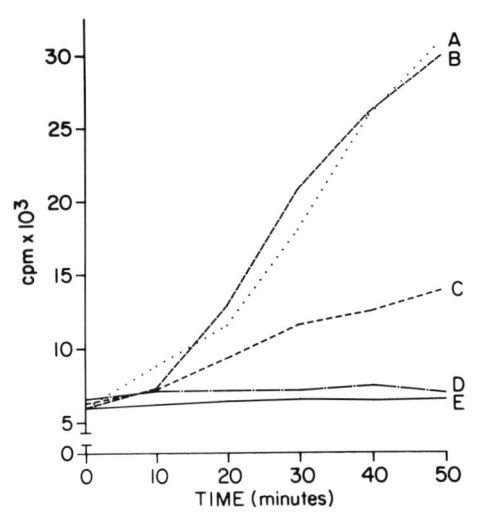

FIG. 16. Time course of neutrophil respiratory burst induced by IgG isolated from a C-ANCA-positive serum (A), MPO-ANCA-positive serum (B), and Goodpasture's syndrome patient serum (D). Curve E shows the lack of response of neutrophils from a chronic granulomatous disease patient to MPO-ANCA IgG. Curve C is the response of neutrophils to MPO-ANCA F(ab')$_2$ plus TNF. [From Falk *et al.* (1990a) with permission.]

ROS by 70% in chemiluminescence assays. Additionally, PMNs from a patient with chronic granulomatous disease failed to produce ROS in response to ANCAs (Fig. 16), but did induce degranulation. Together the catalase and chronic granulomatous disease IgG data confirm that the chemiluminescence produced in response to ANCAs is not due to nonspecific emission of light from mixed-function oxidases that are not involved in the inflammatory response.

2. *Superoxide Release Assay*

To confirm the stimulation of a respiratory burst by ANCAs, a second method was employed. ANCA-induced superoxide production was analyzed by measuring superoxide dismutase-inhibitable reduction of ferricytochrome C (Falk *et al.*, 1990a). TNF proved to be an important facilitator in these studies. In a continuous assay, both C-ANCA and P-ANCA (MPO-ANCA) IgG stimulated superoxide release from TNF-primed neutrophils, but control IgG did not (Fig. 17). We have preliminary data indicating that ANCA IgG can similarly stimulate release of superoxide by primed monocytes.

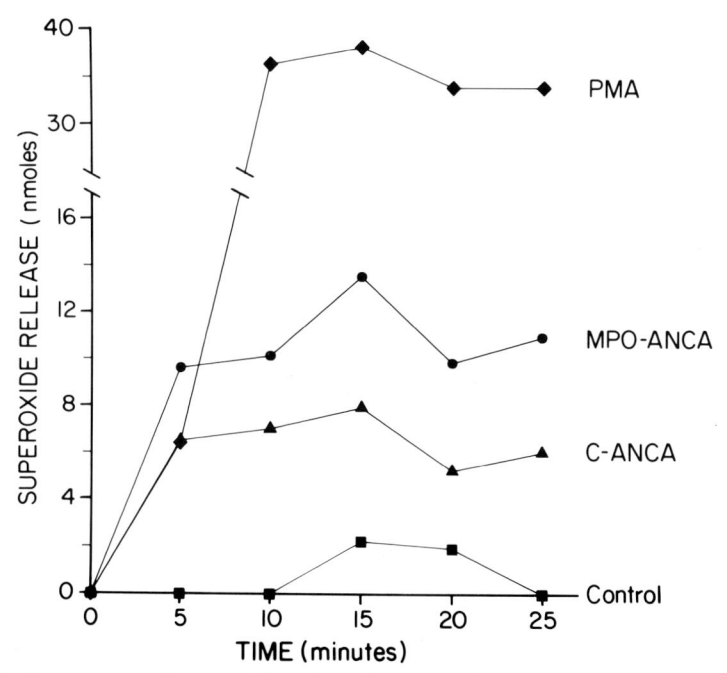

FIG. 17. Time course of superoxide release by neutrophils exposed to phorbol myristate acetate (PMA), or IgG isolated from MPO-ANCA-positive sera, C-ANCA-positive sera, or ANCA-negative control sera. [From Falk *et al.* (1990a) with permission.]

The capacity of autoantibodies specific for neutrophil granule proteins to activate neutrophils also is supported by our observation that heterologous antibodies specific for neutrophil granule proteins can activate neutrophils and cause the release of superoxide (Charles et al., 1990b). Polyclonal and monoclonal antibodies specific for neutrophil granule constituents were used to stimulate superoxide production. As negative controls, a series of nongranule antibodies were also tested. Rabbit antihuman MPO, sheep antihuman elastase, sheep antihuman cathepsin G, rabbit antihuman lactoferrin, rabbit antihuman lysozyme, mouse antihuman PR3, and mouse antihuman CAP57 were all tested as potential activators. Negative control antibodies included rabbit antihuman alkaline phosphatase, rabbit antihorse ferritin, rabbit antihuman α_2-macroglobulin, rabbit antihuman platelet-derived growth factor, goat antihuman C5, rabbit antimouse albumin, and mouse antihuman double-stranded DNA. Induction of superoxide release by each antibody was assayed in the presence and absence of 100 pg/ml recombinant TNF. Doses of 50, 10, and 5 μg/ml of heterologous antigranule antibodies caused the production of superoxide when measured at an end point of 45 minutes. Higher doses of antibody generally did not require priming by TNF, but superoxide generation with lower antibody doses was significantly enhanced by TNF. Evaluation of the kinetics of superoxide production showed that pretreatment of neutrophils with TNF allowed superoxide production to occur sooner. When the reaction with antigranule antibodies was allowed to proceed for up to 60 minutes, significant superoxide production occurred even without the presence of TNF, probably as a result of eventual release of granule antigens at the neutrophil surfaces during the prolonged incubation. TNF alone at the dose used in these experiments (100 pg/ml, 2 U) caused only a slight release of superoxide. Antibodies against nongranule antigens failed to stimulate neutrophils either with or without TNF. The facilitated superoxide release following TNF priming was most likely caused by the slight degranulation that occurs in response to cytokines (as described in Section IV,A), making granule antigens available to interact with their respective antibodies.

C. ANCA-Induced Degranulation

Along with the release of ROS, degranulation is the other major destructive event carried out by activated neutrophils and monocytes. Neutrophils and monocytes release ROS and lytic granule constituents into phagocytic vacuoles, as well as into the extracellular fluid. The latter is a major cause for tissue injury at sites of inflammation.

ANCA-induced neutrophil degranulation was assessed *in vitro* by measuring β-glucuronidase and *N*-acetyl-β-glucosaminidase (NAG) secretion.

1. *β-Glucuronidase Release*

β-Glucuronidase was measured indirectly by cleavage of a phenolphthalein glucuronic acid conjugate (Falk *et al.*, 1990a). In the presence of TNF, 10 ANCA IgG specimens (500 µg/ml) triggered neutrophil degranulation, but 6 control IgG specimens failed to produce any significant β-glucuronidase release (17.5 ± 16.6 µg versus 4.9 ± 4.8 µg phenolphthalein, respectively). There was a dose-dependent effect covering a range of 100–500 µg/ml of IgG (Fig. 18). Without the TNF priming, neutrophil stimulation with ANCA IgG was not significantly different from control IgG. TNF alone did not stimulate β-glucuronidase release that was detectable by this assay system.

2. *N-Acetyl-β-Glucosaminidase Release*

To confirm ANCA-induced degranulation, a second assay method was used. ANCA-induced NAG release was measured using a fluorometric assay (Falk *et al.*, 1990a). In the presence of TNF, ANCA IgG (500 µg/ml) induced neutrophil NAG release, but control IgG did not (0.0020 ± 0.0008 µM versus 0.0007 ± 0.0003 µM, respectively). ANCA IgG alone and TNF alone did not induce NAG release by neutrophils.

Therefore, two different assay systems indicate that ANCAs alone and cytokine (i.e., TNF) alone do not induce degranulation, but the two together act synergistically to cause neutrophil activation and degranulation.

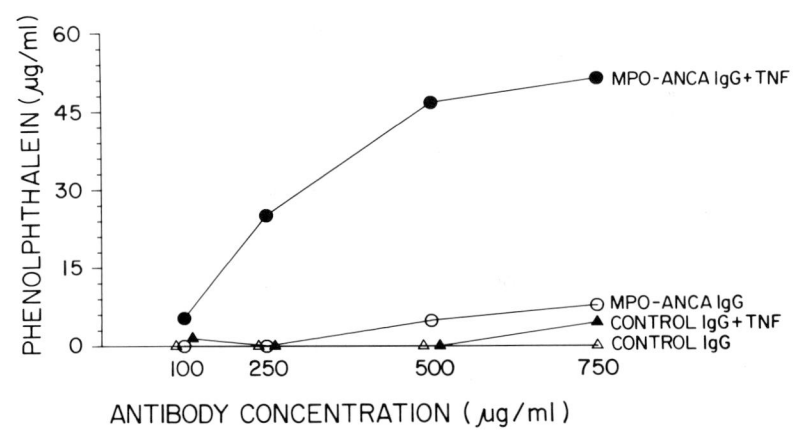

FIG. 18. Dose–response curves demonstrating the amount of β-glucuronidase released from primary granules of neutrophils exposed to MPO-ANCA IgG with or without tissue necrosis factor (TNF), or control IgG with or without TNF. Only the ANCA IgG plus TNF caused significant degranulation. [From Falk *et al.* (1990a) with permission.]

D. PUTATIVE PATHOGENESIS OF ANCA-ASSOCIATED DISEASES

We propose that ANCAs are pathogenic and are responsible for mediating the most common forms of systemic necrotizing vasculitis and crescentic glomerulonephritis. This contention is supported by (1) the high frequency with which ANCAs are found in patients with these diseases, (2) the correlation of ANCA titer with disease activity, and (3) the capacity of ANCAs to activate primed neutrophils and monocytes *in vitro*.

According to our hypothesis, ANCAs alone are not capable of activating unprimed neutrophils or monocytes. As diagrammed in Fig. 19-1, ANCAs in

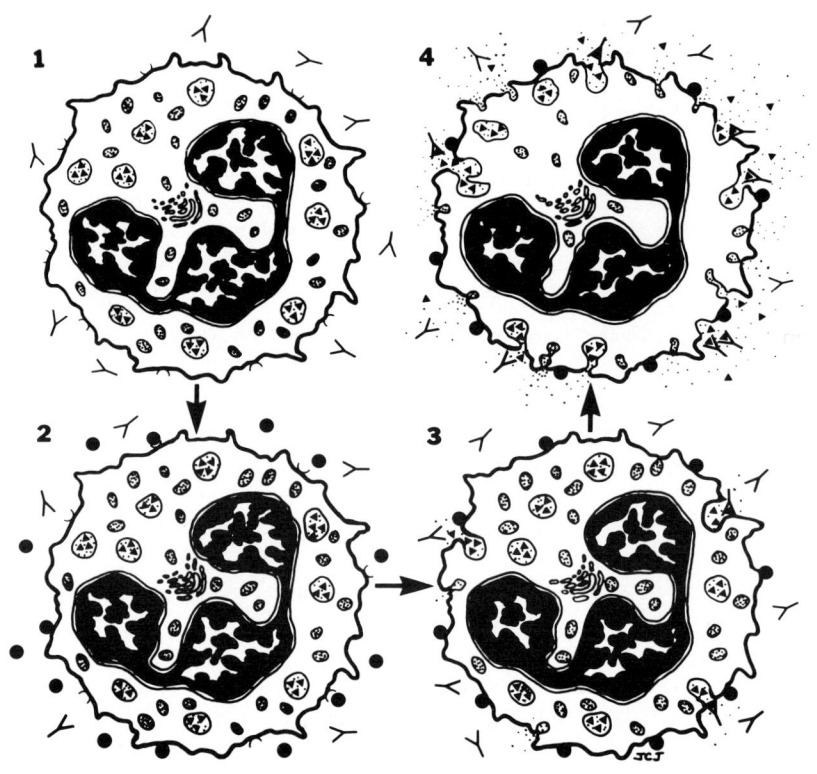

FIG. 19. Diagram depicting the putative sequence of events that would allow ANCAs (Y) to interact with ANCA antigen (▲). The ANCA antigens of totally unactivated neutrophils are within primary granules and therefore are not available to interact with ANCAs in the plasma (1). Priming factors (●), such as cytokines or formyl peptides, would bind to cell surface receptors and cause the release of small amounts of ANCA antigens at the cell surface (2 and 3). This would allow ANCAs to bind to ANCA antigens and cause complete neutrophil activation with respiratory burst and degranulation of primary and secondary granules (4). Such activation within vessels would result in inflammatory injury to the vessel walls.

the plasma would not have access to ANCA antigens within neutrophil granules or monocyte lysosomes. However, up-regulation of neutrophils and monocytes, for example, by cytokines released in response to a viral infection, would result in the release of small amounts of ANCA antigens at the cell surface (Figs. 19-2 and 19-3). This release of small amounts of ANCA antigens would allow for an interaction between ANCAs and ANCA antigens at the cell surface, resulting in total neutrophil or monocyte activation with release of toxic oxygen species and lytic granule and lysosome enzymes (Fig. 19-4). The mechanism of this activation is unknown, but we have preliminary data indicating that it is mediated by channeling of calcium into the cells. Such activation also would cause up-regulation of adhesion molecules on neutrophils and monocytes, allowing them to adhere to endothelial surfaces, especially at sites where leukocytes come into close proximity to vessel walls, such as in glomerular and alveolar capillaries. Activated neutrophils and monocytes adherent to vessel walls would cause vascular necrosis and recruitment of additional inflammatory mediator systems.

This scenario is supported by epidemiologic data (Falk *et al.*, 1990d). Over 90% of patients with ANCA-associated vasculitis or glomerulonephritis report a flulike prodrome prior to the onset of manifestations of vasculitis or nephritis. In addition, the onset of ANCA-associated disease activity is greater than expected in the winter ($p < 0.05$), when infectious processes are most frequent, and is lower than expected in the summer ($p < 0.05$), when infections are least common.

In summary, we hypothesize that circulating ANCAs are tolerated well until an inflammatory event occurs that primes circulating neutrophils and monocytes, allowing them to be activated by the ANCAs. For example, when a patient with circulating ANCAs develops a viral respiratory tract infection, activated T lymphocytes in the respiratory tract would release cytokines into the circulation, as evidenced by the resultant systemic effects (e.g., fever, malaise, and myalgias). These cytokines would also prime circulating and local neutrophils and monocytes, resulting in the release of ANCA antigens at their surfaces. Interaction between these antigens and ANCAs would cause neutrophil and monocyte activation. Because the activated leukocytes are within vessels, the expected phenotype of injury would be vasculitis.

V. Conclusion

ANCAs are useful for diagnosing and assessing the activity of systemic necrotizing vasculitis, including Wegener's granulomatosis and polyarteritis nodosa, and idiopathic crescentic glomerulonephritis. ANCAs may be involved in a previously unrecognized immune-mediated mechanism of tissue injury that involves direct activation of neutrophils and monocytes by autoantibodies.

References

Andrassy, K., Koderisch, J., Waldherr, R., and Rufer, M. (1988). *Nephron* **49,** 257.
Calafat, J., Goldschmeding, R., Ringeling, P. L., Janssen, H., and van der Schoot, C. E. (1990). *Blood* **75,** 242.
Carrington, C. B., and Liebow, A. A. (1966). *Am. J. Med.* **41,** 497.
Charles, L. A., Falk, R. J., and Jennette, J. C. (1989). *Clin. Immunol. Immunopathol.* **53,** 243.
Charles, L. A., Falk, R. J., and Jennette, J. C. (1990a). *FASEB J.* **4,** A2255.
Charles, L. A., Falk, R. J., Terrell, R., and Jennette, J. C. (1990b). *J. Leukocyte Biol.* (submitted).
Churg, J., and Strauss, L. (1951). *Am. J. Pathol.* **27,** 277.
Cohen Tervaert, J. W., Goldschmeding, R., Elema, J. D., van der Giessen, M., Huitema, M. G., van der Hem, G. K., The, T. H., von dem Borne, A. E. G. K., and Kallenberg, C. G. M. (1990). *Kidney Int.* **37,** 799.
Davies, D. J., Moran, J. E., Niall, J. F., and Ryan, G. B. (1982). *Br. Med. J.* **285,** 606.
Deremee, R. A., McDonald, T. J., Harrison, E. G., and Coles, D. T. (1976). *Mayo Clin. Proc.* **51,** 777.
Falk, R. J., and Jennette, J. C. (1988). *N. Engl. J. Med.* **318,** 1651.
Falk, R. J., Terrell, R. S., Charles, L. A., and Jennette, J. C. (1990a). *Proc. Natl. Acad. Sci. U.S.A.* **87,** 4115.
Falk, R. J., Sartor, R. B., Jones, D. A., Jefferies, B. D., and Jennette, J. C. (1990b). *Clin Res.* **38,** 387A (abstr.).
Falk, R. J., Becker, M., Pereira, H. A., Spitznagel, J. K., Hoidal, J., and Jennette, J. C. (1990c). *Blood* (submitted).
Falk, R. J., Hogan, S., Carey, T. S., and Jennette, J. C. (1990d). *Ann. Intern. Med.* **113,** 656.
Gans, R. O. B., Goldschmeding, R., Donker, A. J. M., Hoorntje, S. J., Kuizinga, M. C., Cohen Tervaert, J. W., Kallenberg, C. G. M., and von dem Borne, A. E. G. K. (1989). *Lancet* **1,** 269.
Godman, G. C., and Churg, J. (1954). *Arch. Pathol.* **58,** 533.
Goldschmeding, R., van der Schoot, C. E., ten Bokkel Huinink, D., Hack, C. E., van den Ende, M. E., Kallenberg, C. G. M., and von dem Borne, A. E. G. K. (1989a). *J. Clin. Invest.* **84,** 1577.
Goldschmeding, R., Cohen Tervaert, J. W., van der Schoot, C. E., van der Veen, C., Kallenberg, C. G. M., and von dem Borne, A. E. G. K. (1989b). *Acta Pathol. Microbiol. Immunol. Scand.* **97** (Suppl. 6), 48.
Hall, J. B., Wadham, B. M., Wood, C. J., Ashton, V., and Adam, W. R. (1984). *Aust. N.Z. J. Med.* **14,** 227.
Jennette, J. C., and Falk, R. J. (1988). *N. Engl. J. Med.* **319,** 1417.
Jennette, J. C., and Falk , R. J. (1990a). *Med. Clin. North Am.* **74,** 893.
Jennette, J. C., and Falk, R. J. (1990b). *Am. J. Kidney Dis.* **15,** 517.
Jennette, J. C., Wilkman, A. S., and Falk, R. J. (1989). *Am. J. Pathol.* **135,** 921.
Jennette, J. C., Hoidal, J. H., and Falk, R. J. (1990). *Blood* **78,** 2263.
Kao, R. C., Wehner, N. G., Skubitz, K. M., Gray, B. H., and Hoidal, J. R. (1988). *J. Clin. Invest.* **82,** 1963.
Klinger, H. (1931). *Frankf. Z. Pathol.* **42,** 455.
Kussmaul, A., and Maier, R. (1866). *Dtsch. Arch. Klin. Med.* **1,** 484.
Ludemann, J., Utecht, B., and Gross, W. L. (1990). *J. Exp. Med.* **171,** 357.
Niles, J. L., McCluskey, R. T., Ahmad, M. F., and Arnaout, M. A. (1989). *Blood* **74,** 1888.
Nolle, B., Specks, U., Ludemann, J., Rohrbach, M. S., DeRemee, R. A., and Gross, W. L. (1989). *Ann. Intern. Med.* **111,** 28.

Savage, C. O. S., Winearlsk, C. G., Jones, S., Marshall, P. D., and Lockwood, C. M. (1987). *Lancet* **1,** 1389.
van der Woude, F. J., Rasmussen, N., Lobatto, S., Wiik, A., Permin, H., van Es, L. A., van der Giessen, M., van der Hem, G. K., and The, T. H. (1985). *Lancet* **1,** 425.
Venning, M. C., Arfeen, S., and Bird, A. G. (1987). *Lancet* **2,** 850.
Walters, M. D. S., Savage, C. O. S., Dillon, M. J., Lockwood, C. M., and Barratt, T. M. (1988). *Arch. Dis. Child.* **63,** 814.
Wathen, C. W., and Harrison, D. J. (1987). *Lancet* **1,** 1037.
Wegener, F. (1939). *Beitr. Pathol. Anat. Allg. Pathol.* **102,** 36.

Apoptosis: Mechanisms and Roles in Pathology

MARK J. ARENDS and ANDREW H. WYLLIE

Department of Pathology
University of Edinburgh Medical School
Edinburgh EH8 9AG, Scotland

I. Introduction
   Incidence

II. Morphology

III. Mechanisms
   A. Cell Density Increase
   B. Intracellular Signaling Pathways
   C. Chromatin Cleavage
   D. Transglutaminase Activation
   E. Cell Surface Alterations

IV. Roles in Pathology
   A. Inflammation
   B. Immune Killing
   C. Neoplasia

V. Conclusions
   References

I. Introduction

Cell death plays a major role in the organization of the cell associations that we call tissues. Sometimes it is conspicuous and clearly pathologic. Sheets of cells die in synchrony, for example, on restriction of their vascular supply during infarction. This usually elicits an inflammatory reaction, itself capable of inflicting more cell damage and at the same time initiating digestion of the dead cells by neutrophil polymorphs. Sometimes death is inconspicuous but essential for normal regulation of tissue cell number. The "programmed death" of development falls into this category. There is no inflammatory reaction, and often the occurrence of death is perceived more readily from the reduction in cell number than from visualization of the dying cells. Cell death of great biologic significance occurs within the lymphoid system. Examples include the clonal selection of specifically reactive populations of lymphocytes of both T and B lineages, and also the death of target cells attacked by killer cells of various types. A whole science—toxicology—has grown up around the study of agents that injure and kill cells, but it is not always clear whether the end points observed by toxicologists are similar to the physiologic or the pathologic processes of cell death described above.

This article is about a cell death process, apoptosis, found in a great variety of circumstances. Originally recognized because of its distinctive morphology, apoptosis has since been shown to incorporate several characteristic biochemical events. It is the purpose of this article only to summarize the incidence and morphology of apoptosis, as these have been often reviewed (Wyllie, 1987a, 1988; Walker *et al.*, 1988b), and to enlarge on newer information on its mechanism and regulation. The roles of apoptosis in pathology are then discussed. It will be evident that exciting new therapeutic approaches to inflammatory and neoplastic disease would open up, were apoptosis to prove regulable by pharmacologic means.

INCIDENCE

Apoptosis occurs frequently (though not exclusively) in circumstances to which the term "programmed cell death" has often been applied (Table I). It is the major mode of death observed, from the modeling of embryonic and fetal tissue from the early blastocyst (Handyside and Hunter, 1986) to fine tuning of the organization of the central nervous system (O'Connor and Wyttenbach, 1974). It is activated in invertebrate and amphibian metamorphosis (Kerr *et al.*, 1974). Cell loss by apoptosis is seen in gland atrophy following duct obstruction (Walker, 1987; Walker and Gobe, 1987), in the involution of experimentally induced hyperplasia (Fesus *et al.*, 1987), and in resolution of hypercellular glomerular disease (Harrison, 1988). In mammals it accounts for hormone-dependent cell death in the breast (Ferguson and Anderson, 1981a,b; Walker *et al.*, 1989), adrenal (Wyllie *et al.*, 1973a,b), prostate (Kerr and Searle, 1973), endometrium (Rotello *et al.*, 1989), and ovary (O'Shea *et al.*, 1978; Zeleznik *et al.*, 1989). Apoptosis is observed following the removal of specific growth factors, including lymphocytes deprived of IL-2 (Duke and Cohen, 1986), hemopoietic precursors deprived of IL-3 (Williams *et al.*, 1990), and fibroblasts deprived of serum (M. J. Arends, unpublished observations). It can also be caused by physiologic regulatory hormones, such as glucocorticoids applied to lymphocytes (Van Haelst, 1967a,b;

TABLE I

Incidence of Apoptosis[a]

Circumstance	Example
Normal embryonic/fetal development	Blastocyst inner cell mass modeling
	Palatal fusion
	Interdigital web deletion
	Avian wing development—"posterior necrotic zone"
	Müllerian duct regression in the presence of fetal testis
	Supernumerary motor neuron deletion in the absence of end-plate formation
Normal tissue turnover	Intestinal villo-cryptal modeling
	Adrenal zona reticularis
Metamorphosis	Amphibian tail regression
	Caterpillar labial feeding gland regression
Atrophy	Pancreatic duct obstruction
Hormone-dependent atrophy	Endometrium cyclic proliferation and deletion
	Breast cyclic proliferation and deletion
	Ovary corpus luteum regression
	Adrenal atrophy after ACTH withdrawal
	Prostate atrophy after castration
Growth factor-dependent survival	IL-2 withdrawal from thymocytes
	IL-3 withdrawal from hemopoietic precursors
	Serum withdrawal from fibroblasts
Involution of hyperplasia	Atrophy of lead nitrate-induced rat liver hyperplastic foci
	Restitution of hypercellular glomeruli
Immune cell ontogeny	Autoreactive T cell clone deletion
	B cell deletion in the absence of antigen-driven centrocyte selection
Immune killing	Cytotoxic T cell killing
	Natural killer cell killing
	K cell killing
	Lymphotoxin-mediated killing
Toxin exposure	Gliotoxin-induced macrophage death
	TCD-dioxin-induced thymocyte death
	DMBA-induced adrenocortical cell death
Teratogenesis	Polycyclic hydrocarbon-induced teratogenesis
Irradiation	Thymic cortical cell death
	Intestinal mucosal crypt cell death
	Neonatal renal cortical nephrogenic cell death
Resolution of inflammation	Disposal of unstimulated senescent neutrophil polymorphs
Tumor cell deletion	Basal and squamous cell skin carcinomas
	Antibody-induced leukemic cell death
	Regression of endocrine-dependent tumors
	Treatment with cancer chemotherapeutic agents

[a] A reference list is given in the text [see, in particular, Kerr et al. (1972), Wyllie et al. (1980), and Wyllie (1981, 1987a,b)].

Wyllie and Morris, 1982). In the ontogeny of the immune system it occurs in deletion of autoreactive T cell clones during thymic maturation (Smith et al., 1989; Shi et al., 1989, 1990), and in B cell deletion in germinal centers in the absence of antigen-driven positive selection of centrocytes (Liu et al., 1990). Apoptosis is found in cells attacked by cytotoxic T lymphocytes (CTLs) (Russell, 1981, 1983) and natural killer (NK) cells (reviewed by Duvall and Wyllie, 1986). It occurs in cells exposed to moderate doses of toxins (Currie et al., 1962; Barker and Smuckler, 1973; Wyllie, 1987b; Waring et al., 1988; McConkey et al., 1988) or ionizing radiation (Skalka et al., 1976; Umanksy et al., 1981; Ijiri and Potten, 1983; Yamada and Ohyama, 1988; Gobe et al., 1988). During resolution of acute inflammation, unstimulated senescent neutrophil polymorphs are disposed of by undergoing apoptosis and phagocytosis by macrophages (Savill et al., 1989a, 1990). Apoptosis occurs in growing and regressing tumors (Kerr et al., 1972; Moore, 1983; Wyllie, 1985; Sarraf and Bowen, 1986; Bowen et al., 1988) and influences the rate of tumor cell population expansion via the balance of cell gain and loss (Wyllie, 1985). It has often been observed as the mode of tumor cell death following cytotoxic therapy (Searle et al., 1975) and recently has been induced in experimental B and T leukemic cells by treatment with monoclonal antibodies to a specific surface epitope (APO-1) (Trauth et al., 1989; Debatin et al., 1990). In all these circumstances, apoptosis is delineated by a series of strikingly similar morphologic changes.

II. Morphology

The morphologic changes of apoptosis occur in three phases (Kerr et al., 1972; Wyllie et al., 1980; Wyllie, 1987a, 1988; Walker et al., 1988b) (Figs. 1–3). In the first, there is reduction in nuclear size, condensation of chromatin into toroids or crescentic caps at the nuclear periphery, and nucleolar disintegration with dissociation of the transcriptional complexes from the fibrillar center. Cells dying by apoptosis detach themselves from their neighbors and from culture substrata. There is loss of specialized surface structures, such as microvilli and contact regions. The cell adopts a smooth contour. Cell volume shrinks, cytoplasmic organelles become compacted, and the smooth endoplasmic reticulum dilates. The dilated cisternae fuse with the cell membrane, giving rise to a bubbling appearance at the surface (Fig. 3c). Cytoskeletal filaments aggregate in side-to-side arrays, often parallel to the cell surface, and ribosomal particles clump in semicrystalline formations, but otherwise the organelles remain intact. In contrast to necrosis, the other major type of cell death (Trump et al., 1981), mitochondria do not show "high-amplitude swelling," the cell membrane does not become permeable to vital dyes at this

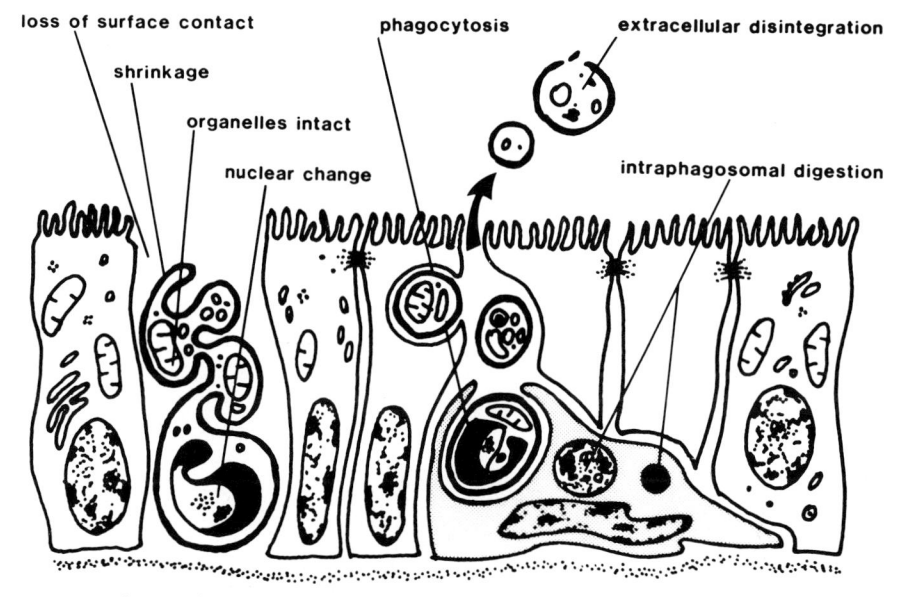

FIG. 1. Scheme of events in apoptosis within an epithelium. Dying cells lose surface contact with their neighbors and undergo cell shrinkage, but retain intact organelles. Chromatin condensation occurs with eventual fragmentation of nucleus and cytoplasm into multiple, small "apoptotic bodies." These may be lost from the epithelial surface and undergo extracellular degeneration, or be phagocytosed by neighbors or macrophages and experience intraphagosomal digestion.

stage, and apoptotic cells within tissues do not elicit an acute inflammatory reaction (Wyllie, 1981).

In the second phase (which may overlap with the first), there is blebbing at the cell surface (Fig. 3b) and crenation of the nuclear outline. Both nucleus and cytoplasm may split into fragments of various sizes. Typically, the cell becomes a cluster of round, smooth, membrane-bounded "apoptotic bodies," some containing nuclear fragments, others without. These bodies may be shed from epithelial surfaces or phagocytosed by neighboring cells or macrophages. In glandular tissues in particular, intraepithelial macrophages are prominent in this activity (Walker, 1987; Walker and Gobe, 1987).

In the third phase, there is progressive degeneration of residual nuclear and cytoplasmic structures. In cultured cells, this is manifested as membrane rupture, producing permeability to vital dyes. In tissues, these changes (sometimes termed "secondary necrosis") usually occur within the phagosome of the ingesting cell. Eventually membranes disappear, organelles become unrecognizable, and the appearance is that of a lysosomal residual body. The majority of apoptotic bodies seen in tissues studied with the light

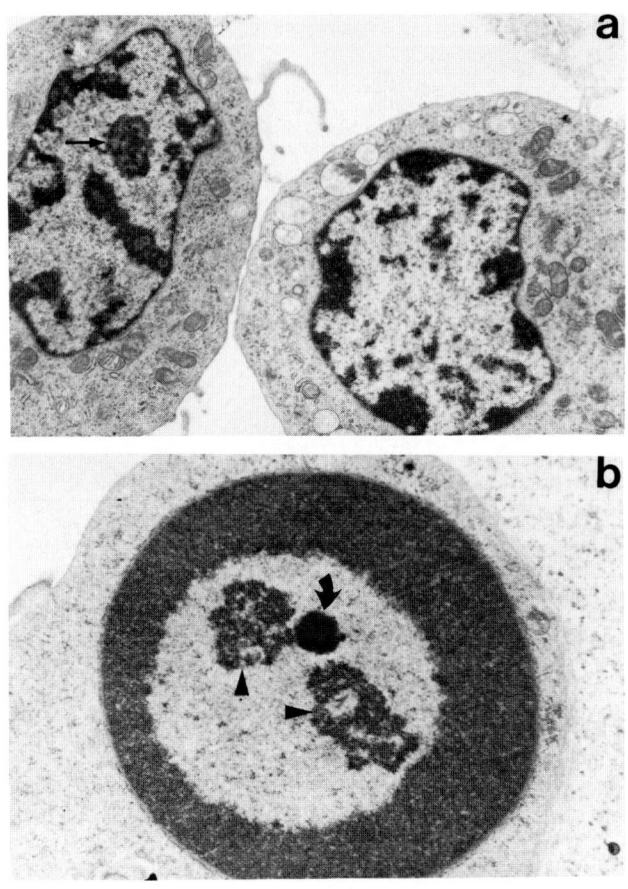

FIG. 2. Apoptosis in rodent fibroblast cell lines. (a) Normal cell nuclei display euchromatin and heterochromatin, with one or more nucleoli (arrow) (×5100). (b) In apoptosis, the chromatin condenses around the periphery of the nucleus, forming either toroids or crescentic caps, and the nucleolus undergoes a characteristic pattern of disintegration. The fibrillar center is conserved (arrow) following dissociation of the dense fibrillar (arrowheads) and granular components (×6700). (c) The apoptotic nuclear membrane invaginates around crescents of condensed chromatin (×8500) as the nucleus fragments (d), forming multiple, small chromatin spheres. Ribosomes detached from the endoplasmic reticulum often aggregate into semicrystalline arrays and vesicles of endoplasmic reticulum swell up and fuse with the plasma membrane (×4300). (e) Following cell fragmentation, "apoptotic bodies" may be phagocytosed by their viable neighbors; they are seen with a surrounding phagosome membrane (×5100). (f) Silver staining demonstrates conservation of the nucleolar fibrillar center (arrowheads) (×27000).

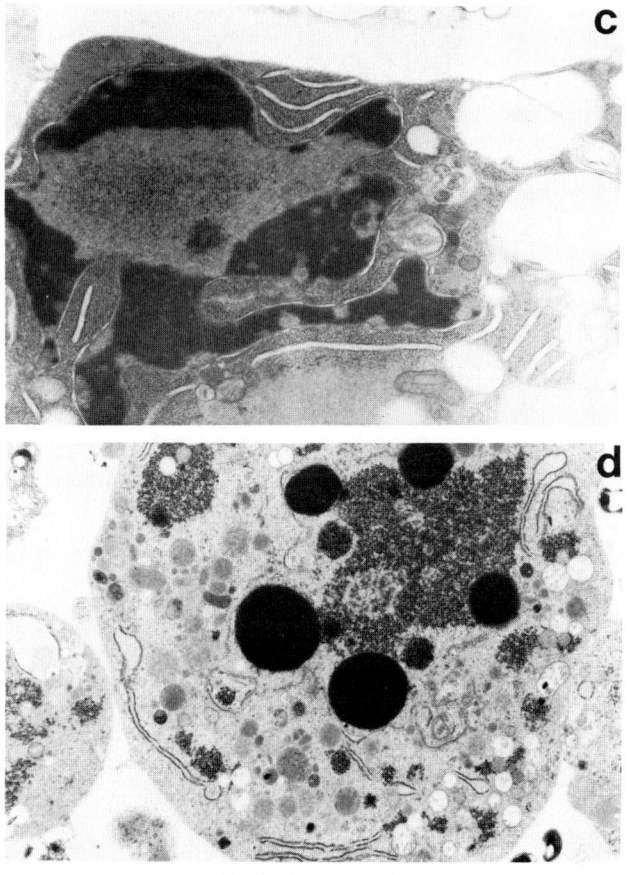

FIG. 2. (*continued*)

microscope are in this phase, and sometimes the smooth outline of the ingesting phagosome can be seen around them, but earlier phases can also be recognized by their rounded contours and deeply hyperchromatic and often fragmented nuclei. The histological appearance familiar to pathologists as "melanosis coli" is the accumulation in the lamina propria of macrophages laden with apoptotic bodies derived from mucosal cells (Walker *et al.*, 1988a). "Tingible body macrophages" in lymph node reactive centers are similar, being laden with the apoptotic residues of lymphocytes.

Time-lapse cinematographic studies of apoptosis reveal the sudden onset of cell shrinkage, with surface blebbing and bubbling, as cells enter phases 1 and 2, after a variable time, from exposure to the lethal stimulus. This initial

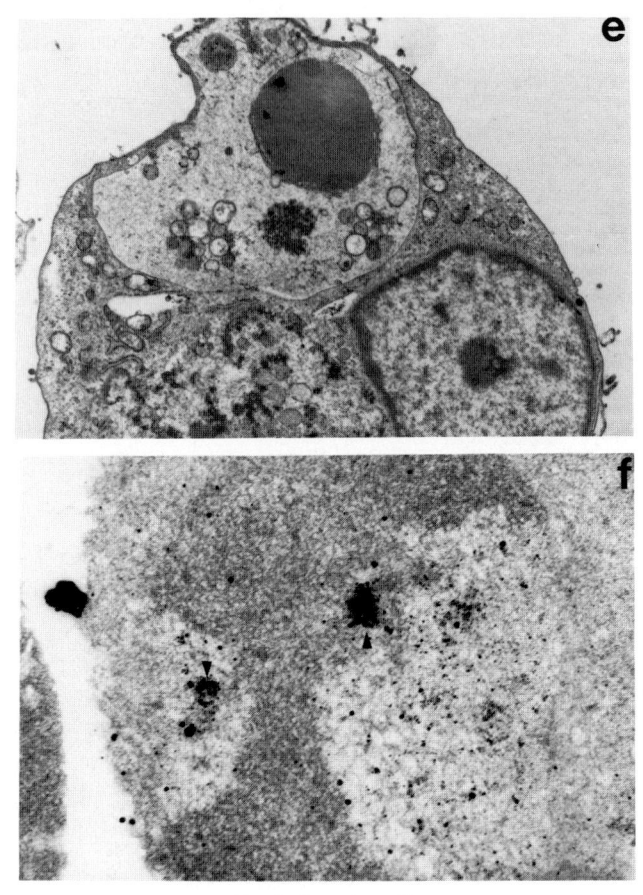

FIG. 2. (*continued*)

response lasts for only a few minutes and generates small, dense apoptotic cells. If not phagocytosed immediately, these cellular particles undergo a gradual loss of cell density (Wyllie, 1985), coinciding with loss of membrane integrity, shown ultrastructurally and by failure to exclude vital dyes. Apoptotic cells remain recognizable within tissues for 4–9 hours, a time course that coincides with that of complete degradation of other large biological structures within the phagosomes of macrophages. This relatively short period ensures that high rates of apoptosis produce only small increases in the proportion of apoptotic cells observed in tissue sections. Very simple calculations show, for example, that if a tissue were to undergo involution to half its cell number over 3 days, by a steady rate of apoptosis, each apop-

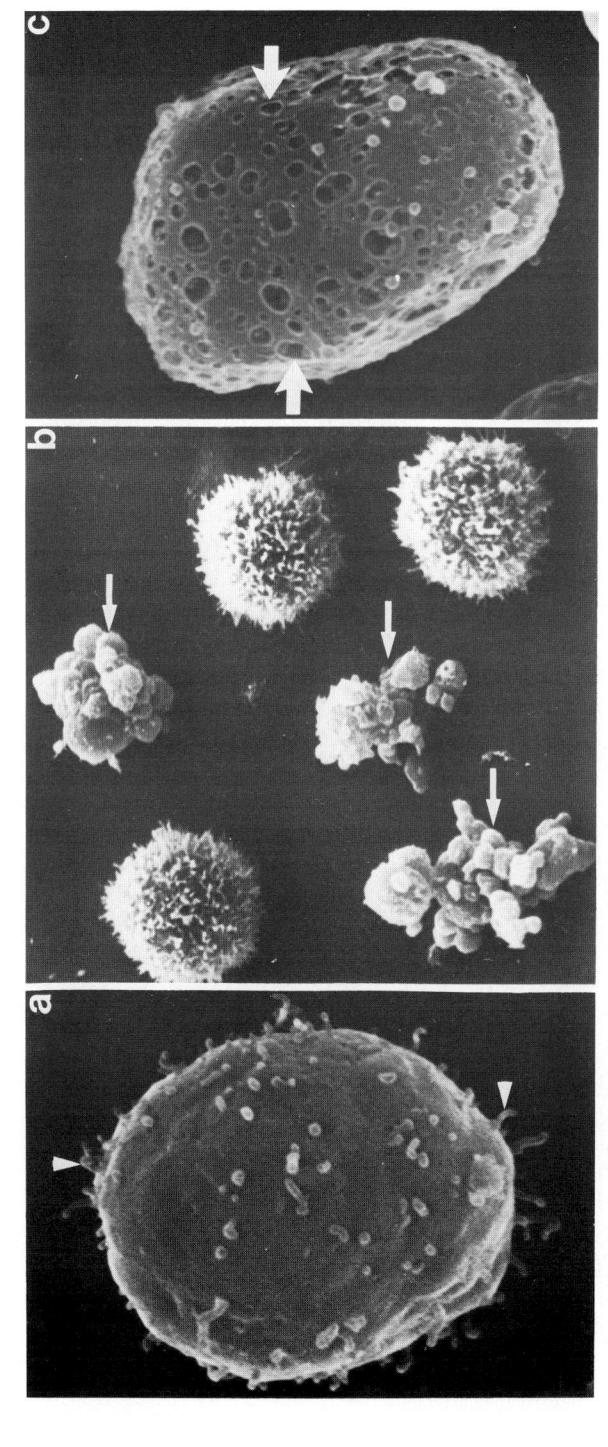

FIG. 3. Cell surface changes in apoptosis. Scanning electron micrographs of (a) normal thymocyte with microvilli (arrowheads), (b) apoptotic mouse sarcoma 180 cells with surface blebbing and budding (arrows), and (c) apoptotic thymocyte with surface blisters (arrows) due to fusion of dilated vesicles of endoplasmic reticulum with the membrane. (Courtesy of Dr. C. Bishop and Mr. R. Morris.)

totic body remaining recognizable for 6 hours, then the proportion of apoptotic cells evident on microscopy would rise in the first 6 hours by just over 4%, and thereafter more slowly to just over 8% by the end of the third day.

III. Mechanisms

The biochemistry of apoptosis is less well defined than its morphology, probably because this process characteristically involves scattered single cells within tissues, surrounded and outnumbered by viable neighbors. Nonetheless, six major events are known. Cell density rises abruptly (Wyllie and Morris, 1982; Wyllie, 1985). Intracellular calcium concentration undergoes a moderate but sustained rise (in necrosis, intracellular calcium rises rapidly several thousandfold) (McConkey et al., 1989a). Total protein and RNA synthesis are shut down (Wyllie and Morris, 1982). Chromatin is cleaved at internucleosomal sites, apparently by an endogenous endonuclease (Wyllie, 1980). Previously cryptic glycan groups become exposed on the cell membrane and act as recognition signals, permitting binding and engulfment by phagocytes (Morris et al., 1984; Duvall et al., 1985). Cytoskeletal elements become less readily deformable, perhaps as a result of transglutaminase activity (Fesus et al., 1987, 1989).

A. Cell Density Increase

The conspicuous volume reduction of apoptotic cells initially led to this type of death being called "shrinkage necrosis" (Kerr et al., 1972). In thymocytes, this is associated with a pronounced single step-wise increase in buoyant density, suggesting that proportions of intracellular water and ions are lost, without corresponding loss of macromolecules or organelles (Ohyama et al., 1981; Wyllie and Morris, 1982). In apoptotic cells, endoplasmic reticulum (ER) dilates, forming vesicles that fuse with the plasma membrane, voiding their contents extracellularly (Morris et al., 1984). This rapid and selective export of fluid and intracellular ions into the ER may be mediated by an ionic transporter system. Recently a sodium–potassium–chloride cotransporter has been described, inhibition of which leads to net loss of sodium and water from affected cells (Wilcock et al., 1988). At this time, apoptotic cells show no evidence of increased permeability to vital dyes or increased loss of previously accumulated radioactive chromium. At a more pragmatic level this density increase allows purification of intact apoptotic cells by density centrifugation for experimental purposes (Wyllie and Morris, 1982).

B. Intracellular Signaling Pathways

Perception of physiologic lethal stimuli is presumably mediated by cell type- and stimulus-specific receptors. Possible intracellular signaling mechanisms in the initiation of apoptosis include ion fluxes, phosphoinositide hydrolysis, changes in activity of protein kinases, and altered expression or activity of oncogenes. Although there is shutdown of total protein and RNA synthesis early in apoptosis (Wyllie and Morris, 1982), in some cell types initiation of the process appears dependent upon protein synthesis and can be abrogated by application of inhibitors such as cycloheximide or actinomycin D, shortly after the lethal stimulus (Wyllie *et al.*, 1984b; Wyllie, 1985).

An interesting example of cell type- and stage-specific signal transduction is the response of T cells to CD3 ligand binding: in postthymic cells the response is proliferation, whereas in the immature intrathymic cells it is apoptosis (Smith *et al.*, 1989; McConkey *et al.*, 1989b). Similar observations have been made in T cell clones, in which apoptosis is blocked by cyclosporine A and inhibitors of protein and RNA synthesis (Shi *et al.*, 1989). As in the apoptosis induced by glucocorticoid, the response to CD3 binding is preceded by a sustained rise in cytosolic Ca^{2+} (McConkey *et al.*, 1989a,b). Apoptosis in thymocytes can also be induced using low doses of calcium ionophore (Wyllie *et al.*, 1984b). Endonuclease activation (in intact cells or even in isolated thymocyte nuclei incubated in Ca^{2+}) is inhibited by the phorbol ester 12-O-tetradecanoylphorbol-13-acetate (TPA), an agent that stimulates endogenous protein kinase C (PKC), and this can be reversed by H-7, a supposedly specific PKC inhibitor (McConkey *et al.*, 1989b,c). Thus calcium mobilization without commensurate stimulation of PKC may trigger apoptosis in suitably primed cells. Direct measurement of PKC, diacylglycerol, and phosphoinositides in apoptotic cells has not yet been reported, however, and it is therefore still uncertain whether the different responses of intrathymic and postthymic cells reflect differences in signaling pathways or in the downstream effectors.

In prostatic epithelium, castration initiates a cascade of transcriptional activation involving c-*fos*, c-*myc*, and *hsp-70* genes prior to the onset of apoptosis (Buttyan *et al.*, 1988), and novel RNA transcripts have been observed (Montpetit *et al.*, 1986). Withdrawal of certain specific growth factors (e.g., IL-2 or bcl-2 protein) from lymphoid cell lines in culture, or serum withdrawal from fibroblasts, initiates apoptosis, although the factors do not necessarily stimulate proliferation (Duke and Cohen, 1986; Vaux *et al.*, 1988). It appears likely that the oncogene and growth factor-dependent signal transduction pathways, long interpreted rather single-mindedly in terms of cell proliferation, will be shown to play additional important roles in the regulation of cell survival and death.

C. Chromatin Cleavage

Internucleosomal chromatin cleavage is associated almost exclusively with the morphology of apoptosis. This association was first demonstrated in glucocorticoid-treated rat thymocytes in 1980 (Wyllie, 1980). Cleavage of internucleosomal linker DNA generates well-organized chains of oligonucleosomes, with DNA lengths that are integer multiples of 180–200 bp—the size of DNA wrapped around a single histone octamer—observed as a ladder on gel electrophoresis (Fig. 4). The typical "chromatin ladder" has now been reported along with morphologic chromatin condensation of apoptosis in

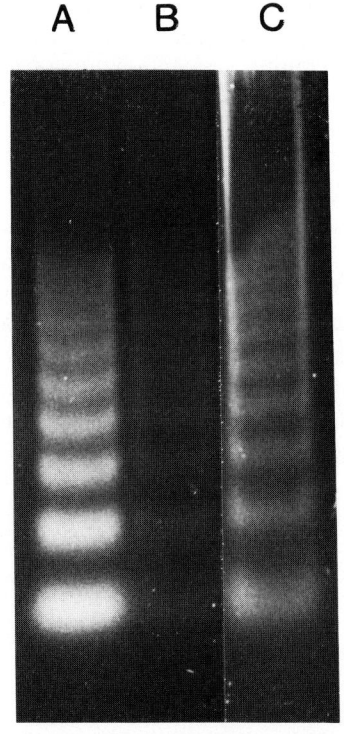

FIG. 4. Agarose gel electrophoresis of DNA recovered from the 27,000g supernatant lysates of two L5178 lymphoma cell sublines after incubation with methyl prednisolone sodium succinate at 10^{-5} M for 48 hours. The L5178 subline, which is positive for glucocorticoid receptors (track A), displays the DNA band pattern characteristic of apoptosis—a "chromatin ladder" of DNA fragments, with lengths that are integer multiples of 180–200 bp. This is consistent with cleavage of chromatin into oligonucleosomes, as produced by micrococcal nuclease digestion of the same nuclei as a control (track C). The glucocorticoid receptor negative L5178 subline, isolated by subculture in increasing concentrations of steroid over 3 months, shows only minimal DNA cleavage (track B).

many cell systems (Rotello *et al.*, 1989; Zeleznik *et al.*, 1989; Vaux *et al.*, 1988; Baxter *et al.*, 1989). The only known circumstances in which endogenous chromatin cleavage is not accompanied by the complete morphology of apoptosis are normoblast maturation and the differentiation of the lens epithelium (reviewed by Wyllie, 1987a). In both of these, although some of the cytoplasmic changes are atypical, nuclear chromatin undergoes widespread condensation entirely similar to that of apoptosis. In contrast, cell death by necrosis is not associated with internucleosomal DNA cleavage (Russell, 1983).

It has recently been demonstrated that DNA cleavage in apoptosis occurs selectively, without associated chromatin proteolysis (Arends *et al.*, 1990). The nuclear matrix appears normal in terms of structural organization and the presence of the most abundant protein species. DNA cleavage is at widely dispersed sites: the apoptotic nucleus has a normal content of acid-precipitable DNA. Two classes of chromatin fragments are generated (Arends *et al.*, 1990): 70% of DNA exists as oligonucleosome fragments bound to the nucleus, and 30% is unattached. Although the bound chromatin includes fragments as short as dinucleosomes, the majority are long; in contrast, the free chromatin comprises mono- and short oligonucleosome fragments only. This minority class probably derives from chromatin in a transcriptionally active configuration, as the chromatin-bound proteins are depleted in histone H1 and enriched in high-mobility groups (HMGs) 1 and 2—changes associated with active gene transcription (Tremethick and Malloy, 1988). Whereas inactive heterochromatin is thought to be tightly wound in a solenoid (Finch and Klug, 1976), transcriptionally active chromatin is not compacted in this way, which would allow better access to enzymes in the nucleoplasm and produce more complete digestion. The pattern of chromatin digestion in apoptosis, therefore, is consistent with activation of an endonuclease in solution in the nucleoplasm, rather than a constituent of the matrix itself.

Brief digestion of normal nuclei with a purified exogenous endonuclease (micrococcal nuclease) in the presence of protease inhibitors reproduces the nuclear morphologic changes of apoptosis, in step with generation of the typical DNA ladder (Arends *et al.*, 1990). Interestingly, these changes include those observed in the apoptotic nucleolus: segregation and dispersal of the dense fibrillar and granular components with preservation of an intact fibrillar center. These may be explained in terms of cleavage of the transcriptionally active ribosomal genes within the dense fibrillar component, with conservation of the inactive ribosomal DNA protected within the nucleolin-rich fibrillar center.

Thus, there is good evidence that the characteristic morphologic condensation of chromatin in apoptosis is due to DNA cleavage. It is more difficult to be certain that DNA change in apoptosis is due to an endogenous endonuclease. It has been suggested that in some circumstances similar chromatin cleavage might be the result of damage by reactive oxygen intermediates (Balkwill, 1989). Three observations, however, make this improbable. First, cells dying by necrosis (in which there is at least as much precedent for generation of reactive oxygen intermediates as in apoptosis) do not show the characteristic chromatin ladder (Russell, 1983). Second, the DNA cleavage in apoptosis is predominantly double stranded, with no single-strand nicks or gaps detectable by incubation with S1 nuclease (Arends *et al.*, 1990), whereas free radical damage would be expected to generate a high proportion of single-strand breaks. Third, in thymocytes subjected to ionizing radiation, wherein free radicals are known to mediate many biological effects, the evolution of apoptosis shows a different time scale compared to the ionization events that generate free radicals (reviewed by Wyllie, 1985). Within seconds of radiation exposure, cellular DNA undergoes multiple single-strand breaks, with consequent relaxation of supercoiling, characteristic of ionization damage (Filippovich *et al.*, 1982). These breaks are repaired within minutes and at this stage there is no apoptosis. About an hour later, however, the cells begin to show morphologic apoptosis, together with internucleosomal double-strand chromatin cleavage, processes that can be abrogated by treatment (after the radiation) with inhibitors of protein synthesis (Yamada and Ohyama, 1988).

Early experiments with thymocyte nuclei suggested that they contained an enzyme capable of cleaving chromatin in apoptosis. If incubated at neutral pH with both calcium and magnesium, such nuclei quickly developed multiple double-strand DNA breaks, generating the familiar ladder on electrophoresis (Duke *et al.*, 1983; Cohen and Duke, 1984). Endonucleases with suitable features are known to be present within the nuclei of many cell types (Ishida *et al.*, 1974; Nakamura *et al.*, 1981; Liu *et al.*, 1980) and it seemed plausible that the raised calcium levels within apoptotic cells might be sufficient to activate this enzyme. Attempts to purify an enzyme with properties of the thymocyte neutral nuclease have been reported (Wyllie *et al.*, 1986b; Dykes *et al.*, 1987).

The thymocyte nuclease cleaves chromatin of a target system (nuclei from cells labeled during growth with tritiated thymidine) to release labeled oligonucleosomes. This nuclease activity is optimum at pH 7.5, in contrast to contaminating acid nucleases, which also differ in cleaving DNA to much smaller (acid soluble) fragments. The neutral calcium–magnesium endonuclease is maximally eluted from normal thymocyte nuclei at 300 mM NaCl, and appears to be an anionic protein of around 130 kDa (A. H. Wyllie, unpublished observations). This is substantially larger than other candidates reported previously (Compton and Cidlowski, 1987) and now disputed (Al-nemri and Litwack, 1989), but is close to the size of one subunit of topoisomerase II (Halligan *et al.*, 1985). Topoisomerase II is known to be present in thymocytes and would be capable of engendering double-strand DNA cleavage under appropriate conditions (e.g., low ATP) (Udvardy et al., 1986; Chow and Ross, 1987). Normally, however, it is a constituent of the matrix and there is no evidence that it is ever free in the nucleoplasm. It is not at present clear whether the thymocyte Ca–Mg endonuclease is identical with topoisomerase II, or indeed whether either is responsible for the chromatin changes in apoptosis.

In thymocytes, the Ca–Mg endonuclease is constitutively present (Alnemri and Litwack, 1989). In contrast, when certain human and murine lymphoid cell lines underwent apoptosis *in vitro* in response to glucocorticoid, the extractable Ca–Mg endonuclease activity rose from low levels, peaking as endogenous chromatin cleavage and the morphology of apoptosis appeared (Wyllie et al., 1986a). None of these changes occurred in sublines selected for glucocorticoid resistance. Similar nuclease activity has been observed in an entirely different cell system, the physiologic death of ovarian corpus luteum cells (Zeleznik et al., 1989). Thus, endogenous endonucleases remain interesting candidates among the effectors of apoptosis, but their induction can precede the event of apoptosis.

D. Transglutaminase Activation

Coincident with the onset of apoptosis during the involution of liver hyperplasia and in glucocorticoid-treated thymocytes, there is induction and activation of tissue transglutaminase (Ca^{2+}-dependent protein–glutamine γ-glutamyltransferase) (Fesus et al., 1987). Transglutaminases cross-link proteins through ε-(γ-glutamyl) lysine bonds and mediate both formation of cornified envelopes by epidermal keratinocytes (Green, 1980) and cross-linking of fibrin and 2-plasmin inhibitor in the final stages of thrombus stabilization (Tanaka and Aoki, 1982). In apoptosis there is an increase in transglutaminase mRNA and protein, enzyme activity, and protein-bound (γ-glutamyl) lysine (Fesus et al., 1987). The probable consequence of transglutaminase activation is an extensive cross-linking of cytoplasmic and membrane proteins. In fact, apoptotic cells contain protein shells insoluble in detergents and chaotropic agents (Fig. 5). These shells, which are not extractable from normal cells, appear in scanning electron micrographs as wrinkled, spherical structures with some morphologic similarities to epidermal cornified envelopes (Fesus et al., 1989).

E. Cell Surface Alterations

It is characteristic of apoptotic cells that they are rapidly recognized and phagocytosed by their neighbors or by macrophages. The recognition pro-

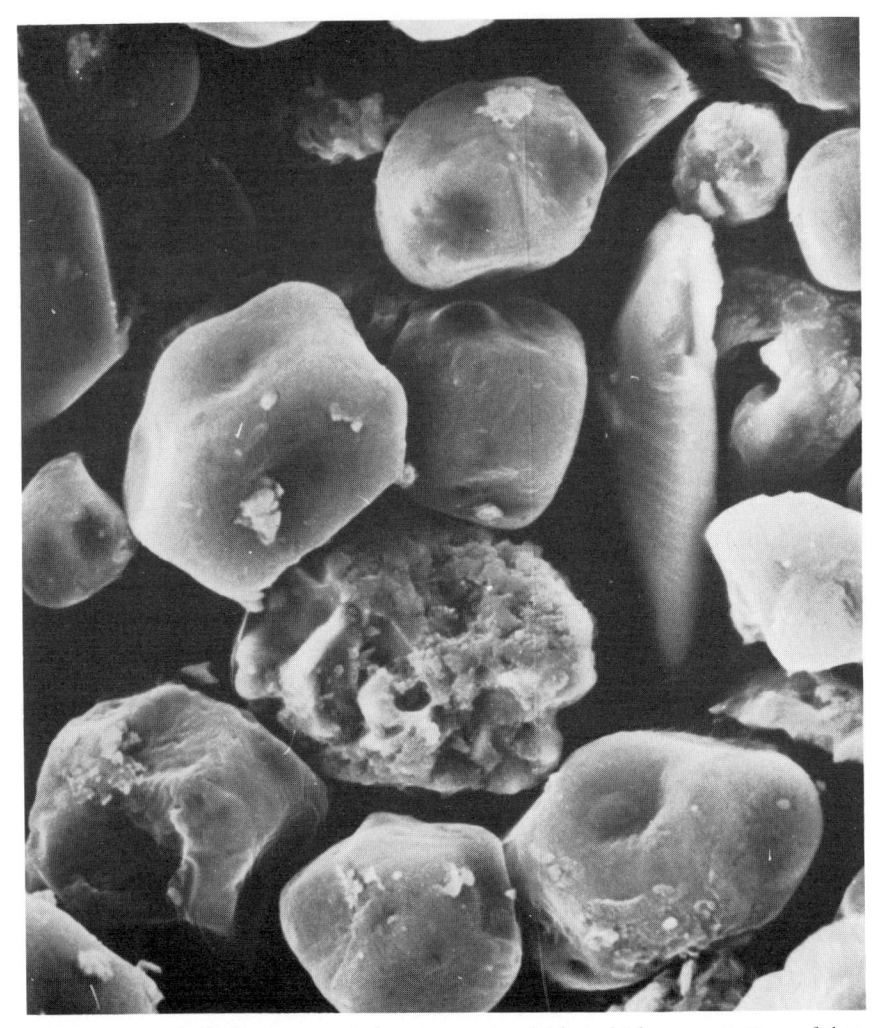

FIG. 5. Protein shells from apoptotic hepatocytes, insoluble in high concentrations of detergents and chaotropic agents, appear in scanning electron micrographs as wrinkled, irregularly globular structures with some similarities to epidermal cornified envelopes. (Courtesy of Dr. M. Piacentini and Dr. L. Fesus.)

cess has been reproduced *in vitro* in two isologous systems. Macrophages bound preferentially to apoptotic cells compared with normal cells. Recognition of apoptotic rodent thymocytes was mediated by a sugar-dependent mechanism, inhibited in this test system by *N*-acetylglucosamine (GlcNAc) or its dimer, *N,N'*-diacetylchitobiose, but not by mannose or fucose, and only to a slight extent by other monosaccharides, including galactose (Duvall et al., 1985). A similar sugar-dependent binding was demonstrated in the recognition of apoptotic, aging human neutrophils by isogeneic macrophages, although here glucosamine, galactosamine, and mannosamine inhibited recognition, as did the basic amino acids L-lysine and L-arginine; the inhibition reactions were pH sensitive and localized to the apoptotic neutrophil surface (Savill et al., 1989b). This sugar inhibition pattern suggests a lectin-type interaction of the apoptotic thymocyte with a receptor-like molecular complex on the surface of rodent macrophages capable of recognizing exposed glycan groups on the surface of apoptotic cells. GlcNAc, the sugar recognized in rodent thymocyte apoptosis, is present only in deep positions within glycan structures of mature glycoproteins and glycolipids. Other sugars, including galactose and charged sialyl groups, are added superficially during processing in the Golgi apparatus (Fig. 6a and b). There is independent evidence that these superficial groups may be lost in apoptosis, based on the observed reduction in cell surface charge density measured by microelectrophoretic mobility (Morris et al., 1984). Apoptotic cell surfaces lose existing cell membrane due to surface blebbing and budding, with shedding of microvilli, and gain new membrane through fusion of vesicles of dilated ER (Wyllie et al., 1980; Wyllie, 1987a) (Figs. 3 and 6c). Although other mechanisms are possible, including the expression of specific cell surface receptors (Wyllie et al., 1984a), this membrane loss and replacement could explain the change from the normal population of mature surface glycan groups to one containing some immature glycan groups, leading to focal exposure of sugars normally found in the interior of glycan structures, such as GlcNAc (Morris et al., 1984; Wyllie, 1987a) (Fig. 6). Macrophages and hepatocytes are also known to clear blood glycoproteins (gps) that have lost terminal sugar residues, either asialo-gp (galactose terminated) or asialoagalacto-gp (GlcNAc terminated). In each case the clearance was found to be mediated by specific cell receptors on the phagocytic cells (Ashwell and Hartford, 1982; Drickamer, 1988).

Macrophage recognition and phagocytosis of apoptotic human neutrophils and lymphocytes can also be inhibited by the RGDS tetrapeptide (Arg-Gly-Asp-Ser), RGD-bearing proteins vitronectin and fibronectin, or monoclonal antibodies specific for the vitronectin receptor polypeptide subunits (Savill et al., 1990) (Fig. 7). The inhibitory effect was localized to the macrophage cell surface, from which the vitronectin receptor polypeptide subunits were immunoprecipitated, demonstrating that recognition of apoptotic cells involves the vitronectin receptor (Savill et al., 1990), a member of the β_3 cytoadhesin family of integrins (Hynes, 1987).

Thus, it is likely that recognition of apoptotic cells by macrophages or neighboring cells involves existing specific receptors on acceptor cells binding to newly exposed ligands on apoptotic cells by integrin–peptide and

RER

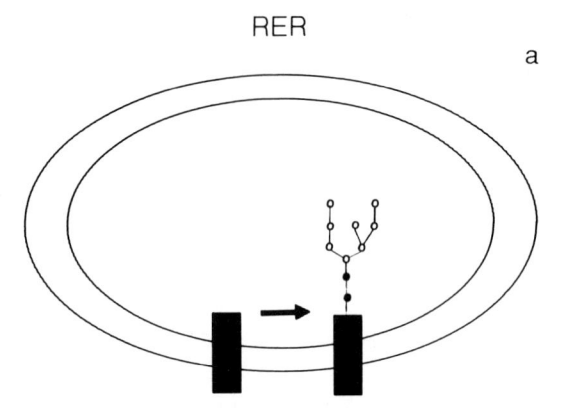

nascent polypeptide   N-glycosidically linked oligosaccharide

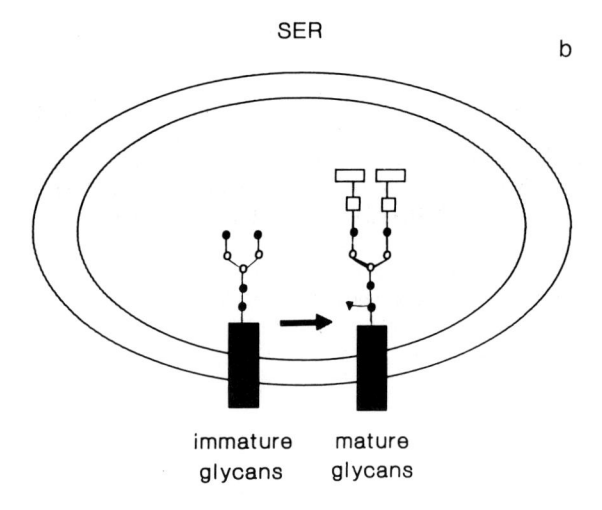

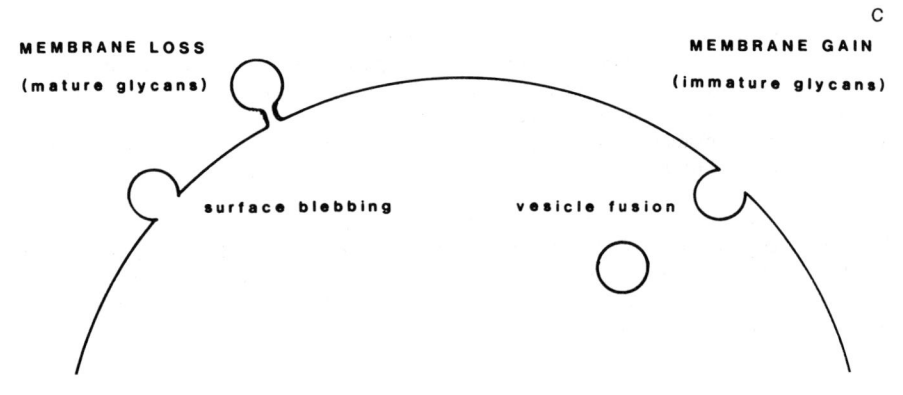

SER

immature glycans   mature glycans

MEMBRANE LOSS (mature glycans)   **MEMBRANE GAIN** (immature glycans)

surface blebbing   vesicle fusion

Macrophage ingestion

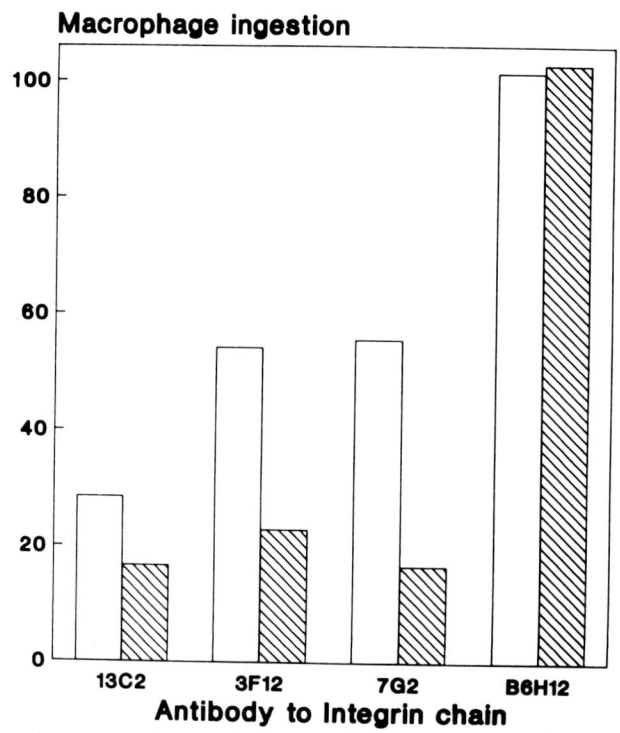

FIG. 7. Macrophage recognition and ingestion of apoptotic human neutrophils (open bars) and apoptotic human lymphocytes (cross-hatched bars) are inhibited by monoclonal antibodies that specifically bind the vitronectin receptor (VnR). 13C2 and 3F12 bind the VnR α_V chain, and 7G2 binds the VnR β_3 chain. No inhibition is observed using a monoclonal antibody; B6H12, to the chain of the VnR-like integrin LRI. [Redrawn from Savill et al. (1990).]

FIG. 6. A simplified schematic pathway of oligosaccharide processing on newly synthesized glycoproteins. (a) Oligosaccharide precursor is transferred from lipid donor to nascent polypeptide during its vectorial transport across the rough endoplasmic reticulum (RER) membrane, and some terminal sugars are removed. (b) Following transport to the Golgi stack, or smooth endoplasmic reticulum (SER), some mannose residues (○) are trimmed and other sugars are added to produce mature glycan groups (●, N-acetylglucosamine; □, galactose; □, sialic acid; ▼, fucose). Some immature glycan groups within the trans-Golgi cisternae have terminal N-acetylglucosamine sugars, and these may be exposed in apoptosis. (c) A model is presented that may explain the exposure of immature glycan groups by apoptotic cells. Mature glycan groups linked to glycoproteins are sited in the cell membrane, some of which is lost during cell surface budding and blebbing in apoptosis. This may be partially replaced by the membrane of dilated ER vesicles, containing immature glycan groups, which fuse with the cell surface. [Redrawn from Kornfield and Kornfield (1985).]

lectin–carbohydrate types of interactions. It is not known whether there is a direct interaction between acceptor cell receptors and apoptotic cell ligands, or whether adherence is mediated via a molecular bridge, such as occurs during platelet aggregation in which fibrinogen bridges GPIIb–IIIa integrins on platelet surfaces (Phillips et al., 1988). Molecular bridging would be compatible with the inhibition data, as lectin–carbohydrate interactions may occur between one end of the bridge and the apoptotic cell surface, and integrin–peptide interactions may occur between the other end of the bridge and the macrophage cell surface (Savill, 1990). It is also not known whether single or multiple receptor–ligand or receptor–bridge–ligand interactions are required for recognition and adherence. Diverse mechanisms might be expected, however, as apoptotic cells can be phagocytosed by neighboring parenchymal cells as well as macrophages. There are precedents for multiple, and sometimes synergistic, receptor recognition mechanisms in other cell–cell interactions mediated by integrins (Hynes, 1987; Dransfield et al., 1990).

IV. Roles in Pathology

A. Inflammation

Migration of large numbers of neutrophil polymorphs is the major cellular event at the onset of acute inflammation. Neutrophil granule contents are not only able to damage inflammation-inducing agents such as bacteria, but can amplify the inflammatory response by enzymatic cleavage of matrix proteins (Vartio et al., 1981) and are potentially histotoxic (Henson and Johnston, 1987). Leukocyte depletion experiments have shown that neutrophils play an important role in mediating reperfusion injury following ischemia of the heart and kidney (Romson et al., 1983; Mullane et al., 1987; Olof et al., 1989; Klausner et al., 1989). Before resolution can occur at an inflamed site, neutrophils must therefore be removed. Disintegration in situ with disgorgement of granule contents would cause tissue injury, however, and amplify inflammation. Recently it has been shown that human neutrophils from blood or inflamed joints, aged in culture, undergo the morphologic changes and chromatin fragmentation of apoptosis, and that this closely correlates with the degree of macrophage recognition and phagocytosis in vitro at a stage when their cell membrane appears functionally intact (Savill et al., 1989a). In acute experimental peritonitis induced by Corynebacterium parvum (Chapes and Haskill, 1983) or by thioglycollate (Sanui et al., 1982), massive waves of neutrophil phagocytosis by macrophages were observed, indicating that this is the major pathway of neutrophil disposal in vivo. Thus, apoptosis in unstimulated, senescent neutrophils represents a mechanism for their disposal without degranulation, and hence a control point in the resolution of inflammation (Haslett *et al.*, 1989). In theory, minor changes in the activation of apoptosis in senescent neutrophils could lead to significant alterations in the limitation of tissue injury associated with inflammation. It will therefore be of great interest to determine whether there are abnormalities in the kinetics of neutrophil apoptosis in disorders in which tissue destruction is associated with prolongation of inflammatory processes, such as rheumatoid arthritis.

B. IMMUNE KILLING

There are multiple mechanisms of immunologically mediated cytodestruction. Complement attack inserts transmembrane channels of polymerized, activated C9, of approximately 10 nm in internal diameter (Tschopp *et al.*, 1982). Complement-injured cells die by necrosis rather than apoptosis (Hawkins *et al.*, 1972), and it is probable that the ultimate lethal event is Ca^{2+} influx to high intracellular concentrations via such channels. Other effectors of immune killing—cytotoxic T lymphocytes (CTLs), natural killer (NK) cells, antibody-dependent cytotoxic cells (K cells), and tumor necrosis factors (TNFs)—induce typical apoptosis in their target cells, as evidenced by both morphology and DNA fragmentation (Russell, 1981, 1983; Stacey *et al.*, 1985; reviewed by Duvall and Wyllie, 1986; Allbritton *et al.*, 1988; Martz and Howell, 1989). The two types of death may coexist, as TNF-induced endothelial apoptosis may result in necrosis in the tissues supplied by affected vessels.

CTL and NK cells kill targets by an efficient contact-dependent mechanism (Martz, 1977; Berke, 1980). Killing occurs in three stages: recognition, programming for death, and disintegration (reviewed by Duvall and Wyllie, 1986). CTL specificity resides in the recognition stage ($t_{\frac{1}{2}} = 1$ minute), and living cytotoxic cells must also be present for the stage of programming for death ($t_{\frac{1}{2}} = 5$ minutes), during which target cell DNA is cleaved. Disintegration ($t_{\frac{1}{2}} = 100$ minutes), essentially an *in vitro* phenomenon and akin morphologically to "secondary necrosis," does not require continuing cytotoxic cell contact.

Several mechanisms of lymphocyte-mediated killing have been proposed (Young *et al.*, 1988). The observation that CTL targets die by apoptosis without requirement for protein synthesis suggests that T lymphocytes possess, and transfer into their targets, a complete mechanism for the execution of apoptosis (Golstein, 1987). It is not surprising that they should possess such a mechanism: it is well developed within intrathymic T cells and triggered there during deletion of autoreactive clones. CTLs, however, transfer this mechanism into their targets without suffering damage themselves. This paradox, for which several explanatory hypotheses have been constructed (Muller-Eberhard, 1988; Young *et al.*, 1988), is not unexpected if apoptosis of the target cell is initiated from within, by material transferred by the CTL. Attention has therefore focused on what the transferred material might include.

Several agents have been isolated from the cytoplasmic granules of cultured CTL and NK cells. These include perforin (P1), a protein of 70–75 kDa, structurally and functionally homologous to C9 (62–66 kDa). Like polymerized C9, perforins assemble into ringlike structures, creating transmembrane channels of approximately 16 nm in internal diameter (Podack, 1986; Podack *et al.*, 1988). Perhaps the focal distribution of these channels on target cell membranes in CTL killing explains why they are associated with apoptosis rather than necrosis. Necrosis is expected with extensive membrane-destructive lesions, and is apparently always observed in complement-induced killing (Russell, 1983). CTL granules also contain a large family of serine proteases ("granzymes") (Jenne and Tschopp, 1988). Their precise function is unknown, but may include activation of other effectors of apoptosis, such as the nuclease activity implicated in chromatin cleavage (Munger *et al.*, 1988).

A family of interrelated cytotoxins, not necessarily confined to granules, has also been implicated in CTL and NK cell-mediated killing: these include tumor necrosis factor α (TNF-α), lymphotoxin (LT, or TNF-β), NK cytotoxic factor (NKCF), leukalexin, and other less well-characterized factors. Several of these agents, in purified preparations, induce DNA fragmentation in coincubated targets (Young *et al.*, 1988; Joag *et al.*, 1989). TNF-induced DNA fragmentation can be inhibited by Zn^{2+}, suggesting mediation by an endonuclease (Flieger *et al.*, 1989). Cytotoxic cells may use different methods of target killing in different circumstances and the precise mechanisms are still a matter of dispute (Clark *et al.*, 1988).

NK cells are active in limiting viral replication during the early stages of an infection, during which time T lymphocytes undergo clonal selection and proliferation. Once differentiation to effector cells occurs, the CTLs specifically kill virally infected cells, clearing the infection. Because one of the major functions of CTLs and NK cells is control of viruses, and they both induce apoptosis with fragmentation of target cell DNA, Martz and Howell (1989) have suggested the "prelytic halt" hypothesis in which viral DNA is also fragmented. Thus, during target cell apoptosis there may be destruction of viral DNA and disposal of apoptotic bodies by macrophage phagocytosis without rapid cell lysis, efficiently blocking viral replication. In comparison, lysis of target cells with necrosis presumably leaves much viral DNA intact and would allow escape of assembled virion particles.

C. Neoplasia

Cell gain and loss occur concurrently in tumor cell populations. The balance between proliferation by mitosis and loss by exfoliation, differentiation, cell migration, or death determines the net growth rate of tumors, an important parameter in neoplastic aggression. It is possible to calculate the *potential doubling time* (T_p) from estimates of tumor cell production rates (thymidine labeling or mitotic indices), and the *actual doubling time* (T_d) from measurements of tumor volume, and so derive the *cell loss factor* (CLF = 1 − T_p/T_d). The CLF approaches zero with no cell loss, and approaches unity if extensive loss makes the actual doubling time unmeasurably large. In deriving CLFs, errors can arise from several inevitable assumptions, but in almost every tumor studied the CLF is large. In rodent sarcomas and carcinomas and in human bronchial and colorectal carcinomas and a malignant melanoma CLFs of 0.65–0.78 and 0.73–0.96, respectively, were recorded (Steel, 1977; Moore, 1983; Kerr and Lamb, 1984).

Of the modes of cell loss, death appears to be the most numerically significant and can occur by either necrosis or apoptosis. Zones of tumor necrosis are usually the result of hypoxia, in some tumors occurring at a strikingly constant distance from blood vessels (Thomlinson and Gray, 1955; Tozer *et al.*, 1990). High CLFs, however, can occur in tumors with almost no necrosis (Lala, 1972). There is evidence that apoptosis accounts for regression not only of nonneoplastic tissues (Wyllie *et al.*, 1973a,b; Kerr and Searle, 1973) and preneoplastic focal proliferations of hepatocytes (Bursch *et al.*, 1984), but also of hormone-dependent carcinomas (Gullino, 1980) and experimental pancreatic carcinomas after treatment with peptide hormone analogs (Szende *et al.*, 1989). The paradoxically slow growth of basal cell carcinomas, which have a high mitotic index, but no necrosis (Kerr and Searle, 1972) is also attributable to apoptosis.

Recently we have asked whether the "spontaneous" rates of apoptosis in tumors are influenced by oncogene expression, and the extent to which apoptosis determines tumor cell population growth. Oncogene-expressing rodent fibroblast lines transfected with c-*myc*, or mutationally-activated c-Ha-*ras*l (from the T24 bladder cancer cell line, with a point mutation at codon 12) or the c-Ha-*ras*l protooncogene, formed malignant tumors in immune-suppressed mice (Spandidos, 1985; Wyllie *et al.*, 1987, 1989) (Fig. 8a). The immortalized 208F parent cell line gave rise to small, nonprogressive indolent tumors. About half of the mice injected with c-*myc* transfectants developed primary tumors that grew slowly and were weakly tumorigenic and nonmetastatic at 14 days. Within these tumors apoptosis was conspicuous, occurring at high levels similar to those of mitosis. In contrast, over 90% of the mice injected with cells expressing activated T24-*ras* developed aggressive, large, metastasizing tumors in which apoptosis was seldom seen, although mitoses occurred at high frequency. Cells expressing the c-Ha-*ras*l protooncogene were intermediate in properties. Net tumor growth can be viewed as a balance of cell gain and loss, which may be manifested in the

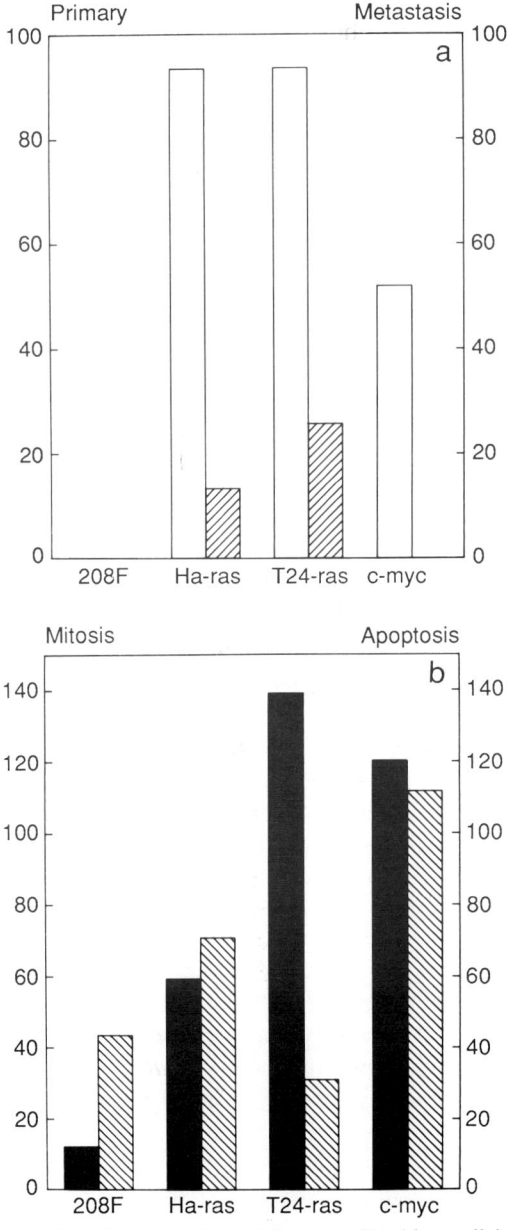

FIG. 8. Growth properties of tumors derived from rat fibroblast cell lines expressing the human oncogenes c-*myc*, c-Ha-*ras1*, and mutationally activated T24-*ras*. (1) Mean percentages of immune-suppressed mice injected with 10^7 cells that develop progressively growing primary tumors (open bars), and either lymphatic or hematogenous metastases after 14 days (cross-

differing frequencies of mitosis and apoptosis (Fig. 8b). The T24-*ras*-expressing cells differed from the others, both in combining low apoptosis with high mitosis and in producing more aggressive tumors. *In vitro*, the patterns of rates of tumor cell apoptosis were similar to those observed *in vivo* for these lines (Wyllie *et al.*, 1989) and were inversely correlated with the rates of population expansion (M. J. Arends, unpublished observations). Thus, *ras* and *myc* oncogenes apparently differentially regulate the relative rates of cell gain and loss within tumor cell populations: *ras* activation and its interaction with other oncoprotein-mediated transduction pathways may expand a population of neoplastic cells through inhibiting cell death as well as inducing cell proliferation. This not only permits rapid tumor growth, but also survival of potentially aggressive variants. Tumor cell apoptosis may also occur via mechanisms other than endogenous activation of internal programs, including attack by CTLs, NK and K cells, and triggering of apoptosis-prone cells by therapeutic agents, toxins, or relative hypoxia around necrotic zones.

V. Conclusions

Three broad conclusions can be drawn from this review of the mechanisms and roles of apoptosis.

1. Apoptosis is Fundamentally Different from Necrosis. Necrosis differs from apoptosis in structure, mechanism, and sequelae (Wyllie, 1981; Trump *et al.*, 1981). Structurally, necrotic cells show critically damaged organelles (e.g., mitochondria with "high-amplitude swelling"), ruptured plasma membranes, and dispersal of cytoplasmic elements into the extracellular space. The mechanisms are various, but do not depend upon continuing synthetic activity. There is no evidence that specific signaling pathways are involved. There is breakdown of membrane homeostasis and net flow of water into the necrotic cell, whose density falls. Intracellular calcium rises uncontrollably to equilibriate with the millomolar concentrations in the extracellular space. The process results in an acute inflammatory reaction, perhaps triggered by complement-activating factors emanating from mitochondria that have escaped from the damaged cell (Kagiyama *et al.*, 1989). Alternatively, leukotrienes and other arachidonate chemotaxins may be generated from partially

---

hatched bars). The established parent line, 208F, formed nonprogressive, indolent nodules. (b) Mitosis (solid bars) and apoptosis (cross-hatched bars) within apparently viable regions of tumors were scored as figures per 10 high-power fields. The T24-*ras*-expressing cell line formed the most aggressive tumors, which display high mitotic but low apoptotic rates, whereas the c-*myc*-expressing cell line was much less aggressive and showed a markedly higher rate of apoptosis in comparison with the rate of mitosis. [Redrawn from Wyllie *et al.* (1987).]

degraded cell membranes (Denzlinger et al., 1985). The arrival of neutrophil polymorphs permits digestion and phagocytosis of the constituents of the necrotic cells, but brings with it the risk of further tissue damage (Romson et al., 1983). In all these features, the cell biology of necrosis contrasts strongly with that of apoptosis.

2. *Two Classes of Event are Required for Apoptosis.* Apoptosis depends upon the availability of certain key proteins. These include the calcium–magnesium endonuclease and the glutamyl transferases. It is probable that there are several more. Neither the endonuclease nor the transglutaminases are normally present in every cell in a tissue; they accumulate before apoptosis takes place. Their coordinate expression is presumably regulated by specific controller genes. We call this *priming* for apoptosis (Fig. 9). Some tissues include a high proportion of primed cells (e.g., thymus cortex) (Van Haelst, 1967a), but in most (e.g., liver) (Zajicek et al., 1985) they normally represent a small minority. Only within the primed subpopulation can apoptosis occur. In these, the initiation of apoptosis is the result of a distinct set of events that we call *triggering*. Triggering mechanisms include the controlled influx of calcium into the cell and cause activation of the endonuclease, transglutaminases, and other putative effectors of apoptosis. It is probable that triggered cells proceed inevitably into apoptosis, but priming is reversible. One of the actions of the activated *ras* oncogene, in this scenario, would be to prevent or reverse the priming of cells.

One of the interesting implications of this distinction between priming and triggering is that triggering stimuli need not be as specific as those involved in priming. Mild cellular injury, for example, which generates a temporary influx of calcium, could constitute a triggering stimulus to a primed cell, although it would have no such effect on an unprimed one. Two predictions follow: primed cells should be vulnerable to apoptosis in response to a wide variety of minor injury stimuli, and apoptosis of this sort should occur *exclusively* in those regions of tissues in which primed cells lie. In fact there is evidence supporting both these predictions. Thymocytes undergo apoptosis in response to specific stimuli as diverse as glucocorticoid or CD3 ligands, and to nonspecific stimuli such as low to moderate doses of ionizing radiation, TCD-dioxin, or calcium ionophore (Van Haelst, 1967b; Umansky et al., 1981; Wyllie et al., 1984b; Yamada and Ohyama, 1988; Smith et al., 1989; McConkey et al., 1988, 1989b). The death is always in the thymus cortex, not in the medulla (Van Haelst, 1967a). Intestinal mucosal cells in the lower third of the crypt (but not including the stem cells near the crypt base) occasionally undergo apoptosis spontaneously (Searle et al., 1975) and so are presumptively "primed," and are also the main targets for death by apoptosis in response to a diverse range of chemotherapeutic agents, to ionizing radia-

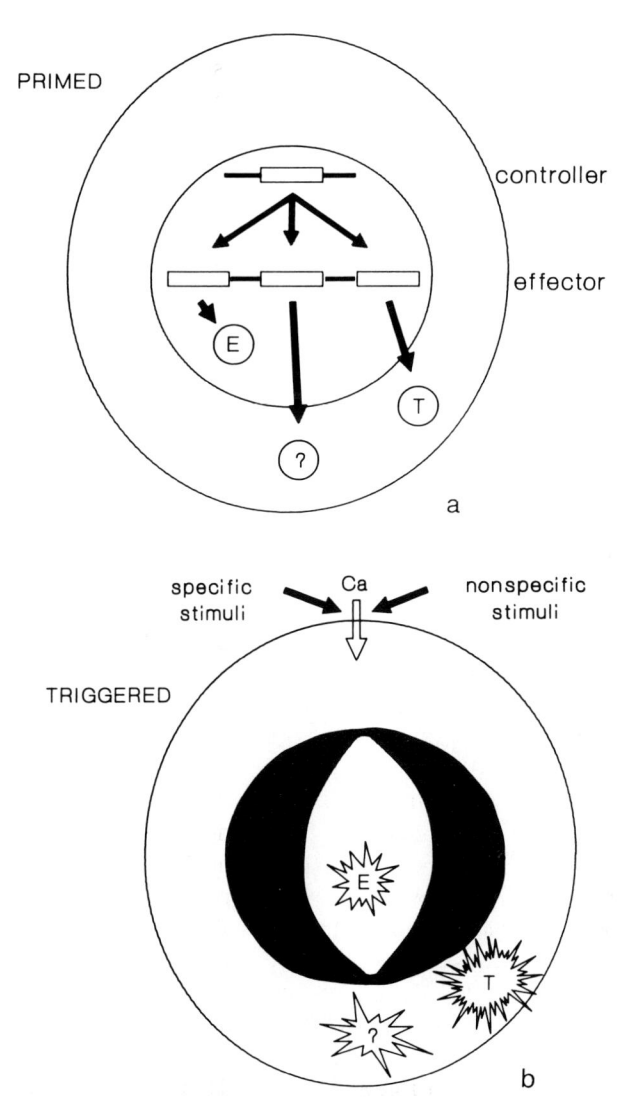

FIG. 9. Two-stage model for induction and activation of the effectors of apoptosis. (a) Cells become primed for apoptosis, presumably in response to cell type-specific signals, by expression of inactive precursor effector proteins, such as the endonucleases (E), transglutaminases (T), and other putative effectors (?). Effector expression may be coordinately regulated by specific controller genes. (b) Apoptosis is initiated in primed cells, through activation of effector molecules, by triggering mechanisms. In thymocytes, these include the controlled influx of calcium, without activation of protein kinase C, and occur in response either to specific stimuli, such as glucocorticoid or CD3 ligands, or to nonspecific stimuli, such as calcium ionophore, TCD-dioxin, or low to moderate doses of irradiation.

tion, and to zinc deprivation (Ijiri and Potten, 1983, 1987; Elmes, 1977). Adrenal cortical epithelial cells of the innermost region of the gland, the zona reticularis, are exclusively the cells sensitive to apoptosis in response to adrenocorticotropic hormone (ACTH) withdrawal (Wyllie et al., 1973a,b) and to low doses of the toxic carcinogen 9,10-dimethyl-1,2-benzanthracene (DMBA) (Currie et al., 1962). The zona reticularis includes the oldest postmitotic cells in the adrenal cortex. Spontaneous apoptosis is seen in late fetal and neonatal kidney cells in the rapidly proliferating nephrogenic zone in the outer renal cortex, but not in the zone of slow cell turnover in the medulla. Greatly increased cell deletion by apoptosis occurs in response to low to moderate doses of irradiation and follows the same spatial distribution (Gobe et al., 1988). It is of course part of the definition of cellular aging, that vulnerability increases to a broad variety of stimuli. When antibodies become available for the proteins characteristic of primed cells, it should be possible to visualize their distribution within tissues and to test these predictions more directly.

One interesting suggestion stimulated by the provocative paper by Servoma and Rytomaa (1988) is that part of the triggering mechanism of apoptosis may involve activation of the long interspersed repetitive DNA (LINE-1) transposon-like element, present in all mammalian cells. LINE-1 activation was observed in rat chloroleukemic cells that had reached a critical level (about half maximal) of population density in suspension culture, at which point growth was inhibited. Within 1–2 days, after the population had reached maximal density, all cells died by apoptosis. LINE-1 activation and apoptosis were associated with repression of c-Ki-*ras* expression, supporting the view that ras may inhibit apoptosis. The activation involved sudden transcription of LINE-1 to an RNA intermediate at half-maximal density, followed by apparent reverse transcription to DNA and integration of hundreds of thousands of copies of the LINE-1 element into random locations in the genome. This explosive integration of LINE-1 elements conferred irreversibility on the process leading to death, but up to this point subculturing the chloroleukemic cells reversed the phenomena of LINE-1 transcription, c-Ki-*ras* repression, and growth inhibition. It is not known whether LINE-1 integration is associated with chromatin cleavage, or indeed whether this dramatic series of events is a peculiarity of chloroleukemic cells.

3. *Immune Cell Killing by Apoptosis Requires Special Interpretation.* In contrast to the preceding discussion, apoptosis in response to attack from cytotoxic T cells and NK cells does not appear to be restricted to primed cells. Nor do the attacked cells engage in protein synthesis before entering apoptosis. The implication of this might be that CTL and NK cell killing involve the transfer to the target of not only a triggering stimulus, but also the key priming molecules. As the contents of CTL and NK cell granules are explored,

it will be illuminating to establish whether similar proteins appear within cells primed for apoptosis. Such proteins and their regulation could revolutionize current approaches to chemotherapy of tumors.

Acknowledgments

For the provision of scanning electron micrographs we wish to thank Dr. M. Piacentini, Dr. L. Fesus, Dr. C. Bishop, and Mr. R. Morris, and also Mr. A. McGregor for some of the transmission electron micrographs. The material reviewed included experimental work supported by the Cancer Research Campaign and the Wellcome Trust. M.J.A. is a Medical Research Council Training Fellow.

References

Allbritton, N., Verret, C. R., Wolley, R. C., and Eisen, H. N. (1988). *J. Exp. Med.* 167, 514–527.
Alnemri, E. S., and Litwack, G. (1989). *J. Biol. Chem.* 264, 4104–4111.
Arends, M. J., Morris, R. G., and Wyllie, A. H. (1990). *Am. J. Pathol.* 136, 593–608.
Ashwell, G., and Hartford, J. (1982). *Annu. Rev. Biochem.* 51, 531–554.
Balkwill, F. R. (1989). *Br. Med. Bull.* 45, 389–400.
Barker, E. A., and Smuckler, E. A. (1973). *Am. J. Pathol.* 71, 409–418.
Baxter, G. D., Collins, R. J., Harmon, B. V., Kumar, S., Prentice, R. L., Smith, P. J., and Lavin, M. F. (1989). *J. Pathol.* 158, 123–129.
Berke, G. (1980). *Prog. Allergy* 27, 69–133.
Bowen, I. D., Bowen, S. M., Sarraf, C. E., and Britton, S. L. (1988). *In* "The Contribution of Science to Cancer Medicine" (T. J. Deeley, D. Lloyd, and W. H. Sutherland, eds.), pp. 60–71. CRC Press, Boca Raton, Florida.
Bursch, W., Lauer, B., Timmermann-Trosiener, I., Barthel, G., Schuppler, J., and Schulte-Hermann, R. (1984). *Carcinogenesis* 5, 453–458.
Buttyan, R., Zakeri, Z., Lockshin, R., and Wolgemuth, D. (1988). *Mol. Endocrinol.* 2, 650–657.
Chapes, S. K., and Haskill, S. (1983). *Cell. Immunol.* 75, 367–377.
Chow, K.-C., and Ross, W. E. (1987). *Mol. Cell. Biol.* 7, 3119–3123.
Clark, W., Ostergaard, H., Gorman, K., and Torbett, B. (1988). *Immunol. Rev.* 103, 37–51.
Cohen, J. J., and Duke, R. C. (1984). *J. Immunol.* 132, 38–42.
Compton, M. M., and Cidlowski, J. A. (1987). *J. Biol. Chem.* 262, 8288–8292.
Currie, A. R., Hefelstein, J. E., and Young, S. (1962). *Lancet* 2, 1199–1200.
Debatin, K.-M., Goldmann, C. K., Bamford, R., Waldmann, T. A., and Krammer, P. H. (1990). *Lancet* 1, 497–500.
Denzlinger, C., Rapps, S., Hagmann, W., and Keppler, D. (1985). *Science* 230, 330–332.
Dransfield, I., Buckle, A.-M., and Hogg, N. (1990). *Immunol. Rev.* 114, 29–44.
Drickamer, K. (1988). *J. Biol. Chem.* 263, 9557–9560.
Duke, R. C., and Cohen, J. J. (1986). *Lymphokine Res.* 5, 289–299.
Duke, R. C., Chervenak, R., and Cohen, J. J. (1983). *Proc. Natl. Acad. Sci. U.S.A.* 80, 6361–6365.
Duvall, E., and Wyllie, A. H. (1986). *Immunol. Today* 7, 115–119.
Duvall, E., Wyllie, A. H., and Morris, R. G. (1985). *Immunology* 56, 351–358.
Dykes, T. A., McCall, C., Weiner, L., Duke, R., and Cohen, J. J. (1987). *Clin. Res.* 35, 139A.
Elmes, M. E. (1977). *J. Pathol.* 123, 219–223.
Ferguson, D. J. P., and Anderson, T. J. (1981a). *Virchows Arch. A: Pathol. Anat. Histol.* 393, 193–203.

Ferguson, D. J. P., and Anderson, T. J. (1981b). *Br. J. Cancer* **44,** 177–181.
Fesus, L., Thomazy, V., and Falus, A. (1987). *FEBS Lett.* **224,** 104–108.
Fesus, L., Thomazy, V., Autuori, F., Ceru, M. P., Tarcsa, E., and Piacentini, M. (1989). *FEBS Lett.* **245,** 150–154.
Filippovich, I. V., Sorokina, N. I., Soldatenkov, V. A., and Romantzev, E. F. (1982). *Int. J. Radiat. Biol.* **42,** 31–44.
Finch, J. T., and Klug, A. (1976). *Proc. Natl. Acad. Sci. U.S.A.* **73,** 1897–1901.
Flieger, D., Riethmuller, G., and Ziegler-Heitbrock, H. W. L. (1989). *Int. J. Cancer* **44,** 315–319.
Gobe, G. C., Axelsen, R. A., Harmon, B. V., and Allan, D. J. (1988). *Int. J. Radiat. Biol.* **54,** 567–576.
Golstein, P. (1987). *Nature (London)* **327,** 12.
Green, H. (1980). *Harvey Lect.* **74,** 101–155.
Gullino, P. (1980). *Prog. Cancer Res. Ther.* **14,** 271–279.
Halligan, B. D., Edwards, K. A., and Liu, L. F. (1985). *J. Biol. Chem.* **260,** 2475–2482.
Handyside, A. H., and Hunter, S. (1986). *Wilhelm Roux's Arch. Dev. Biol.* **195,** 519–526.
Harrison, D. J. (1988). *Histopathology* **12,** 679–683.
Haslett, C., Savill, J. S., and Meagher, L. (1989). *Curr. Opin. Immunol.* **2,** 10–18.
Hawkins, H. K., Ericsson, J. L. E., Biberfield, P., Trump, B. F. (1972). *Am. J. Pathol.* **68,** 255–287.
Henson, P. M., and Johnston, R. B. (1987). *J. Clin. Invest.* **79,** 669–674.
Hynes, R. O. (1987). *Cell* **48,** 549–554.
Ijiri, K., and Potten, C. S. (1983). *Br. J. Cancer* **47,** 175–185.
Ijiri, K., and Potten, C. S. (1987). *Br. J. Cancer* **55,** 113–123.
Ishida, R., Akiyoshi, H., and Takahoshi, T. (1974). *Biochem. Biophys. Res. Commun.* **56,** 703–710.
Jenne, D. E., and Tschopp, J. (1988). *Immunol. Rev.* **103,** 53–71.
Joag, S., Zychlinksy, A., and Young, D.-E. (1989). *J. Cell. Biochem.* **39,** 239–252.
Kagiyama, A., Savage, H. E., Michael, L. H., Hanson, G., Entmon, M. L., and Rossen, R. D. (1989). *Circ. Res.* **64,** 607–615.
Kerr, J. F. R., and Searle, J. (1972). *J. Pathol.* **107,** 41–44.
Kerr, J. F. R., and Searle, J. (1973). *Virchow's Arch. B* **13,** 87–102.
Kerr, K. M., and Lamb, D. (1984). *Br. J. Cancer* **50,** 343–349.
Kerr, J. F. R., Wyllie, A. H., and Currie, A. R. (1972). *Br. J. Cancer* **26,** 239–257.
Kerr, J. F. R., Harmon, B., and Searle, J. (1974). *J. Cell Sci.* **14,** 571–585.
Klausner, J. M., Paterson, I. S., Goldman, G., Kobzik, L., Rodzen, C., Lawrence, R., Valeri, C. R., Shepro, D., and Hechtman, H. B. (1989). *Am J. Physiol.* **256,** F794–F802.
Kornfield, R., and Kornfield, S. (1985). *Ann. Rev. Biochem.* **54,** 631–664.
Lala, P. K. (1972). *Cancer* **29,** 261–266.
Liu, L. F., Liu, C. C., and Alberts, B. M. (1980). *Cell* **19,** 697–707.
Liu, Y.-J., Joshua, D. E., Williams, G. T., Smith, C. A., Gordon, J., and MacLennan, I.C. M. (1989). *Nature (London)* **342,** 929–931.
Martz, E. (1977). *Contemp. Top. Immunobiol.* **4,** 301–361.
Martz, E., and Howell, D. M. (1989). *Immunol. Today* **10,** 79–86.
McConkey, D. J., Hartzell, P., Duddy, S. K., Hakansson, H., and Orrenius, S. (1988). *Science* **242,** 256–259.
McConkey, D. J., Nicotera, P., Hartzell, P., Bolloma, G., Wyllie, A. H., and Orrenius, S. (1989a). *Arch. Biochem. Biophys.* **269,** 365–370.
McConkey, D. J., Hartzell, P., Amador-Perez, J. F., Orrenius, S., and Jondal, M. J. (1989b). *J. Immunol.* **143,** 1801–1806.
McConkey, D. J., Hartzell, P., Jondal, M., and Orrenius, S. (1989c). *J. Biol. Chem.* **264,** 13399–13402.
Montpetit, M. L., Lawless, K. R., and Tenniswood, M. (1986). *Prostate* **8,** 25–36.
Moore, J. V. (1983). *In* "Cytotoxic Insult to Tissue" (C. S. Potten and J. H. Hendry, eds.), pp. 368–404. Churchill Livingstone, Edinburgh, Scotland.

Morris, R. G., Duvall, E. D., Hargreaves, A. D., and Wyllie, A. H. (1984). *Am. J. Pathol.* **115,** 426–436.
Mullane, K. M., Salmon, J. A., and Kraemer, R. (1987). *Fed. Proc., Fed. Am. Soc. Exp. Biol.* **46,** 2422–2433.
Muller-Eberhard, H. J. (1988). *Immunol. Rev.* **103,** 87–98.
Munger, W. E., Berrebi, G. A., and Henkart, P. A. (1988). *Immunol. Rev.* **103,** 99–109.
Nakamura, M., Sakaki, Y., Watanabe, N., and Takagi, Y. (1981). *J. Biochem. (Tokyo)* **89,** 143–152.
O'Connor, T. M., and Wyttenbach, C. R. (1974). *J. Cell Biol.* **60,** 448–459.
Ohyama, H., Yamada, T., and Watanabe, I. (1981). *Radiat. Res.* **85,** 333–339.
Olof, P., Hellberg, A., and Kallskog, T. O. K. (1989). *Kidney Int.* **36,** 555–561.
O'Shea, J. D., Hay, M. F., and Cran, D. G. (1978). *J. Reprod. Fertil.* **54,** 183–187.
Phillips, D. R., Charo, I. F., Parise, L. V., Fitzgerald, L. A. (1988). *Blood* **71,** 831–843.
Podack, E. R. (1986). *J. Cell. Biochem.* **30,** 133–170.
Podack, E. R., Lowrey, D. M., Lichtenheld, M., Olsen, K. J., Aebischer, T., Binder, D., Rupp, F., and Hengartner, H. (1988). *Immunol. Rev.* **103,** 203–211.
Romson, J. L., Hook, B. G., Kunkel, S. L., Abrams, G. D., Schork, M. A., and Lucchesi, B. R. (1983). *Circulation* **67,** 1016–1023.
Rotello, R. J., Hocker, M. B., and Gerschenson, L. E. (1989). *Am. J. Pathol.* **134,** 491–495.
Russell, J. H. (1981). *Biol. Rev.* **56,** 153–197.
Russell, J. H. (1983). *Immunol. Rev.* **72,** 97–118.
Sanui, H., Yoshida, S.-I., Nomoto, K., Ohhara, R., and Adachi, Y. (1982). *Br. J. Exp. Pathol.* **63,** 278–285.
Sarraf, C. E., and Bowen, I. D. (1986). *Br. J. Cancer* **54,** 989–998.
Savill, J. S. (1990). Ph.D. thesis. University of London, London.
Savill, J. S., Wyllie, A. H., Henson, J. E., Walport, M. J., Henson, P. M., and Haslett, C. (1989a). *J. Clin. Invest.* **83,** 865–875.
Savill, J. S., Henson, P. M., and Haslett, C. (1989b). *J. Clin. Invest.* **84,** 1518–1527.
Savill, J., Dransfield, I., Hogg, N., and Haslett, C. (1990). *Nature (London)* **343,** 170–173.
Searle, J., Lawson, T. A., Abbott, P. J., Harmon, B., and Kerr, J. F. R. (1975). *J. Pathol.* **116,** 129–138.
Servomaa, K., and Rytomaa, T. (1988). *Cell Tissue Kinet.* **21,** 33–43.
Shi, Y., Sahai, B. M., and Green, D. R. (1989). *Nature (London)* **339,** 625–626.
Shi, Y., Bissonnette, R. P., Parfrey, N., Szalay, M., and Green, D. R. (1991). Manuscript in preparation.
Skalka, M., Matyasova, J., and Cejkova, M. (1976). *FEBS Lett.* **72,** 271–274.
Smith, C. A., Williams, G. T., Kingston, R., Jenkinson, E. J., and Owen, J. J. T. (1989). *Nature (London)* **337,** 181–184.
Spandidos, D. A. (1985). *Anticancer Res.* **5,** 485–498.
Stacey, N. H., Bishop, C. J., Halliday, J. W., Halliday, W. J., Cooksley, W. G., Powell, L. W., and Kerr, J. F. (1985). *J. Cell Sci.* **74,** 169–179.
Steel, G. G., ed. (1977). "Growth Kinetics of Tumours." Oxford Univ. Press, Oxford, England.
Szende, B., Zalatna, A., and Schally, A. V. (1989). *Proc. Natl. Acad. Sci. U.S.A.* **86,** 1643–1647.
Tanaka, Y., and Aoki, N. J. (1982). *J. Clin. Invest.* **69,** 536–542.
Thomlinson, R. H., and Gray, L. H. (1955). *Cancer* **9,** 539–549.
Tozer, G. M., Lewis, S., Michalowsky, A., and Aber, V. (1990). *Br. J. Cancer* **61,** 250–257.
Trauth, B. C., Klas, C., Peters, A. M. J., Matzku, S., Moller, P., Falk, W., Debatin, K.-M., and Krammer, P. H. (1989). *Science* **245,** 301–305.
Tremethick, D. J., and Molloy, P. L. (1988). *Nucleic Acids Res.* **16,** 11107–11123.
Trump, B. F., Berezesky, I. K., and Osornio-Vargas, A. R. (1981). *In* "Cell Death in Biology and Pathology" (I. D. Bowen and R. A. Lockshin, eds.), pp. 209–242. Chapman and Hall, London.
Tschopp, J., Muller-Eberhard, H. J., and Podack, E. R. (1982). *Nature (London)* **298,** 534–537.
Udvardy, A., Schedl, P., Sander, M., and Hsieh, T. S. (1986). *J. Mol. Biol.* **191,** 231–246.

disease of childhood. During the 1960s, measles virus was identified as the etiologic agent in a slowly progressive fatal central nervous system (CNS) disease, subacute sclerosing panencephalitis (SSPE). SSPE has been recognized as a disease entity since the 1930s, when Dawson (1933) described a clinical and pathological entity distinct from encephalitis lethargica and Van Bogaert (1945) identified a disease with similar clinical manifestations, but with primarily white matter pathology. Measles virus antigen was demonstrated in brain tissue of SSPE patients in 1967 (Connolly *et al.*, 1967), and the virus was first cultured from infected brain tissue by three independent laboratories in 1969 (Chen *et al.*, 1969; Horta-Barbosa *et al.*, 1969; Payne *et al.*, 1969). Subsequently, it was recognized that measles virus is also responsible for CNS disease in immunosuppressed individuals. This form of measles encephalitis has been called measles inclusion body encephalitis (MIBE), immunosuppressive measles encephalitis (IME), or subacute measles encephalitis (SME).

II. Clinical and Epidemiological Features

A. Subacute Sclerosing Panencephalitis

SSPE is a rare consequence of measles infection. It most frequently occurs in individuals who had measles at less than 2 years of age (Halsey *et al.*, 1980; Moodie *et al.*, 1980; Aaby *et al.*, 1984). The mean incubation period is 6–7 years and 85% of cases occur between the ages of 5 and 14 years, although SSPE has been reported in individuals over 30 years old (Cape *et al.*, 1973). Effective measles vaccination programs have dramatically reduced the incidence of SSPE in the United States and Western Europe, but large numbers of cases continue to occur in developing countries.

SSPE is a disease with insidious onset; decline in school performance or behavioral problems are frequently the first symptoms. The clinical course has been divided into stages of disability, which begin with progressive mental and behavioral changes, and progress to myoclonic jerks, ataxia, decorticate posturing, and coma (Jabbour *et al.*, 1969). The events may occur over a period as short as 4 weeks or may last for several years, and result in death in 95% of cases. The usual duration is 9 months to 3 years, although long-term stabilization or improvement has very occasionally been reported (e.g., Risk *et al.*, 1978).

Antibody titers to measles virus are elevated in serum and cerebrospinal fluid (CSF) of SSPE patients, and may be dramatically increased. Over 50% of CSF IgG represents antibodies to measles virus proteins (Link *et al.*, 1973; Vandvik *et al.*, 1976), and is synthesized intrathecally (Tourtellotte *et al.*,

1981). The measles-specific IgG is oligoclonal on agarose electrophoresis, signifying synthesis by expanded clones of cells (Vandvik and Norrby, 1973).

B. Measles Inclusion Body Encephalitis

MIBE occurs in individuals who are immunocompromised. Most cases have occurred in children with leukemia (Booss and Esiri, 1986), but cases have also been reported in adults with Hodgkin's disease (Wolinsky *et al.*, 1977) or renal allograft (Agamanolis *et al.*, 1979). There is usually a history of exposure to measles in the months preceeding the onset of encephalitis, but acute illness may never have been apparent or may have been very mild. The clinical course may last up to 15 months, with 90% of individuals succumbing within 4 months (Kipps *et al.*, 1983). Serum and CSF antibodies to measles are present in some cases, but may be absent due to the immunosuppressed status of the individual.

III. Pathology of Measles-Infected Brain Tissue

Most areas of the brain may be infected in SSPE, although the cerebellum is rarely involved, and the infection may be focal or widespread (Ohya *et al.*,

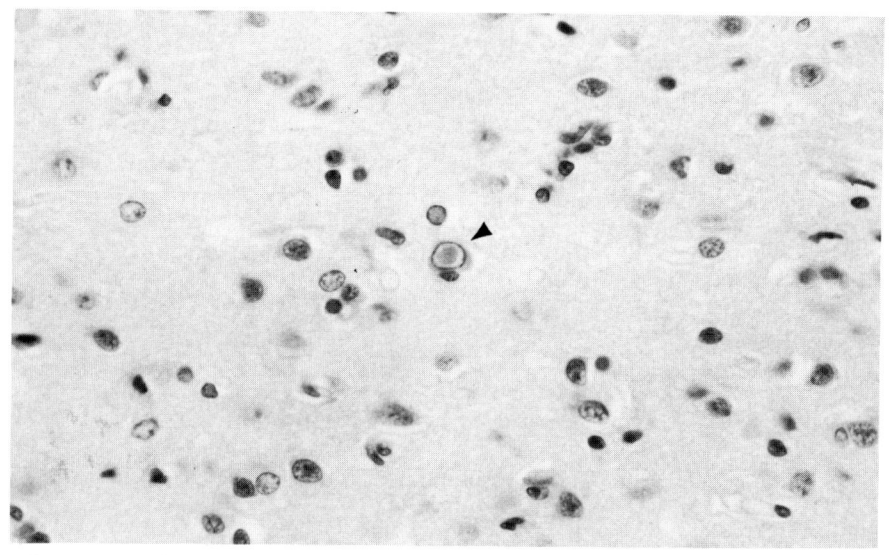

Fig. 1. Cortical gray matter of SSPE brain tissue. An intranuclear inclusion (arrowhead) is prominent in a neuron. Hematoxylin and eosin stain (×450).

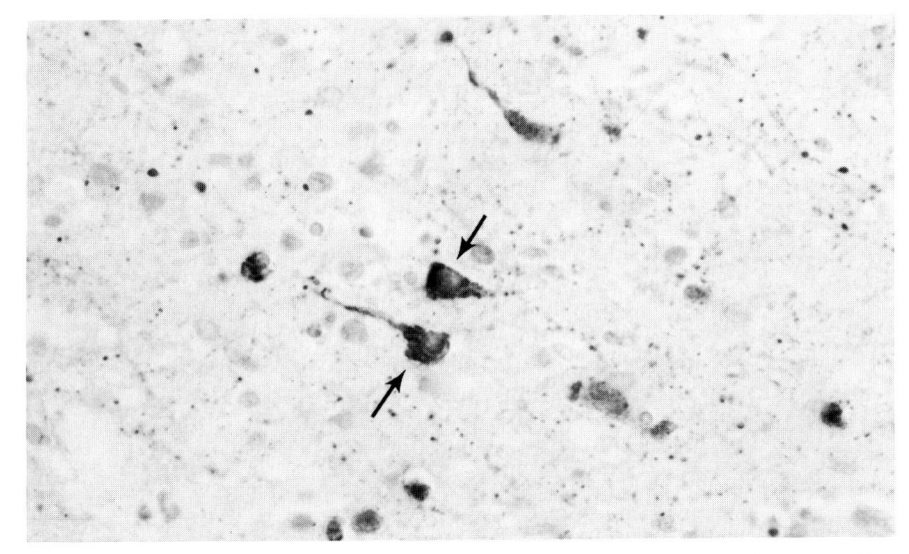

FIG. 2. A region of cortex comparable to Fig. 1, immunocytochemically labeled with rabbit antimeasles serum and peroxidase-coupled avidin–biotin complex, counterstained with hematoxylin. Several infected neurons are labeled (arrows) (×450).

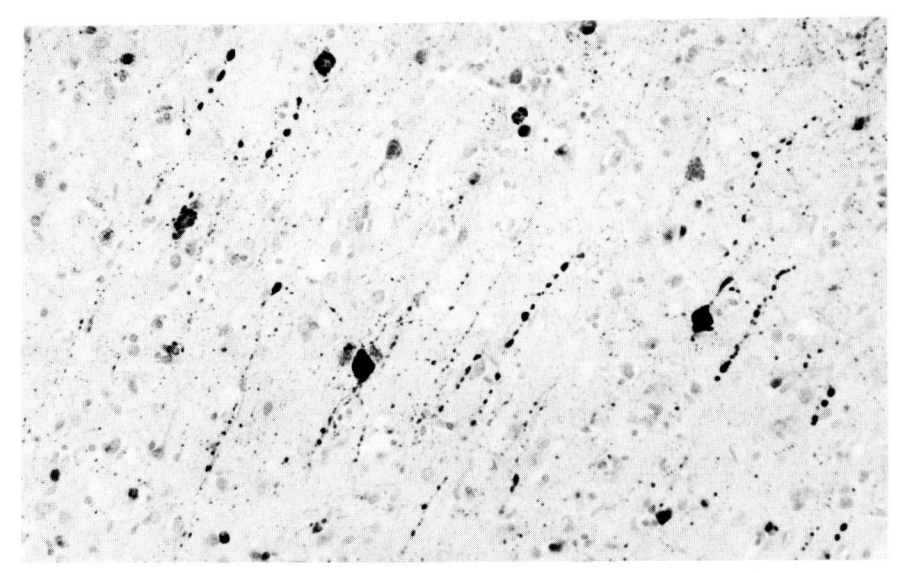

FIG. 3. SSPE brain tissue immunocytochemically labeled with rabbit antimeasles serum. Numerous infected neurons and neuronal processes containing measles virus antigen can be seen (×180).

1974). Mild to moderate inflammatory infiltrates are common in both gray and white matter. Eosinophilic intranuclear and cytoplasmic inclusions can be found in neurons and oligodendrocytes (Fig. 1), although immunocytochemical labeling for measles antigens reveals many more infected cells than can be identified by the presence of inclusions (Fig. 2). Viral antigen can be visualized in neuronal processes extending long distances from the cell body (Fig. 3). Infected cells can usually be found in both gray and white matter, but either neurons or oligodendrocytes may be the predominant cell type infected in an individual brain. Reactive astrocytes are abundant in affected areas, but rarely if ever contain viral antigen (Fig. 4). Demyelination may be severe in cases in which oligodendrocytes are infected. Neuronal loss may be pronounced in cases of long duration. However, virus infection does not appear to be rapidly lytic to cells, because many cells appear morphologically intact despite the presence of viral antigen.

One striking morphologic feature that distinguishes measles virus in SSPE from wild-type virus in tissue culture is the incomplete assembly of viral particles in the brain as seen by electron microscopy. Whereas measles virus

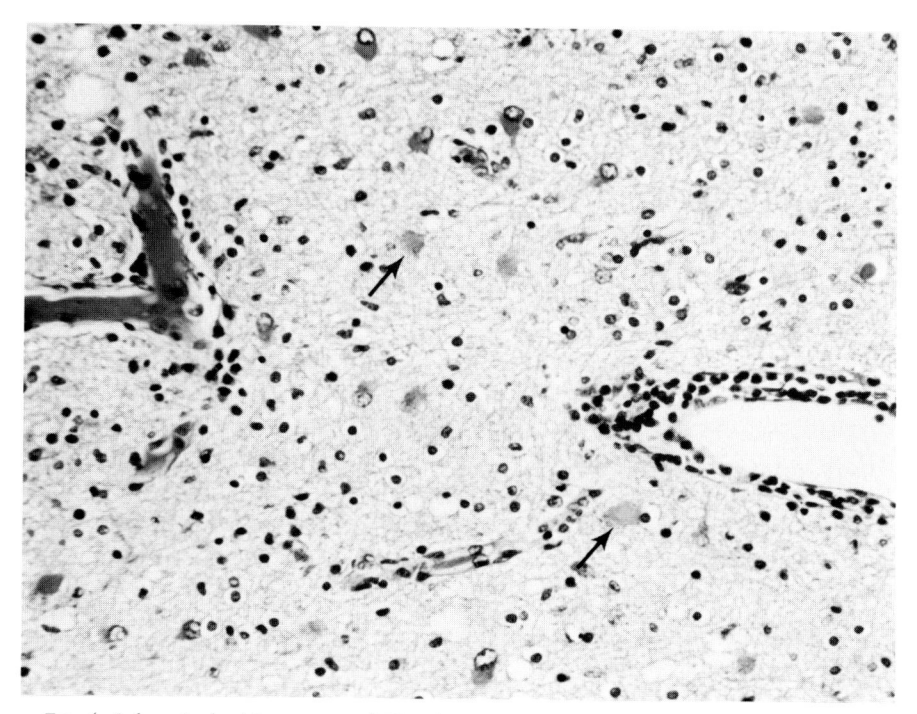

FIG. 4. Subcortical white matter of SSPE brain with perivascular infiltrates and numerous reactive astrocytes (arrows). Hematoxylin and eosin stain (×225).

nucleocapsids are normally enveloped by modified cell membranes and bud from the cell surface, in SSPE viral nucleocapsids accumulate in cytoplasmic inclusions, but are not aligned with the cell membrane and no budding virions are observed (Herndon and Rubinstein, 1967; Jenis *et al.*, 1973; Dubois-Dalcq *et al.*, 1974).

MIBE is pathologically distinguished from SSPE by the absence of or minimal perivascular infiltration by T and B lymphocytes. Intranuclear and cytoplasmic inclusions have the same appearance as in SSPE, as do the intranuclear nucleocapsid profiles (Roos *et al.*, 1981).

The combined features of prolonged clinical course, continued spread of infection in the presence of a robust antibody response and morphologically incomplete virus assembly, have been the hallmarks of persistent measles virus infection of the CNS in SSPE. MIBE has similar features in the absence of a pronounced immune response. These initial observations have led to many studies to identify the molecular mechanisms for viral persistence within the central nervous system.

IV. Properties of Measles Virus

A. BIOLOGICAL PROPERTIES

Measles virus is a negative-strand RNA virus in the family Paramyxoviridae and genus *Morbillivirus* (Kingsbury *et al.*, 1978). The nucleocapsid is of helical symmetry and the pleomorphic virions range in size from 150 to 300 nm. Measles virus is closely related to canine distemper virus and rinderpest virus of cattle, and is less closely related to mumps, Newcastle disease, Sendai, and parainfluenza viruses (Rima, 1989).

In a lytic infection, the viral replication cycle takes approximately 24 hours. Infectious virions enter the cell by binding to the cell surface, fusing with the cell membrane, and releasing the viral nucleocapsid into the cytoplasm. After synthesis of viral proteins and RNA, virions are assembled at the cell surface and infectious virus particles bud from the cell membrane.

In lytic infections of cells in culture or in animal brains, cytoplasmic nucleocapsids have a "fuzzy" morphology (Fig. 5a). However, in SSPE or persistently infected animal brains, where budding virions are not observed, the nucleocapsid profile is "smooth" (Fig. 5b). Intranuclear nucleocapsids always have the smooth profile.

B. MEASLES VIRUS PROTEINS

The structural proteins of measles virus were identified and characterized by a number of groups during the 1970s (Mountcastle and Choppin, 1977;

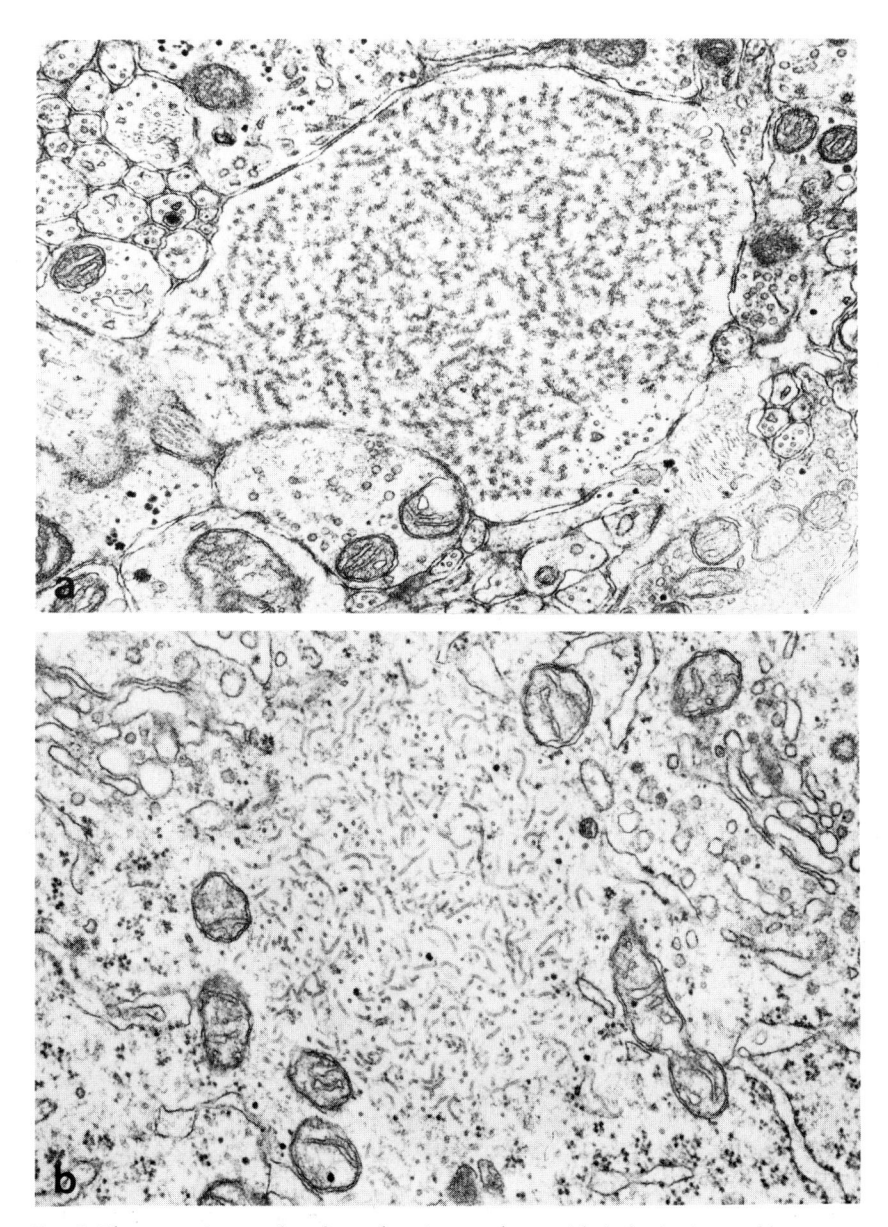

FIG. 5. Electron micrographs of measles virus nucleocapsids in brain tissue of hamsters infected with the HBS strain of virus. (a) "Fuzzy" nucleocapsids in a neuronal process of a newborn hamster brain 5 days postinoculation. (b) "Smooth" nucleocapsids in the cytoplasm of a neuron from a weanling hamster 16 days postinoculation (×29,200).

Graves et al., 1978; Wechsler and Fields, 1978). The viral proteins include the large (L; >200 kDa), hemagglutinin (H; 78 kDa), phosphoprotein (P; 70 kDa), nucleocapsid (N; 62 kDa), matrix (M; 38 kDa), and fusion (F_0; 62 kDa) proteins, in addition to the F_0 proteolytic cleavage products, two disulfide bonded fragments F_1 (42 kDa) and F_2 (20 kDa). The N, P, and L proteins are closely associated with the viral nucleocapsid and participate in polymerase functions. In addition, N functions as a structural support for the viral RNA. The matrix protein is an intermediary between the nucleocapsid and the cell membrane, localized on nucleocapsids and on the inner aspect of the cell membrane (Johnson et al., 1981). H and F are both glycoproteins that are inserted into the cell membrane. The H protein is named for its property of agglutinating red blood cells from some species. It functions as the virion attachment protein by interaction with a cell surface receptor. H is synthesized as a 65-kDa apoprotein (Kohama et al., 1985) that is rapidly translocated across the endoplasmic reticulum membrane and is glycosylated, modified, and transported to the cell surface by cellular pathways (Bellini et al., 1983). The fusion protein is named for its functional property of fusing membranes. This function is essential for fusing the virus envelope to cell membrane for viral entry into cells; infected cells also fuse with adjacent cells, resulting in multinucleated giant cells. Nucleotide sequence analysis of the P gene revealed the possible presence of an additional gene product (Bellini et al., 1985). Antibodies made to synthetic peptides verified that this peptide designated C is present in the nucleus and cytoplasm of infected cells. It is not found in virions, and therefore is presumed to be a nonstructural protein with an unknown function. A third protein designated V has been found to be the product of gene editing (Cattaneo et al., 1989) and will be discussed later.

Viral genomic RNA is surrounded by N, P, and L proteins to form the nucleocapsid. Infectious virions are assembled at and bud from the cell surface. They are composed of nucleocapsids enveloped in modified cell membranes with H and F protein spikes protruding from the virion surface.

C. Measles Virus RNA

Sequencing the measles genome has been the combined effort of several groups. The genome contains 15,892 nucleotides, with allowance for minor variations among virus strains (Crowley et al., 1988). The gene order from the 3' end of the genome is N-P-M-F-H-L (Dowling et al., 1986). The 3' and 5' ends of the genome contain untranslated sequences of 52 and 37 nucleotides, respectively (Billeter et al., 1984; Crowley et al., 1988). Intergenic regions have been sequenced by Cattaneo et al. (1987b). The genome is shown diagrammatically in Fig. 6.

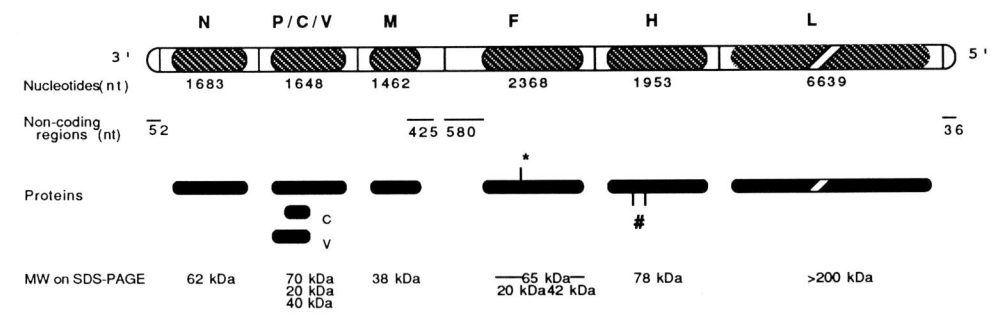

FIG. 6. Genome and gene products of the measles virus; *, F₀ cleavage site; #, region of glycosylation.

The N gene is composed of 1983 nucleotides and codes for a 523-amino acid protein (Rozenblatt et al., 1985; Buckland et al., 1988). The P gene contains 1657 nucleotides and codes for a 507-amino acid protein. The sequence of the P gene revealed the possible presence of a second protein coded in a different reading frame (Bellini et al., 1985). As noted earlier, the second protein designated C has been identified in infected cells. Both P and C are the products of a single mRNA, which is read in two independently initiated overlapping reading frames. A third product of the P gene has been identified, a 46-kDa protein designated V (Cattaneo et al., 1989). This protein contains the amino-terminal region of P, but has a different carboxy-terminal region and occurs because of the insertion of one nucleotide, causing a switch in reading frame. This protein is synthesized in *in vitro* translation reactions using RNA from measles-infected cells, but, like C, its function is unknown.

The M gene codes for a 335-amino acid protein (Bellini et al., 1986). There is a long (425 nucleotide) noncoding region at the 3' end of the mRNA. It has been speculated that this noncoding region provides the secondary structure necessary for stability of the genome or mRNA. However, the noncoding region in its entirety is not essential for transcription and translation, because it has been shown that *in vitro* and *in vivo* translation of M mRNA produce normal products in the absence of the terminal 146 nucleotides (Wong et al., 1987).

The F mRNA contains 2377 nucleotides and codes for a 550- to 553-amino acid protein (Richardson et al., 1986; Buckland et al., 1987). This gene contains a long (580 nucleotide) 5' noncoding region that is GC rich. There is extensive stem–loop secondary structure in the noncoding region that may reduce translational efficiency. The predicted amino acid sequence is highly hydrophobic, which is consistent with the protein property of fusing membranes.

The sequence of the H gene (1953 nucleotides; 617-amino acid protein) reveals five potential N-linked glycosylation sites closely grouped in the amino portion of the molecule (Alkhatib and Briedis, 1986; Gerald *et al.*, 1986). The hydrophobic transmembrane region is near the amino terminus.

The L gene is the largest gene, and its corresponding protein is the least abundant of the measles virus gene products. Its 6639 nucleotides could code for a protein of approximately 247 kDa (Blumberg *et al.*, 1988). Significant homology in the L proteins among the paramyxoviruses suggests a highly conserved ancestral role for L in the polymerase function of paramyxoviruses (Rima, 1989).

V. Viral Protein Expression

A. SSPE Virus Isolates

The accumulated information on the proteins and genes of measles virus have provided the groundwork for addressing many issues related to mechanisms of viral persistence within the CNS. One of the early issues was whether SSPE virus isolates were inherently different from wild-type or vaccine measles strains. Several virus isolates from SSPE brain tissue remain largely cell associated, producing little or no infectious virus in tissue culture. The virus spreads by fusion of adjacent cells, resulting in syncytia formation, but no infectious virus particles mature and bud from the cell surface. However, numerous other virus isolates from SSPE brain tissue undergo a complete replication cycle and produce infectious virions. Therefore, SSPE viruses cannot be easily distinguished from wild-type virus based on progression through the replication cycle *in vitro*. It should be noted, however, that all cell-associated strains have been derived from SSPE brain tissue.

Viral proteins have been analyzed by sodium dodecyl sulfate and polyacrylamide gel electrophoresis (SDS–PAGE) and monoclonal antibody panels. SDS–PAGE reveals minor variations in the migration rate of some viral proteins among virus strains, but no pattern unique to SSPE strains (reviewed by Wechsler and Meissner, 1982). Panels of monoclonal antibodies have been used to compare viral proteins from wild-type virus isolates, vaccine strains, and productive SSPE isolates. The most extensive analyses have been done with monoclonal antibodies against epitopes on the H and M proteins (Sheshberadaran *et al.*, 1983; ter Meulen *et al.*, 1981). Variation in antibody binding to H proteins of different virus strains was demonstrated by radioimmunoassay (RIA), hemagglutination inhibition, and virus neutralization. Reactivity of M monoclonal antibodies also varied among strains. These results show that antigenic variation occurs among virus strains. Though variation in reactivity was encountered, no pattern of reactivity emerged to distinguish the groups of viruses.

Monoclonal antibody labeling reveals restricted expression of some viral proteins in cell-associated virus strains (Johnson *et al.*, 1982). In contrast to N and P, which are always abundant, M, F, and H proteins are less intensely labeled or are nondetectable. In a cell line persistently infected with one of these cell-associated strains, IP-3, M protein is synthesized but is rapidly degraded intracellularly (Sheppard *et al.*, 1986).

B. SSPE and MIBE Brain Tissue

Because no distinctive differences can be discerned among wild-type and productive SSPE viruses, but differences in expression of viral proteins occur in cell-associated strains, attention has turned to the virus in the brain itself. Early observations suggested that absence of M protein was the viral defect responsible for SSPE (Hall and Choppin, 1981). Two studies have examined viral proteins in SSPE brain tissue using monoclonal antibodies (Norrby *et al.*, 1985; Liebert *et al.*, 1986). Four cases were included in each study, with ages ranging from 9 to 16 years and duration of disease ranging from 3 to 18 months. In all cases, N and P were present and gave strong labeling. In the Norrby series, M protein was visible in all four cases, but labeling with nine different monoclonal antibodies resulted in fluorescence intensity ranging from negative to strong. The Liebert series showed M protein in only one of four brains. All five major viral proteins could not be demonstrated in any of the brains; one or more of the three 5' proteins (M, F, or H) were nondetectable in each case. Cells labeled with antibodies to F were present in three out of four brains, whereas H was present in two out of four. In addition, the percentage of infected cells labeling for M, F, and H was greatly reduced, with antigen found in less than 12% of infected cells. Detection of H relative to N has also been shown to be variable in formalin-fixed SSPE brain tissue, with greater H expression in cases of short duration (<4 months) than in long duration (Swoveland *et al.*, 1989) (Fig. 7). In several cases, extensive infection was present with no detectable H antigen in the cells.

C. Experimental Animal Studies

Several studies in experimental animals reproduce the pattern of restricted viral protein expression observed in SSPE and provide useful models for analyzing mechanisms of viral persistence. Persistent measles virus infections of the CNS have been produced in hamsters (Johnson and Byington, 1977), rats (Liebert and ter Meulen, 1987), mice (Rammohan *et al.*, 1980), and

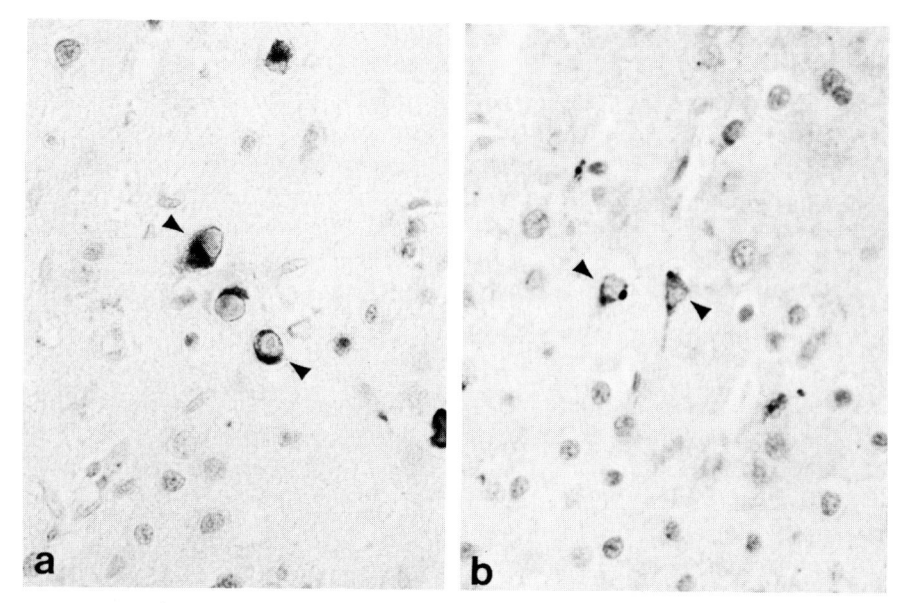

FIG. 7. SSPE brain tissue immunocytochemically labeled with rabbit antihemagglutinin (H) serum and counterstained with hematoxylin. (a) An area from a brain with many infected neurons containing abundant cytoplasmic H protein (arrowheads). (b) Area from a heavily infected brain with only occasional neurons containing limited amounts of H protein (arrowheads) (×450).

monkeys (Albrecht et al., 1977; Ueda et al., 1975). Different virus strains have been adapted to each species, but a common theme in hamsters, mice, and rats is that age at infection is a critical parameter for outcome of infection. The HBS virus strain is a hamster-brain-adapted derivative of the Mantooth SSPE isolate (Byington and Johnson, 1972). Newborn hamsters develop a rapidly progressing encephalitis that kills all animals within 5 days. Weanling (21–24 days old) hamsters develop an acute encephalitis in 5–7 days; 50–70% of animals survive the acute phase and are persistently infected. Cell-free virus can be recovered from brain homogenates of newborn animals and weanling animals during the acute phase of infection. By 16 days postinoculation, cell-free virus can no longer be recovered, although virus can be isolated by cocultivation of brain tissue with susceptible cell lines.

A similar disease course occurs in Lewis and Brown Norway (BN) rats infected with the CAM strain of virus (Liebert and ter Meulen, 1987). CAM is a Japanese vaccine virus strain that has been adapted for growth in rat brains (Kobune et al., 1983). In both rat strains, newborn animals develop a rapidly fatal encephalitis with virus recoverable from brain homogenates. Lewis rats inoculated after 28 days of age develop a subacute measles encephalomyelitis

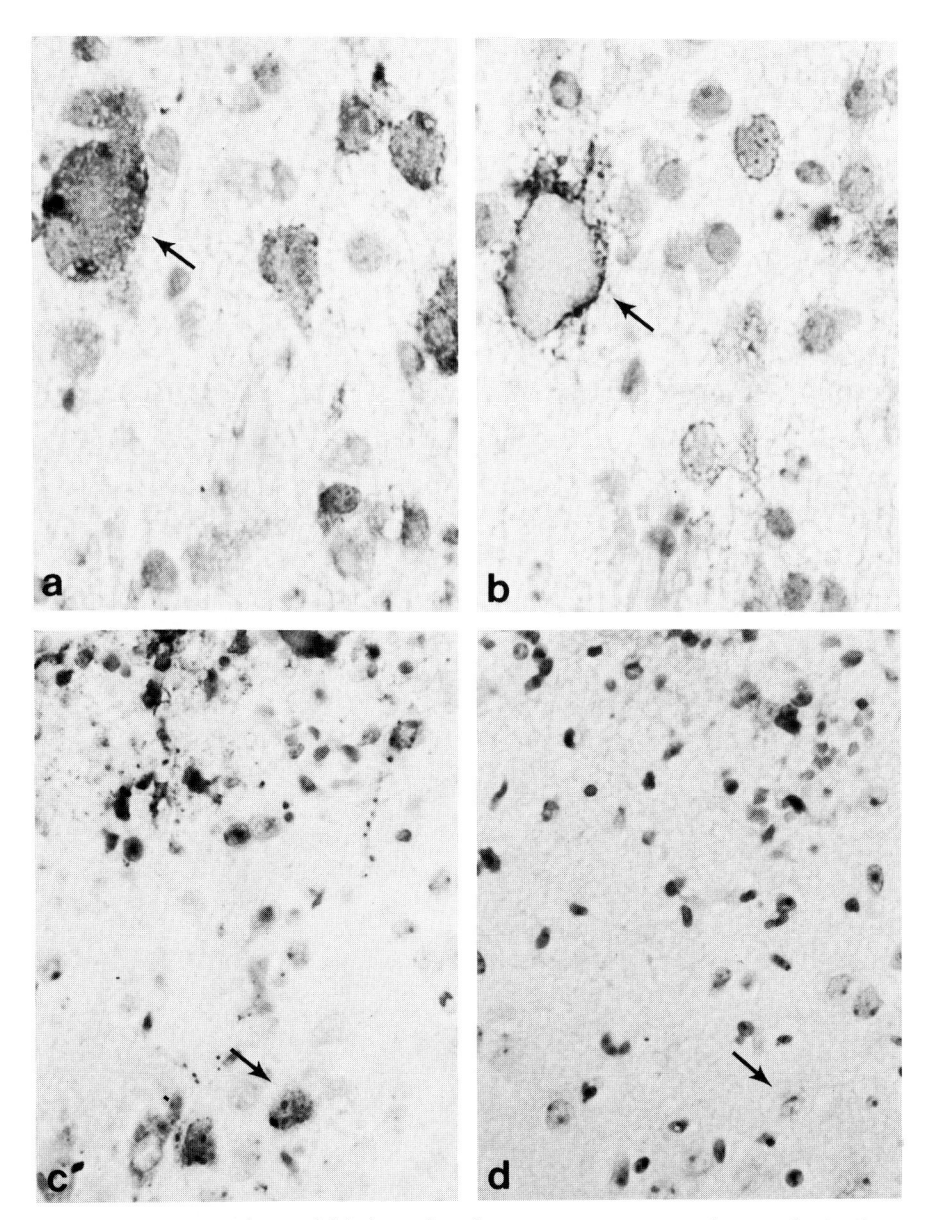

FIG. 8. Immunocytochemical labeling of viral antigens in neurons in hamster brains from suckling (a and b) and weanling (c and d) animals. Adjacent sections are labeled for NP (a and c) and H (b and d) proteins. Arrows identify corresponding areas in adjacent sections. [From Swoveland and Johnson (1989) with permission of Academic Press.]

(SAME) with virus occasionally recoverable by cocultivation. BN rats develop a clinically silent encephalitis (CSE) with no virus recoverable.

In both the hamster and rat models, all viral proteins examined can be identified in brains of newborn animals. However, restricted expression, much as in SSPE, is demonstrable in animals infected as weanlings or young adults. In weanling hamsters infected with HBS virus, N and P are always abundant by immunocytochemical labeling or Western blots. Immunofluorescence and electron microscopic immunocytochemistry for M identify the protein in the acute phase of infection (6–12 days postinoculation), but not at later times, even though abundant infected cells are present (Johnson *et al.*, 1981). Studies on H expression show reduction to undetectable levels in weanling animals, even during the acute infection (Swoveland and Johnson, 1989). Whereas H protein is labeled on cell membranes of infected cells in newborn brain (Fig. 8a and b), infected cells in weanling brains occasionally contain cytoplasmic H, but none is detectable by light microscopic immunocytochemistry on the cell surface (Fig. 8c and d). The exception to this pattern is on occasional infected ependymal cells; H antigen can be demonstrated on the ventricular surface of these cells. This restricted expression has been confirmed on Western blots of viral proteins from infected brain tissue (Fig. 9 and Table I).

In Lewis rats with SAME, a similar pattern of viral protein expression is

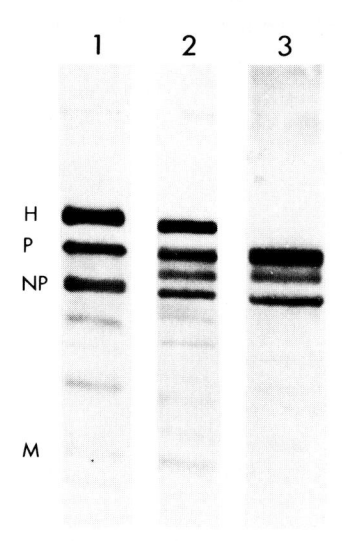

FIG. 9. Immunoblot of SDS–PAGE separated measles virus proteins, labeled with rabbit anti-measles serum. Affinity-isolated viral proteins from purified LEC strain of measles virus (lane 1), 1 mg suckling hamster brain (lane 2), and 15 mg weanling hamster brain (lane 3). [From Swoveland and Johnson (1989) with permission of Academic Press.]

TABLE I

CHARACTERISTICS OF HBS VIRUS GROWN IN CELL CULTURE OR HAMSTER BRAIN

HBS growth medium	Virus titer[b] (Log_{10} $TCID_{50}$)	Viral proteins[c]			
		NP	P	M	H
Vero cells	5.40 ± 0.25	1.0	1.2	0.10	1.4
Suckling hamsters (4)	5.27 ± 0.53	1.0	1.4	0.17	1.8
Weanling hamster—acute (4)	3.10 ± 0.28	1.0	2.9	0.03	<0.01
Weanling hamster—immunosuppressed (4)	3.19 ± 0.40	1.0	2.2	0.02	<0.01
Vero + brain cocultivated (4)	5.16 ± 0.43	1.0	2.5	0.15	1.1
Purified LEC virus[d]	NA[e]	1.0	2.1	0.12	1.9

[a] The number of specimens is given in parentheses.
[b] Mean titer ± SD/g tissue.
[c] Amount relative to NP (1.0) on densitometer scans of Western blots.
[d] 0.5 μg purified LEC strain of measles virus.
[e] NA, Not applicable.

seen. M and F are detected in less than 1% of infected cells, and H is identified in 2.3% of cells. Interestingly, more cells express all viral proteins in BN rats, although there is a threefold attenuation of M, F, and H in these animals.

One possible explanation for the restricted expression of viral proteins in weanling and young adult animals is that a virus has been selected with altered properties. However, the virus recovered from weanling hamster brains 20 days postinoculation by cocultivation with Vero cells produced cytopathic effects (CPEs), virus titers, and viral protein profile identical to those of the input virus (Swoveland and Johnson, 1989). Viral H protein is not masked by antibodies because the identical restriction is observed in immunosuppressed animals (Table I).

VI. Viral Gene Expression

A. SSPE Brain Tissue

Observations of restricted expression of viral proteins in SSPE and experimental animals lead to questions regarding the viral genome and transcription of viral mRNAs in brain tissue. Haase et al. (1985) showed by *in situ* hybridization that copies of viral genome per infected cell were several hundredfold lower in SSPE brain tissue than in permissive cells in culture, and that M transcripts were present at lower concentrations than were N transcripts. Cattaneo et al. (1987a) examined mRNA for the five major genes from

SSPE and measles inclusion body encephalitis brains, and compared these with mRNA from lytically infected cell cultures. In lytic cell culture infections, there is attenuation of transcription at each gene boundary, resulting in a gradient of transcripts from the N to the H genes; N mRNA is approximately sevenfold more abundant than H mRNA. In SSPE and MIBE brains, a much steeper gradient is observed, with N being 100–250 times more abundant than H. Because the overall rate of transcription is reduced and the transcript gradient is exaggerated, the 5' mRNAs are present at a very low copy number.

The attenuation in transcription from the 3' to 5' end of the genome could explain the decreased expression of M, F, and H proteins. However, it is also possible that mutations occur more frequently in these genes. In one SSPE brain in which all viral proteins except M were detectable (Baczko et al., 1984), M monocistronic transcripts were not present, but were substituted by P–M bicistronic mRNA (Cattaneo et al., 1986). In addition to the bicistronic nature of the transcripts, a point mutation in the M gene introduced an early stop codon, which may account for the absence of M.

Localized hypermutations have been found in the M gene from cell-associated SSPE isolates and in RNA extracted from SSPE brains (Wong et al., 1989; Cattaneo et al., 1989). Extensive mutations have also been encountered in the F gene, leading to premature termination of the C terminus, and in the H gene, resulting in loss or addition of glycosylation sites.

Measles virus RNA extracted from formalin-fixed paraffin-embedded tissues contains mRNA of the appropriate size, and can be amplified by polymerase chain reaction (PCR) (Godec et al., 1990). This method may provide the opportunity to examine RNA from many more SSPE cases.

Obligate intracellular virus strains undoubtedly have more serious defects than those that produce infectious virus. One such strain, IP3-CA, has been shown to produce an M protein that is rapidly degraded intracellularly (Sheppard et al., 1986). Substrains that have regained the capacity to produce limited amounts of infectious virus produce a more stable M protein (Cattaneo et al., 1988). The M gene of the substrains contains one mutation resulting in a nucleotide substitution that appears to account for the increased protein stability. Other strains and some SSPE isolates contain M, F, and H transcripts that cannot be translated in *in vitro* reactions (Baczko et al., 1986, 1988), or M transcripts that are not translated at elevated temperatures, though N, P, and H are translated (Ogura et al., 1987).

B. Viral Gene Expression in Experimental Infection

Transcription of viral genes in infected Lewis rats has been examined by Schneider-Schaulies *et al.* (1989). Transcriptional attenuation was more extreme in all animals than in infected Vero cells. Animals of all ages (newborn to weanling) and with any outcome of infection (acute or subacute disease) had an exaggerated gradient of transcripts, with F and H mRNA most significantly reduced. *In vitro* translation did not yield detectable H or M proteins in animals with subacute disease.

VII. Role of Antibodies in Viral Persistence

Because measles virus persists in the CNS in the presence of antiviral antibodies, do antibodies have a role in establishing or maintaining viral persistence? There is evidence for and against antibodies as important participants in modulating viral infection.

In SSPE, the persistence of virus in the presence of high CSF antibody titers has long suggested a role for antibodies in modulating the infection. On the other hand, MIBE cases have been reported with no CSF antibodies detectable by hemagglutination inhibition (HI), complement fixation (CF), or neutralization tests. RNA transcripts from one MIBE case, in which CSF antibodies to N only were present by immunoprecipitation (Roos *et al.*, 1981), showed exaggerated transcript attenuation, just as in SSPE cases (Cattaneo *et al.*, 1987a). These results suggest that antibodies are not essential for selecting neurotropic viral mutants or modulating the antigenic expression in infected cells, even though they may participate in the process when present.

Four-week-old BALB/c mice inoculated with the HNT strain of virus die from an acute encephalitis. However, animals injected with a neutralizing monoclonal anti-H antibody are either protected from infection or develop a prolonged encephalitis (Rammohan *et al.*, 1983). Nonneutralizing anti-H antibodies did not protect the animals from acute infection. Similar results have been reported with Lewis rats (Liebert *et al.*, 1990). Rats inoculated with anti-N, -M, or -F antibodies develop acute disease, but anti-H antibodies protect animals from fatal infection and the animals develop subacute disease. Transcriptional attenuation is more extreme in animals receiving anti-H antibodies than in brains from animals receiving nonneutralizing antibodies.

Fujinami and Oldstone (1979) reported that exposure of infected cells to polyclonal antimeasles antibodies or monoclonal anti-H antibodies resulted in the decreased presence of all intracellular viral proteins, with the greatest decrease in P and M proteins. Barrett *et al.* (1985) studied C6 glioma cells persistently infected with measles virus. In the presence of SSPE serum or anti-H neutralizing monoclonal antibodies, all viral antigens disappeared from infected cells. Removal of antiserum resulted in reappearance of viral antigens. However, spontaneous reappearance took as long as 5 months after removal of antiserum, and in some instances required freezing in liquid nitrogen and thawing to facilitate antigen reexpression. Persistently infected cells of nonneural origin did not lose intracellular viral antigens in the presence of antibody. These interesting experiments show that measles virus gene expression within cells of neural origin can be repressed for prolonged periods and can subsequently "reactivate."

VIII. CNS Damage by Measles Virus

Finally, consideration should be given to the mechanisms by which measles virus causes clinical disease and damage to the cells of the CNS. CNS damage may be a direct result of structural or functional damage to infected cells, it may be immunopathologically mediated, or it may be a combination of both.

Virus infection of neurons may affect neuronal functions. Human neuroblastoma cells persistently infected with measles virus show disruption in cAMP synthesis by neuromodulatory molecules (R. Ziegler, personal communication). The cAMP synthesis is increased in the presence of prostaglandin E_1 and is decreased in the presence of vasoactive intestinal peptide (VIP). These studies demonstrate that persistent virus infection can affect cellular functions, possibly leading to neuronal dysfunction.

Because the virus persists for months or years in the brains of individuals with SSPE, it is clear that infected cells are not readily recognized and killed either by antibody and complement or by cytotoxic T cells. However, there is a subacute inflammatory response to the infection. It has been shown that Lewis rats with subacute encephalitis have splenic T cells that proliferate in the presence of myelin basic protein (MBP), one of the major components of myelin (Liebert *et al.*, 1988). This suggests that some of the demyelination associated with SSPE may be autoimmune. Small regions of amino acid sequence homology have been identified among measles virus N and C proteins and encephalitogenic regions of human MBP (Jahnke *et al.*, 1985). It is not clear whether these homologous regions are responsible for stimulation of MBP-reactive T cells or whether viral damage to oligodendrocytes releases immunogenic MBP.

Induction of cytokines by virus infection has also been proposed as a means by which immune responses are stimulated and cells are damaged in infected areas. Cells positive for interferon γ (IFN-γ), tumor necrosis factor β (TNF-β), and interleukin 6 (IL-6) have been identified within lesions in SSPE (Nagano *et al.*, 1990). IFN-γ has been shown to increase class II MHC antigens on astrocytes (Massa *et al.*, 1987a), and TNF amplifies class II MHC expression on measles-infected astrocytes (Massa *et al.*, 1987b). These cytokines may participate in the local immune stimulation that leads to immunopathologic damage.

IX. Concluding Remarks

The combined information on expression of measles virus RNA and proteins in human SSPE and MIBE brain tissue, in experimental animals, and in cell cultures helps us to understand events resulting in persistent virus infection in the CNS. Host factors, immune system interactions, and viral gene mutations may all participate at various stages in the process. There is strong evidence that restricted expression of measles RNA and proteins occurs within the CNS. Studies of animal models support the idea that the restriction is a function of the host environment, which sets the stage for initiation of persistent infection. It is not clear whether the mutations encountered in viral genes from SSPE tissue are essential for maintaining the persistent infection or are by-products of prolonged survival of genes nonessential for virus replication and cell-to-cell spread.

References

Aaby, P., Bukh, J., Lisse, I. M., and Smits, A. J. (1984). *Rev. Infect. Dis.* **6,** 239.
Agamanolis, D. P., Tan, J. S., and Parker, D. L. (1979). *Arch. Neurol.* **36,** 636.
Albrecht, P., Burnstein, T., Kutch, M. J., Hicks, J. T., and Ennis, F. A. (1977). *Science* **195,** 64.
Alkhatib, G., and Briedis, D. L. (1986). *Virology* **150,** 479.
Baczko, K., Carter, M. J., Billeter, M., and ter Meulen, V. (1984). *Virus Res.* **1,** 585.
Baczko, K., Liebert, U. G., Billeter, M., Cattaneo, R., Budka, H., and ter Meulen, V. (1986). *J. Virol.* **59,** 472.
Baczko, K., Liebert, U. G., Cattaneo, R., Billeter, M. A., Roos, R. P., and ter Meulen, V. (1988). *J. Infect. Dis.* **158,** 144.
Barrett, P. N., Koschel, K., Carter, M., and ter Meulen, V. (1985). *J. Gen. Virol.* **66,** 1411.
Bellini, W. J., Silver, G. D., and McFarlin, D. E. (1983). *Arch. Virol.* **75,** 87.
Bellini, W. J., Englund, G., Rozenblatt, S., Arnheiter, H., and Richardson, C. D. (1985). *J. Virol.* **53,** 908.
Bellini, W. J., Englund, G., Richardson, C. D., Rozenblatt, S., and Lazzarini, R. A. (1986). *J. Virol.* **58,** 408.
Billeter, M. A., Baczko, K., Schmid, A., and ter Meulen, V. (1984). *Virology* **132,** 147.
Blumberg, B. M., Crowley, J. C., Silverman, J. I., Menonna, J., Cook, S. D., and Dowling, P. C. (1988). *Virology* **164,** 487.
Booss, J., and Esiri, M. M. (1986). "Viral Encephalitis Pathology, Diagnosis and Management." Blackwell, London.
Buckland, R., Gerald, C., Barker, D., and Wild, T. F. (1987). *J. Gen. Virol.* **68,** 1695.
Buckland, R., Gerald, C., Barker, D., and Wild, T. F. (1988). *Nucleic Acids Res.* **16,** 821.
Byington, D. P., and Johnson, K. P. (1972). *J. Infect. Dis.* **127,** 1.
Cape, C., Martinez, A. J., Robertson, J. T., Hamilton, R., and Jabbour, J. T. (1973). *Arch. Neurol.* **28,** 124.
Cattaneo, R., Schmid, A., Rebmann, G., Baczko, K., ter Meulen, V., Bellini, W. J., Rozenblatt, S., and Billeter, M. A. (1986). *Virology* **154,** 97.
Cattaneo, R., Rebmann, G., Baczko, K., ter Meulen, V., and Billeter, M. A. (1987a). *Virology* **160,** 523.

Cattaneo, R., Rebmann, G., Schmid, A., Baczko, K., ter Meulen, V., and Billeter, M. A. (1987b). *EMBO J.* **6**, 681.
Cattaneo, R., Schmid, A., Billeter, M. A., Sheppard, R. D., and Udem, S. A. (1988). *J. Virol.* **62**, 1388.
Cattaneo, R., Kaelin, K., Baczko, K., and Billeter, M. A. (1989). *Cell* **56**, 759.
Chen, T. T., Watanabe, I., Zeman, W., and Mealey, J. (1969). *Science* **163**, 1193.
Connolly, J. H., Allen, I. V., Hurwitz, L. J., and Miller, J. H. D. (1967). *Lancet* **1**, 542.
Crowley, J. C., Dowling, P. C., Menonna, J., Silverman, J. I., Schuback, D., Cook, S. D., and Blumberg, B. M. (1988). *Virology* **164**, 498.
Dawson, J. R. (1933). *Am. J. Pathol.* **9**, 7.
Dowling, P. C., Blumberg, B. M., Menonna, J., Adamus, J. E., Cook, P., Crowley, J. C., Kolakofsky, D., and Cook, S. D. (1986). *J. Gen. Virol.* **67**, 1987.
Dubois-Dalcq, M., Coblentz, J. M., and Pleet, A. B. (1974). *Arch. Neurol.* **31**, 355.
Fujinami, R. S., and Oldstone, M. B. A. (1979). *Nature (London)* **279**, 529.
Gerald, C., Buckland, R., Barker, R., Freeman, G., and Wild, T. F. (1986). *J. Gen. Virol.* **67**, 2695.
Godec, M. S., Asher, D. M., Swoveland, P. T., Eldadah, Z. A., Feinstone, S. M., Goldfarb, L. V., Gibbs, C. J., and Gajdusek, D. C. (1990). *J. Med. Virol.* **30**, in press.
Graves, M. C., Silver, S. M., and Choppin, P. W. (1978). *Virology* **86**, 254.
Haase, A. T., Gantz, D., Eble, B., Walker, D., Stowring, L., Ventura, P., Blum, H., Wietgrefe, S., Zupancie, M., Tourtellotte, W., Gibbs, C. J., Norrby, E., and Rozenblatt, S. (1985). *Proc. Natl. Acad. Sci. U.S.A.* **82**, 3020.
Hall, W. W., and Choppin, P. W. (1981). *N. Engl. J. Med.* **304**, 1152.
Halsey, N. A., Modlin, J. F., Jabbour, J. T., Dubey, L., Eddins, D. L., and Ludwig, D. D. (1980). *Am. J. Epidemiol.* **111**, 415.
Herndon, R. M., and Rubinstein, L. J. (1967). *Neurology* **18**, 8.
Horta-Barbosa, L., Fucillo, D. A., London, W. T., Jabbour, J. T., Zeman, W., and Sever, J. L. (1969). *Proc. Soc. Exp. Biol. Med.* **132**, 272.
Jabbour, J. T., Garcia, J. G., Lemmi, H., Ragland, J., Duenas, D. A., and Sever, J. L. (1969). *JAMA, J. Am. Med. Assoc.* **207**, 2248.
Jahnke, U., Fischer, E. H., and Alvord, E. C. (1985). *Science* **229**, 282.
Jenis, E. M., Knieser, M. R., Rothouse, P. A., Jensen, G. S., and Scott, R. M. (1973). *Arch. Pathol.* **95**, 81.
Johnson, K. P., and Byington, D. P. (1977). *In* "Microbiology" (D. Schlesinger, ed.), pp. 511–515. Am. Soc. Microbiol., Washington, D.C.
Johnson, K. P., Norrby, E., Swoveland, P., and Carrigan, D. R. (1981). *J. Infect. Dis.* **144**, 161.
Johnson, K. P., Norrby, E., Swoveland, P., and Carrigan, D. R. (1982). *Arch. Virol.* **73**, 255.
Kingsbury, D. W., Bratt, M. A., Choppin, P. W., Hanson, R. P., Hosaka, Y., ter Meulen, V., Norrby, E., Plowright, W., Rott, R., and Wunner, W. H. (1978). *Intervirology* **10**, 137.
Kipps, A., Dick, G., and Moodie, J. W. (1983). *Lancet* **2**, 1406.
Kobune, K., Kobune, F., Yamanouchi, K., Nagashima, K., Yoshikawa, Y., and Hayami, M. (1983). *J. Exp. Med.* **53**, 177.
Kohama, T., Sato, T. A., Kobune, F., and Sugiura, A. (1985). *Arch. Virol.* **85**, 257.
Liebert, U. G., and ter Meulen, V. (1987). *J. Gen. Virol.* **68**, 1715.
Liebert, U. G., Baczko, K., Budka, H., and ter Meulen, V. (1986). *J. Gen. Virol.* **67**, 2435.
Liebert, U. G., Linington, C., and ter Meulen, V. (1988). *J. Neuroimmunol.* **17**, 103.
Liebert, U. G., Schneider-Schaulies, S., Baczko, K., and ter Meulen, V. (1990). *J. Virol.* **64**, 706.
Link, H., Panelius, M., and Salmi, A. A. (1973). *Arch. Neurol.* **28**, 23.
Massa, P. T., Schimpl, A., Wecker, E., and ter Meulen, B. (1987a). *Proc. Natl. Acad. Sci. U.S.A.* **84**, 7242.
Massa, P. T., ter Meulen, V., and Fontana, A. (1987b). *Proc. Natl. Acad. Sci. U.S.A.* **84**, 4219.
Moodie, J. W., Mackenzie, D. J. M., and Kipps, A. (1980). *S. Afr. Med. J.* **58**, 964.

Mountcastle, W. E., and Choppin, P. W. (1977). *Virology* **78,** 463.
Nagano, I., Nakamura, S., and Kogure, K. (1990). *Neurology* **40,** 456.
Norrby, E., Kristensson, K., Brzosko, W. J., and Kapsenberg, J. G. (1985). *J. Virol.* **56,** 337.
Ogura, H., Baczko, K., Rima, B. K., and ter Meulen, V. (1987). *J. Virol.* **61,** 472.
Ohya, T., Martinez, A. J., Jabbour, J. T., Lemmie, H., and Duenas, D. A. (1974). *Neurology* **24,** 211.
Payne, F. E., Baublis, V. V., and Itabashi, H. H. (1969). *N. Engl. J. Med.* **281,** 585.
Rammohan, K. W., McFarlin, D. E., and McFarland, H. (1980). *J. Infect. Dis.* **142,** 608.
Rammohan, K. W., McFarland, H. F., Bellini, W. J., Gheuens, J., and McFarlin, D. E. (1983). *J. Infect. Dis.* **147,** 546.
Richardson, C., Hull, D., Greer, P., Hasel, K., Berkovich, A., Englund, G., Bellini, W., Rima, B., and Lazzarini, R. (1986). *Virology* **155,** 508.
Rima, B. K. (1989). *In* "Genetics and Pathogenicity of Negative Strand Viruses" (D. Kolakofsky and B. W. J. Mahy, eds.), pp. 254–263. Elsevier, Amsterdam.
Risk, W. S., Haddad, F. S., and Chemali, R. (1978). *Arch. Neurol.* **35,** 494.
Roos, R. P., Graves, M. C., Wollmann, R. L., Chilcote, R. R., and Nixon, J. (1981). *Neurology* **31,** 1263.
Rozenblatt, S., Eizenberg, O., Ben-Levy, R., Lavie, V., and Bellini, W. J. (1985). *J. Virol.* **53,** 684.
Schneider-Schaulies, S., Liebert, U. G., Baczko, K., Cattaneo, R., Billeter, M., and ter Meulen, V. (1989). *Virology* **171,** 525.
Sheppard, R. D., Raine, C. S., Bornstein, M. B., and Udem, S. A. (1986). *Proc. Natl. Acad. Sci. U.S.A.* **83,** 7913.
Sheshberadaran, H., Shou-ni, C., and Norrby, E. (1983). *Virology* **128,** 341.
Swoveland, P. T., and Johnson, K. P. (1989). *Virology* **170,** 131.
Swoveland, P. T., Camenga, D. R., and Dymecki, J. (1989). *Neurology* **39,** 270.
ter Meulen, V., Loffler, S., Carter, M. J., and Stephenson, J. R. (1981). *J. Gen. Virol.* **57,** 357.
Tourtellotte, W. W., Ma, B. I., Brandes, D. B., Walsh, M. J., and Potvin, A. R. (1981). *Ann. Neurol.* **9,** 551.
Ueda, S., Atsuka, T., and Akuno, Y. (1975). *Biken J.* **18,** 179.
Van Bogaert, L. (1945). *J. Neurol., Neurosurg. Psychiatry* **8,** 101.
Vandvik, B., and Norrby, E. (1973). *Proc. Natl. Acad. Sci. U.S.A.* **70,** 1060.
Vandvik, B., Norrby, E., Nordal, J., and Degre, M. (1976). *Scand. J. Immunol.* **5,** 979.
Wechsler, S. L., and Fields, B. N. (1978). *J. Virol.* **25,** 285.
Wechsler, S. L., and Meissner, H. C. (1982). *Prog. Med. Virol.* **28,** 65.
Wolinsky, J. S., Swoveland, P., Johnson, K. P., and Baringer, J. R. (1977). *Ann. Neurol.* **1,** 451.
Wong, T. C., Wipf, G., and Hirano, A. (1987). *Virology* **157,** 497.
Wong, T. C., Ayata, M., Hirano, A., Yoshikawa, Y., Tsuruoka, H., and Yamanouchi, K. (1989). *J. Gen. Virol.* **63,** 5464.

Index

A

N-Acetyl-β-glucosaminidase release, 217
Adenocarcinomatous effusion, 178–179
Adhesion molecules, 65
Adhesives, *in situ* hybridization, 5
Ag-NOR proteins, 169–170
  correlation between quantity and proliferation, 186–187
  tumor lesion diagnosis of malignancy, 176, 179
Aminopropyltriethoxysilane, *in situ* hybridization, 5
Ammoniacal silver technique, 154
Amyloid β-protein precursor, IL-1 upregulation, 132
ANCA-associated diseases
  clinical manifestations, 195
  glomerulonephritis, 202–204
  pathologic lesion, 195–198
  polyarteritis nodosa, 202
  putative pathogenesis, 218–219
  systemic vasculitis, 198–202
  unifying concept, 203, 205
  Wegener's granulomatosis, 199–202
Aneuploidy, nucleolar organizer regions, 184–185
Angiogenesis, endothelial cells, 85–86
Anogenital carcinomas, *in situ* hybridization, 28
Anti-LFA-1 MAb, 69–70
Antineutrophil cytoplasmic autoantibodies, 193–220, *see also* ANCA-associated diseases
  detection of activity, 203–204
  ELISA, 211
    reactivity, 207–209
  immunofluorescence microscopy, 194
  necrotizing glomerulonephritis, 194
  pathogenetic potential, 212–219
    N-acetyl-β-glucosaminidase release, 217
    ANCA-associated diseases, 218–219
    antigen accessibility, 212–213
    chemiluminescence assay, 213–215

β-glucuronidase release, 217
induced degranulation, 216–217
induced respiratory burst, 213–216
superoxide release assay, 215–216
specificity, 193–194, 205–211
  C-ANCAs, 211
  C-ANCA versus P-ANCA, 205
  cell, 206–207
  MPO-ANCAs, 208–210
  organelle, 207–208
  P-ANCAs, 209–210
  PR3-ANCAs, 210–211
AP-1, 130–131
Apoptosis, 223–251
  cell surface changes, 226–227, 231
  difference from necrosis, 247–248
  immune killing, 243–244, 250–251
  incidence, 224–226
  inflammation, 242–243
  mechanisms, 232–242
    cell density increase, 232
    cell surface alterations, 237–242
    chromatin cleavage, 234–237
    intracellular signaling pathways, 233
    transglutaminase activation, 237–238
  morphology, 226–232
  phases, 226–229
  neoplasia role, 244–247
  priming for, 248
  required events, 248–250
  rodent fibroblast cell lines, 228–230
  triggering, 248, 250
  two-stage model for induction and activation, 248–249
Autoradiography, *in situ* hybridization, 12–13

B

Basic fibroblast growth factor, 122
Biotin, endogenous, *in situ* hybridization, 16–17
Biotinylated alkaline phosphatase, *in situ* hybridization, 20
Biotinylated probes
  detection, 13

in situ hybridization, 7
  sensitivity, 19–20
Blood—brain barrier, permeability, 62
Blood coagulation, gene regulation and induction, 104–105
70Z/3 B lymphoid cells, 98
Breast, interphase silver-stained NOR distribution, 179–181
4B4+ T cells, 75–76

C

Calcium—magnesium endonuclease, 236–237
C-ANCA, 211
  versus P-ANCA, 205
Cancerous cells
  cell loss factor, 245
  interphase nucleolar organizer regions, *see* Nucleolar organizer regions
  neoplastic state and interphase NOR distribution, 181–187
CD11/CD18 complex, 108–109
CD44, 67–68
cDNA, double-stranded probes, 7
CD+ T cells, adhesion to IFN-γ—EC, 77
CD4+ T cells, 75–77
Cell death, *see* Apoptosis
Cell loss factor, 245
Cellular oncogenes, RNA detection, 31–33
Central nervous system, measles infection, *see* Measles infection
c-*fms* gene, 31
c-*fos* gene, 32–33
  expression, 128–132
    AP-1 effects, 130–131
    EGF and TGF-β effects, 128–129
    IL-1 and TNF-α effects, 129–130
Chemiluminescence assay, ANCA-induced respiratory burst, 213–215
Chromatin
  intranucleosomal cleavage, 234–237
  ladder, 234–236
  ribosomal
    NORs, 164–168
    structural organization, 165–168
c-*jun* gene, 100, 130–131
Clotting system, importance in immunologically mediated disease, 62

c-*myc* gene, 32–33
  expression, 128–132
    AP-1 effects, 130–131
    EGF and TGF-β effects, 128–129
    IL-1 and TNF-α effects, 129–130
Coagulation control
  cytokine procoagulant effects, 59–60
  interactions between endothelial cells and immune system cells, 58–63
  tissue factor, 60–61
  TNF-α, 60–61
Collagens, differential localization, *in situ* hybridization, 36
Colon adenocarcinoma, 177, 179
Colony-stimulating factors
  consensus sequence, 128–129
  production, 123–125
    IL-1 effects, 123–124
    TNF-α effects, 124
  role in measles virus persistence, 271
  transcription induction, 124
C_{23} protein, as silver-staining protein, 158
c-*sis*
  expression and IFN-γ, 121–122
  mRNA, 120–121
Cytoadhesion family, 70
Cytokines, 96, *see also* Vascular endothelial cells; specific cytokines
  binding of ECs and monocytes, 74
  effect on IL-6 production, 125–126
  PDGF regulation, 123
  procoagulant effects on endothelial cells, 59–60
  produced by cultured endothelial cells, 116
  regulations of endothelial cell expression of MHC antigens, 82–85
  role in EC activation at inflammation sites, 79–80
  T cell adhesion to ECs, 72–73
Cytomegalovirus, *in situ* hybridization, 22–24

D

Degranulation, ANCA-induced, 216–217
Delayed-type hypersensitivity reactions, 59–60
Disseminated intra-vascular coagulation, 105
DNA
  cleavage in apoptosis, 235–236

detection, *in situ* hybridization, 21–30
double-stranded, denaturation, 10
interphasic NORs, 165–166
labeling, *in situ* hybridization, 7
melting temperature, 11
DNA—DNA hybrid
  in situ hybridization, 17
  stability, 11

E

EGF, effect on protooncogene expression, 128–129
ELAM-1, 68–69, 80, 108
  regulation of gene expression, 112
  structure, 111
EL-4 cells, IL-1 receptors, 98–99
Endogenous avidin-binding activity, 16–17
Endothelial cells, *see also* Vascular endothelial cells
  anticoagulant activities, 104–105
  brain vascular, function, 82
  class II expression, 80–81
  culturing, 96–97
  cytokine role in activation at inflammation sites, 79–80
  function as antigen-presenting cells, 80–82
  IL-1
    effects, 61–62
    production, 81
    secretion, 87
  immune system cells interactions
    coagulation control, 58–63
    mononuclear cell migration, 71–79
  inflammation sites, 63
  lymphocyte interactions and recirculation, 63–71
  memory T cell affinity, 77
  MHC antigen
    expression, regulation by cytokines, 82–85
    on surface, 77
  microvascular
    class II expression, 84
    function, 81
  monocyte binding, 74
  plasminogen activator inhibitor and, 61–62
  procoagulant properties, 104
  product effects on immune system cell function, 86–87
  proliferation and angiogenesis, 85–86
  T cell adhesion, 72–75
  thrombin and, 62
  thrombomodulin production, 61
  tissue factor effects, 60–61
  tissue plasminogen activator, 61–62
  von Willebrand factor and, 61
Endothelial leukocyte adhesion molecule 1, *see* ELAM-1
Endothelin, 132–134
Endothelium-derived relaxing factor, 132
Endotoxin, stimulation of endothelin release, 133–134
Eosinophilic granulocytes, unspecific binding of DNA and RNA probes, 17
Epithelial tumors
  EBV and, 27
  human papillomavirus and, 27
Epithelium, scheme of events in apoptosis, 226–227
Epstein—Barr virus
  genome detection, 19–21
  Hodgkin's disease, 26
  in situ hybridization, 24–27
  in lymphoproliferative disorders, 25–26
  nasopharyngeal carcinoma, 26–27
  in oral hairy leukoplakia, 25
  in Sjögren's syndrome pathogenesis, 25
Extracellular matrix protein genes, transcripts, *in situ* hybridization, 35–39
Extractive techniques, disadvantages, 2

F

Fibrinolysis, gene regulation and induction, 105–106
Fibroblast cell lines
  apoptosis, 228–229
  growth properties, 245–246
Fixatives, *in situ* hybridization, 3–5

G

Glomerulonephritis
  algorithm for classifying rapidly progressive, 203–204
  ANCA-associated, 202–204
β-Glucuronidase release, 217
Glycoproteins, oligosaccharide processing on newly synthesized, 239–240

GMP-140, 112
Growth factor genes, RNA detection, 34–35
Gut-associated lymphoid tissue, lymphocyte
　　recirculation, 64

H

H-7, effect on EC adherence to neutrophils,
　　99–100
HBS virus strain, 266, 268–269
Hematopoiesis, CSF effects, 123
Hepatitis B virus, *in situ* hybridization, 29–30
Hepatocytes
　　apoptotic, protein shells, 237–238
　　in situ hybridization, 38–39
Hermes-MAb, 67–68
High endothelial venules
　　in lymph nodes, 72
　　lymphocyte
　　　　adhesion to, 64
　　　　recirculation, 63–65
Histopathology, practical value of *in situ*
　　hybridization, 42–43
HLA-DRA promoter region, 115
Hodgkin cells, *in situ* hybridization, 41
Hodgkin's disease, EBV and, 26
Homeotic genes, RNA detection, 35
2H4+ T cells, 75–76
Human papillomaviruses, *in situ*
　　hybridization, 27–29
Hybridoma growth factor, 125–126
Hyperdiploidy, 184–185
Hypersensitivity response, delayed-type, 105

I

ICAM-1, 80
　　amino acid sequence, 110
　　expression, 108
　　Ig-like domains, 110–111
　　molecular weight, 109–110
ICAM-2, 76
IFN-γ
　　c-sis expression, 121–122
　　effect on EC expression of MHC antigens,
　　　　83–85
　　T cell adhesion to ECs, 72–73
　　vascular EC responsiveness, 102–103

IL-1
　　CSF production effects, 123–124
　　endothelial cells effects, 61–62
　　gene products, 117
　　induction
　　　　endothelial adhesivity, 107
　　　　PCA, 105
　　inhibitory factors, 137
　　leukocyte—endothelial adherence, 107
　　production, 116–119
　　　　by ECs, 81
　　　　mRNA types, 118–119
　　　　TNF-α effects, 117
　　protooncogene expression effect, 129–130
　　receptors
　　　　classes, 98–99
　　　　molecular weights, 98
　　secreted and membrane-associated forms,
　　　　119
　　secretion by ECs, 87
　　upregulation of APP, 132
　　vascular EC responsiveness, 97–101
IL-1β
　　effect on IL-6 production, 125–126
　　mRNA
　　　　accumulation, 117–118
　　　　expression, 137–138
IL-2 gene, IL-1–responsive element, 131
IL-6, production, 125–126
IL-8, production, 126–127
Immune killing, apoptosis, 243–244, 250–251
Immune system cells
　　EC product effect on function, 86–87
　　EC interactions
　　　　coagulation control, 58–63
　　　　mononuclear cell migration, 71–79
Immunofluorescence microscopy, ANCA, 194
　　associated pathologic lesions, 197–198
Immunoglobulin, *in situ* hybridization,
　　40–41
Immunohistology
　　cellular origin of serum proteins, 39
　　combined with *in situ* hybridization,
　　　　14–15
INCAM-110, 78
Inflammation
　　apoptosis role, 242–243
　　sites, endothelial cells at, 63
In situ hybridization, 1–43
　　autoradiography, 12–13

combined with immunohistology, 14–15
DNA detection, 21–30
  cytomegalovirus, 22–24
  Epstein—Barr virus, 24–27
  hepatitis B virus, 29–30
  human papillomaviruses, 27–29
DNA—DNA hybrids, 11, 17
EBV genome, 19–21
EC gene expression, 134–136
grain formation in nuclear track emulsions, 16
history, 2
kinetics, 11–12
mRNA, 18
nucleolar organizer regions, 150
pitfalls and controls, 16–18
practical value for histopathology, 42–43
pretreatment and hybridization conditions, 10–12
probes, 5–10
  concentration, 12
  detection, 12–14
  double-stranded cDNA probes, 7
  gel filtration, 9
  nick translation, 5–6
  nonradioactive reporter molecules, 6–7, 13–14
  oligonucleotides, 9
  radioactively labeled, 6
  random primer extension, 5–6
  RNA, 8–9
  RNA—RNA hybrids, 8
radiolabeled probes, high background, 16
RNA detection, 30–42
  cellular origin of serum proteins, 39–41
  extracellular matrix protein gene transcripts, 35–39
  transcripts of oncogenes, growth factor genes, and homeotic genes, 30–35
  virus genomes, 41–42
sensitivity of radioactive and nonradioactive techniques, 18–21
tissues, fixatives, and adhesives, 3–5
Insulin-like growth factors, detection, *in situ* hybridization, 34–35
Interleukins, *see also* specific interleukins identification, *in situ* hybridization, 34
int-2 gene, 32
Intracellular signaling pathways, apoptosis, 233

K

Ki-67 antibody, immunoreactivity, 187

L

Laminin B1 transcripts, cellular localization, 39
Leukocyte adhesion molecules
  cytokine effect on adherence to vascular ECs, 106–109
  regulation of gene expression, 109–112
  structure, 110
LFA-1
  lymphocytic infiltration, 75–76
  T cell adhesion to ECs, 73–75
Light microscopy, ANCA-associated pathologic lesion, 196–197
LINE-1, activation, 250
Liver fibrosis, *in situ* hybridization, 36–37
LPAM-2, 67
Lymph nodes, HEVs in, 72
Lymphocyte-associated cell surface molecule 1, 68
Lymphocyte/endothelial cell adhesion molecules, 64–65
Lymphocyte function-associated antigen 1, 69–70
Lymphocytes, 58
  apoptotic, macrophage recognition and phagocytosis, 239, 241–242
  homing receptors, 64–66
  infiltration, LFA-1, 75–76
  recirculation, lymphocyte/endothelial cell interactions, 63–71
    endothelial cells, lymphocyte recirculation, 63–71
    high endothelial venules, 63–65
    organ-specific interactions, 63–69
    non-organ-specific interactions, 69–71
Lymphoproliferative disorders, EBV and, 25–26
Lymphotoxin, *see* TNF-β

M

MAb Leu-8, 68
Mab MEL-14, 64–68
  gene encoding core polypeptide, 66
MAb R1-2, 66–67

Mac-1, 70
Macrophages
    activated, angiogenic effect, 85–86
    recognition of apoptotic cells, 239, 241–242
MAG, 110
Major histocompatibility complex antigen
    EC expression, regulation by cytokines, 82–85
    on EC surface, 77
    gene regulation and induction, 112–116
        HLA-DRA promoter region, 115
        IFN-γ effects, 114
        pathological lesion development, 113
        TNF-α effects, 113–114
        TNF-β effects, 114
        umbilical vein ECs, 113–114
        vascular ECs, 113
Measles inclusion body encephalitis, 257, 260
Measles infection, CNS, 255–273, *see also* Subacute sclerosing panencephalitis
    antibody role in persistence, 271–272
    damage, 272
    HBS virus strain, 266, 268–269
    measles inclusion body encephalitis, 257, 260
    pathology, 257–260
    viral gene expression, 269–271
        experimental infection, 270–271
Measles virus
    biological properties, 260–261
    genome and gene products, 262–263
    nucleocapsids, 260–261
    protein expression
        animal studies, 266–269
        brain tissue, 265–266
        SSPE viral isolates, 264–265
    proteins, 260, 262
        immunoblot, 268
    RNA, 262–264
Mel-14, 112
Melanoma growth stimulatory activity, production, 127
Melting temperature, DNA, 11
MIBE, brain tissue, 265
Monocytes, EC binding, 74
Mononuclear cell migration, inflammatory lesions, endothelial cells/immune system interactions, 71–79
MPO-ANCAs, 208–210
MPO-positive lysosomes, ANCA antigens in, 207

mRNA
    cytokine-induced genes, consensus sequence in 3'-untranslated regions, 127–129
    endothelin, 3'-untranslated region, 133
    in situ hybridization, 18
    PDGF and PDGF receptor genes, 135

N

Nasopharyngeal carcinoma, EBV and, 26–27
Natural killer cells, apoptosis role, 243–244
NCAM, 110
Necrosis, difference from apoptosis, 247–248
Necrotizing glomerulonephritis, antineutrophil cytoplasmic autoantibodies, 194
Neoplasia, apoptosis role, 244–247
Neoplastic cells, interphase NOR distribution, 175–179
Neuronal functions, viral infections and, 272
Neutrophils
    activation, ANCAs, 216
    apoptotic, macrophage recognition and phagocytosis, 239, 241–242
Nick translation, 5–6
Nuclear track emulsions, grain formation, 16
Nucleic acid molecules, labeled, as *in situ* hybridization probes, 5
Nucleolar organizer regions, 149–189
    aneuploidy, 184–185
    dense fibrillar component, 163
    distribution in neoplastic cells, 175–179
    factors affecting silver stain specificity, 155–157
        fixatives, 155–157
        pH, 157
        temperature and time, 157
    fibrillar centers, 159, 163
    granular component, 163
    in situ hybridization, 150
    interphase
        cell duplication rate and, 185–187
        distribution, 172–175
        distribution and ribosomal transcriptional activity, 182–183
        high number in cancer cells, 179–181
        relation between distribution and neoplastic state of cell, 181–187
        relation with metaphase, 183–185
    Ki-67 immunoreactivity, 187

localization in interphase nucleoli,
    159–164
  breast cancerous tissue, 162–163
  components, 159–160, 163
  cytochemistry and
    immunocytochemistry, 164
  neuroblastoma cells, 161, 163
molecular components responsible for
    silver staining, 157–159
  silver reactive groups, 157–158
  silver-stained protein identification,
    158–159
not stained by Ag-NOR techniques, 159
nucleolar morphology, 170–171, 173
  types, 170–171
silver staining techniques, 151–155
  affinity for silver, 151–152
  ammoniacal silver technique, 154
  in mitotic chromosomes, 153–154
  one-step silver staining, 154–155
structural changes of ribosomal genes in
    cells stimulated to proliferate,
    188–189
structure and function, 164–170
  Ag-NOR proteins, 169–170
  ribosomal chromatin, 164–168
  RNA polymerase I and topoisomerase I,
    166, 169

O

Oligonucleotide probes, *in situ*
    hybridization, 9
Oligosaccharide, processing on newly
    synthesized glycoproteins, 239–240
Oncogenes, RNA detection, *in situ*
    hybridization, 31–34
One-step silver staining, 154–155
Oral hairy leukoplakia, *in situ*
    hybridization, 25
Organelles, ANCA antigen specificity,
    207–208

P

p150,95, 70
P-ANCA
  versus C-ANCA, 205
  ELISA results, 209–210
  specificity, 209–210

Papillomaviruses, human, *in situ*
    hybridization, 27–29
Pathologic lesion, ANCA-associated, 195–198
  immunofluorescence microscopy, 197–198
  light microscopy, 196–197
PDGF
  gene expression, 134–135
  homodimers, 120
  physiologic role, 120
  production, 120–123
    bFGF effects, 122
    c-*sis* mRNA, 120–121
  regulation by cytokines, 123
pH, effect on silver staining of NORs, 157
Phagocytosis, apoptotic neutrophils and
    lymphocytes, 239, 241
Phosphatidylcholine, hydrolysis, 100
Plasminogen activator, endothelial cells and,
    61–62
Plasminogen activator inhibitor, immune
    system cells and, 61
Platelet-derived growth factor, *see* PDGF
Polyarteritis nodosa, ANCA-associated, 202
Postcapillary venules, HEV-like, 71–72
PR3–ANCAs, 210–211
Probes, *see also* specific probes
  in situ hybridization, 5–10
Procollagen gene probes, *in situ*
    hybridization, 37–38
Proliferation
  interphase NORs and, 185–187
  ribosomal gene structural changes,
    188–189
Pronase, *in situ* hybridization
    pretreatment, 10
Protein kinase C
  in IFN-γ-induced class II antigen
    expression, 103
  participation in endothelial functions, 100
Protein kinase inhibitors, effect on EC
    adherence to neutrophils, 99–100
Protein shells, apoptotic hepatocytes, 237–238
Protooncogene, expression, 128–132
Pulmonary—renal syndrome, 201

R

Random primer extension, 5–6
ras genes, 32–33
Reed—Sternberg cells, *in situ*
    hybridization, 41

Respiratory burst, ANCA-induced, 213–216
Ribosomal genes, structural changes, proliferation, 188–189
Ribosomal transcriptional activity, interphase NOR distribution and, 182–183
RNA
 in situ hybridization, 3–4
 measles virus, 262–264
RNA polymerase I, NORs, 166, 169
RNA—RNA hybrids, in situ hybridization, 8
rRNA
 inhibition of synthesis, 169–170
 synthesis, 171, 182–183

S

Serum proteins, cellular origin, in situ hybridization, 39–41
Shrinkage necrosis, 232
Silver reactive groups, 157–158
Silver-stained proteins, identification, 158–159
Silver staining techniques, nucleolar organizer regions, 151–155
Sjögren's syndrome, EBV in pathogenesis, 25
^{35}S-labeled probes, sensitivity, 19
SSPE
 brain tissue
  cortical gray matter, 257–259
  subcortical white matter, 259
  viral gene expression, 269–270
  viral protein expression, 265–266
  virus isolates, 264–265
Subacute sclerosing panencephalitis, clinical and epidemiological features, 256–257
Sugar, inhibition pattern, 239
Superoxide release assay, ANCA-induced respiratory burst, 215–216
Synovial cells, in situ hybridization, 40
Systemic vasculitis, ANCA-associated, 198–202

T

T cell
 adhesion to ECs, 72–75
 cytotoxic, apoptosis role, 243–244
 memory, 76–77
TGF-β
 angiogenesis effects, 86

 protooncogene expression effect, 128–129
 vascular EC responsiveness, 103–104
TGF-β1, induced expression of endothelin mRNA, 133
Thrombin, endothelial cells effects, 62
Thrombomodulin, production and endothelial cells, 61
Tissue factor
 cDNA, 105
 coagulation control, 60–62
 endothelial cells effects, 60–62
TNF
 angiogenic effect of activated macrophages, 85–86
 effect on kEC expression of MHC antigens, 83–84
 receptors, components, 102
 T cell adhesion to ECs, 72–73
 vascular EC responsiveness, 101–102
TNF-α, 60–61
 c-*jun* mRNA effects, 130
 CSF production effects, 124
 gene activation role of AP-1, 131
 IL-1 production effects, 117
 IL-6 production effect, 125–126
 MHC antigen expression and, 113–114
 protooncogene expression effect, 129–130
TNF-β, MHC antigen expression and, 114
Topoisomerase I, NORs, 169
tPA, activity and vascular ECs, 105–106
tPA1, activity and vascular ECs, 105–106
Transforming growth factor β, see TGF-β
Transglutaminase, activation, 237–238
Tumor necrosis factor, see TNF
Tumors, cell loss factor, 245

V

Vascular cell adhesion molecule 1, 78
Vascular diseases, distribution in patients with C-ANCAs and P-ANCAs, 198
Vascular endothelial cells, cytokine effects, 95–139
 future directions of research, 136–139
 gene regulation and expression
  common nucleotide sequences in 3'-untranslated regions of mRNA, 127–129
  CSF production, 123–125
  endothelin production, 132–134

genes of leukocyte adhesion molecules,
    106–112
genes related to blood coagulation and
    fibrinolysis, 104–106
IL-1 production, 116–119
IL-6 production, 125–126
IL-8 production, 126–127
in vivo and in *in situ* hybridization,
    134–136
melanoma growth stimulatory activity,
    126–127
MHC antigens, 112–116
PDGF production, 120–123
protooncogene expression, 128–132
IFN-γ, 102
IL-1, 97–101
microvascular, 136
PDGF expression, 135–136

TGF-β, 103–104
TNF, 101–102
VCAM-1, 78
Viral genome
    RNA detection, *in situ* hybridization, 41–42
    size and *in situ* hybridization sensitivity,
        20–21
Virus
    biotin-labeled probes, 16
VLA-4, 66, 68, 76, 78
VLA family, 70
von Willebrand factor, endothelial cells
    and, 61

W

Wegener's granulomatosis, ANCA-associated,
    199–202